VIRUS INFECTIONS OF THE GASTROINTESTINAL TRACT

INFECTIOUS DISEASES AND ANTIMICROBIAL AGENTS

Editors

HAROLD C. NEU
Division of Infectious Diseases
College of Physicians and Surgeons
Columbia University
New York, New York

FRIEDRICH DEINHARDT
Max von Pettenkofer Institute for
Hygiene and Medical Microbiology
Munich, Germany

ANDREW WHELTON
School of Medicine
The Johns Hopkins University
Baltimore, Maryland

JULES L. DIENSTAG
Massachusetts General Hospital
Harvard Medical School
Boston, Massachusetts

JOHN D. WILLIAMS
Department of Medical Microbiology
The London Hospital Medical College
London, England

DAVID A. J. TYRRELL
Division of Communicable Diseases
Clinical Research Centre
Harrow, Middlesex, England

Additional volumes in preparation

VIRUS INFECTIONS OF THE GASTROINTESTINAL TRACT

Edited by

David A.J. Tyrrell

Division of Communicable Diseases
Clinical Research Center
Watford Road
Harrow, Middlesex, England

Albert Z. Kapikian

Laboratory of Infectious Diseases
National Institute of Allergy and Infectious Diseases
National Institutes of Health
Bethesda, Maryland

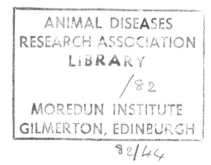

MARCEL DEKKER, INC.   New York • Basel

Dedication to my (D.A.J.T.) wife and family.
My (A.Z.K.) mother and father, wife, children, family,
and to the memory of Jack Zakian.

Library of Congress Cataloging In Publication Data
Main entry under title:

Virus infections of the gastrointestinal tract.

    (Infectious diseases and antimicrobial agents ; v. 3)
    Includes indexes.
    1. Gastroenteritis. 2. Virus diseases. I. Tyrrell,
D. A. J. (David Arthur John) II. Kapikian, Albert Z.,
[date]. III. Series. [DNLM: 1. Gastroenteritis.
2. Diarrhea. 3. Virus diseases. W1 IN406HP v.3 / WI 100
V821]
RC840.G3V57   616.3'307   82-2383
ISBN 0-8247-1567-5   AACR2

MARCEL DEKKER, INC.
270 Madison Avenue, New York, New York 10016

Current printing (last digit):
10 9 8 7 6 5 4 3 2 1

PRINTED IN THE UNITED STATES OF AMERICA

Preface

In all branches of clinical medicine, staying informed of advances made in other scientific areas is imperative. The cause of disease and its modifications, as well as diagnostic measures and the principles and basis of new treatment can be better understood this way. Gastroenterologists are well aware of this and read original articles or reviews on the physiology of the intestine, hematology, endocrinology, pharmacology, electron microscopy, and so on. However, many would think that virology is a subject they could ignore without disadvantage, and until now this was probably true. Nevertheless, in recent years virology has greatly increased our understanding of the acute diarrheal diseases, and it may yet be found that some chronic diseases are also caused by viruses. There is therefore good reason for clinicians to review the basic principles of virology and virus diagnosis and to learn about new and elegant techniques now available and to be brought up to date on what virus infections can do in the human gastrointestinal tract. This book has been put together to make this possible for the nonspecialist and specialist alike, and we are very grateful to the expert authors who have concentrated their detailed knowledge into concise and lucid prose. As often happens, valuable information has also been obtained by the study of animals, though in this case, rather than producing model illnesses in laboratory animals, it is possible to investigate diseases of farm animals produced not only by agents very similar to those that affect humans, but also under experimental conditions by agents that affect humans. Thus some research by veterinarians may answer questions we can never answer by the ethical study of humans, and also suggest where future studies of human disease may lead.

Diarrheal diseases have a striking world-wide impact. It was recently estimated that in Asia, Africa, and Latin America, during a 1 year period, there would be 3 to 5 billion cases of diarrhea and 5 to 10 million deaths. In addition, diarrhea was ranked first in the categories of disease and mortality. Diarrhea is also an important problem in the developed countries. In the Cleveland Family study, which extended over an approximate 10 year period and included some 25,000 illnesses, infectious gastroenteritis was the second most common disease experience accounting for 16% of all illnesses.

In spite of the importance of the problem, attempts to discover the etiologic agents of a large proportion of diarrheal illnesses were unsuccessful prior to the 1970s. Major attempts to find such agents were made in the 1940s and 1950s, when volunteer studies in both the United States and Japan established that filterable agents derived from gastroenteritis outbreaks could induce diarrhea in volunteers, but in spite of this finding, attempts to culture or identify the filterable agents were uniformly unsuccessful. This lack of success was especially disappointing to virologists who, in the 1950s and 1960s, were discovering hundreds of new viruses employing the newly developed tissue culture systems; although many of these viruses were shed in the stool, not one turned out to be the long-sought virus(es) of acute gastroenteritis.

However, in the 1970s, two new groups of viruses were associated with human gastroenteritis—one was the 27 nm Norwalk virus which in 1972 was associated with an epidemic of acute gastroenteritis, and the other was the 70 nm rotavirus which in 1973 was associated with severe infantile gastroenteritis. Ironically, both groups of viruses could have been discovered many years ago, since the methods used for their detection and association with illness were available about 30 years before, when electron microscopes first came into use in the study of viruses. The Norwalk virus was first detected in stools by electron microscopy (EM) employing Norwalk convalescent serum to aggregate the particles, whereas the rotavirus was visualized initially in duodenal biopsies and later in stools. This concept of examining clinical specimens containing viruses by electron microscopy has been termed *direct virology*, a method which bypasses in vitro and in vivo systems for the study of viruses.

This approach of examining specimens directly by electron microscopy for the detection of viruses was previously described in studies involving specimens from animals. The first animal rotavirus was actually detected in 1963, when, by thin-section electron microscopic study of intestinal tissue from mice infected with EDIM (epizootic diarrhea of infant mice) virus, particles were visualized similar to those first observed in humans in 1973. Of course, it was later shown that the EDIM virus was a rotavirus and shared antigens with the human rotavirus. In addition, in 1969, rotavirus particles were visualized in stools of calves with diarrheal illness. This agent is morphologically identical to the human rotavirus visualized in stools of human infants and young children, and of course, it shares antigens with human rotavirus. A further note of historical interest were the studies reported in 1943, in which diarrhea was induced in calves with a filterable agent derived from diarrheal stools obtained from neonates involved in outbreaks of diarrhea in premature or full-term nurseries. Over 30 years later, examination by EM of calf stool obtained from an animal which had developed diarrhea in this study revealed the presence of rotavirus particles. It is not clear whether this represented a true calf rotavirus strain or the human virus. However, over 30 years after this study human rotavirus was shown to induce diarrheal illness in the calf model. Thus, it is clear that others studying animal models had made discoveries which could have provided important leads for the study of disease in humans if their work had been recognized and pursued. In addition, examination of stools by electron microscopy had been pursued by investigators studying human hepatitis viruses in 1970; and in 1973, a year and a few months after the Norwalk virus was visualized in stools by direct virology, hepatitis A virus, another fastidious agent, was also visualized in stools by almost identical techniques.

Neither the Norwalk group of viruses nor the human rotaviruses grow efficiently in cell culture or in a convenient laboratory animal; thus, methods of direct virology have been employed in studying them. However, second and third generation tests have been developed, e.g., radioimmunoassay and immune adherence hemagglutination assay for Norwalk and enzyme-linked immunoabsorbent assay, radioimmunoassay, and a host of other methods for rotaviruses. Most of these methods do not require the in vitro propagation of these agents.

Since the first reports of human gastroenteritis viruses in the early 1970s, there has been a virtual explosion of information about agents associated with this disease. Thus, it was felt that the time was right to gather in a single source the available information on this most important subject. This book attempts to present a description of the field of viral gastroenteritis from an etiologic, epidemiologic, and physiologic perspective. In addition, in an attempt to be complete, we have included a chapter on bacteria associated with gastroenteritis, since much new information has appeared in this area also and no discussion of gastroenteritis would be complete without a presentation of the role of these agents. We have also felt it to be important to present information on the role of viruses in animal gastroenteritis. Certainly, in the field of gastroenteritis, the collaboration of those engaged in human medicine and veterinary medicine has been especially fruitful.

Hopefully, by a following edition, not only the etiology of all or almost all gastroenteritis can be elucidated, but also methods for prevention of at least a portion of the gastroenteritides—especially gastroenteritis of infants and young children—will have been developed.

David A. J. Tyrrell
Albert Z. Kapikian

Contributors

Peter A. Bachmann, Dr. med. vet. Institute of Medical Microbiology, Infections and Epidemic Diseases, Faculty of Veterinary Medicine, University of Munich, Munich, Federal Republic of Germany

Ruth F. Bishop, D.Sc. Department of Gastroenterology, Royal Children's Hospital, Melbourne, Victoria, Australia

Neil R. Blacklow, M.D. Division of Infectious Diseases, Department of Medicine, University of Massachusetts Medical School, Worcester, Massachusetts

E. O. Caul, Ph.D. Public Health Laboratory, Bristol, England

Robert M. Chanock, M.D. Laboratory of Infectious Diseases, National Institute of Allergy and Infectious Diseases, National Institutes of Health, Bethesda, Maryland

George Cukor, Ph.D. Division of Infectious Diseases, Department of Medicine, University of Massachusetts Medical School, Worcester, Massachusetts

Heather A. Davies, MI. Biol. Clinical Research Centre, Section of Histopathology, Electron Microscopy Research Group, Harrow, Middlesex, England

S. I. Egglestone, Ph.D.* Public Health Laboratory, Exeter, England

T. H. Flewett, M.D. Regional Virus Laboratory, East Birmingham Hospital, Birmingham, England

D. Grant Gall, M.D. FRCP(c)[†] Research Institute, The Hospital for Sick Children, and University of Toronto, Toronto, Ontario, Canada

---

*Dr. Egglestone is now with the Public Health Laboratory, Bristol, England.
[†] Dr. Gall is now with the University of Calgary, Calgary, Alberta, Canada

David J. Garwes, Ph.D. Microbiology Department, Agricultural Research Council Institute for Research on Animal Diseases, Compton, Newbury, Berkshire, England

Harry B. Greenberg, M.D. Laboratory of Infectious Diseases, National Institute of Allergy and Infectious Diseases, National Institutes of Health, Bethesda, Maryland

J. Richard Hamilton, M.D. Division of Gastroenterology, Department of Pediatrics, The University of Toronto and the Research Institute, the Hospital for Sick Children, Toronto, Ontario, Canada

R. Guenter Hess, Dr. med. vet. Institute of Medical Microbiology, Infectious and Epidemic Diseases, Faculty of Veterinary Medicine, University of Munich, Federal Republic of Germany

Ian H. Holmes Department of Microbiology, University of Melbourne, Parkville, Victoria, Australia

Walter D. James Laboratory of Infectious Diseases, National Institute of Allergy and Infectious Diseases, National Institutes of Health, Bethesda, Maryland

Anthony R. Kalica, Ph.D. Laboratory of Infectious Diseases, National Institute of Allergy and Infectious Diseases, National Institutes of Health, Bethesda, Maryland

Albert Z. Kapikian, M.D. Laboratory of Infectious Diseases, National Institute of Allergy and Infectious Diseases, National Institutes of Health, Bethesda, Maryland

Charles A. Mebus, D.V.M., Ph.D. United States Department of Agriculture, Agricultural Research Service, Plum Island Animal Disease Center, Greenport, New York

Peter J. Middleton, M.D. Department of Virology, The Hospital for Sick Children, Toronto, Ontario, Canada

M. B. Pepys, Ph.D. F.R.C.P., MRC Path. Immunological Medicine Unit, Department of Medicine, Royal Postgraduate Medical School, London, England

R. Bradley Sack, M.D., Sc.D. Department of Medicine, The Johns Hopkins University School of Medicine and the Baltimore City Hospitals, Baltimore, Maryland

David A. J. Tyrrell, M.D. F.R.S. Medical Research Council Division of Communicable Diseases, Clinical Research Centre, Harrow, Middlesex, England

Gerald N. Woode, B.V.M., D.V.M. Department of Veterinary Microbiology and Preventive Medicine, Iowa State University College of Veterinary Medicine, Ames, Iowa

Richard G. Wyatt, M.D. Laboratory of Infectious Diseases, National Institute of Allergy and Infectious Diseases, National Institutes of Health, Bethesda, Maryland

Robert H. Yolken, M.D. Department of Pediatrics, The Johns Hopkins University School of Medicine, Baltimore, Maryland

Contents

VIRUS INFECTIONS OF THE GASTROINTESTINAL TRACT

1

Some Aspects of the Classification and Basic Biology of Viruses of the Gastrointestinal Tract

David A. J. Tyrrell Clinical Research Centre,
Harrow, Middlesex, England

This chapter is intended to provide an introduction to those that follow. Therefore it includes a general survey of the basic biologic nature of the viruses of the types found in the human alimentary tract, of the ways in which they produce infection and disease, and of the basic principles of virus diagnostic tests. A chapter of this sort can be omitted by any who have a grounding hin human virology, but anyone who has not should read it carefully before embarking on the later, more specialized chapters. Detailed references have been omitted since there are textbooks and reviews that cover the ground fully [1,5].

Structure and Taxonomy of Viruses

A typical virus particle may be thought of as a small piece of genetic information enclosed in a proteinaceous coat to protect it from damage as it passes from one infected cell to another. It would probably be better biologic thinking to consider the virus proper as the organism replicating inside a cell, and the virus particle as the equivalent of the resistant spore form found in many more complex organisms. The genetic information is safely packaged as it passes out of a susceptible cell and is "uncoated" when it reaches a new susceptible cell. There it becomes active and replicates more copies of itself for further packaging.

Whether we start with particles or methods of replication we come to somewhat similar views of the important relationships between different viruses; we shall start by considering the structure and composition of the virus particle.

Viruses contain only one type of nucleic acid, that is, either RNA or DNA, and not both as do higher organisms like bacteria. The nucleic acid may be single- or double-stranded, whether it is RNA or DNA. The single-stranded nucleic acid may be further subdivided according to its "strandedness"—thus, enteroviruses such as poliovirus are "positive stranded" in that the RNA sequence can be, and is, directly translated through the use of the cell's ribosomes into proteins which are used for virus replication. Other viruses, such as influenza, are said to be "negative stranded" because the viral RNA is used to make a complementary copy, and it is this which can be translated to form viral peptides. A further distinction depends on whether the nucleic acid is present as one continuous strand or is segmented into two or more pieces.

All virus particles also contain proteins which surround the nucleic acid in various ways. In some viruses, such as adenoviruses, protein subunits form structural units or *capsomeres* and these in turn form a rigid icosahedral structure, the viral *capsid*; icosahedral symmetry is found in many other viruses as well, though it is particularly easy to recognize in adenoviruses. This type of outer coat may be achieved with a structure composed of a few repeating units, and in some cases it is now known how the various peptides which the virus produces are arranged within the particle. Some are found on the surface and may carry the antigens which are recognized by the immune systems of the host; others are found internally associated with the nucleic acid, and these are particularly likely to be the same in related species and become known as group antigens.

In certain viruses the nucleic acid may be seen to be arranged as a spiral structure in which, for example, in influenza viruses, the RNA is closely associated with a protein. Thus viruses of this sort are said to have helical symmetry.

If viruses bud from the surface of a cell or into the vesicles of the endoplasmic reticulum they gather an envelope of cell membrane around them. However, the peptides in this membrane are largely specified by the virus, although the lipids and glycolipids are the same as those of other normal membranes of the same type in the cell. Viruses with helical symmetry are usually enveloped, but so are some viruses with icosahedral symmetry, such as herpesviruses.

Earlier classifications of viruses referred to their size, and this in fact is still of considerable value when trying to identify an unknown virus. However, it is not a fundamental feature, and in the case of some enveloped viruses, such as coronaviruses, it can be quite variable. Ether lability was also used, and this is still a convenient way of deciding whether a virus is enveloped, since the

Table 1 Some Characteristics of Certain Viruses Found in the Human Intestinal Tract*

Family	Symmetry and size	Essential lipid ether/chloroform sensitivity	Nucleic acid	Virus
Picornaviradae	Icosahedral, 27 nm	0	ssRNA	Poliovirus types 1–3; coxsackie A, B; echoviruses
Reoviridae	Icosahedral, 80 nm	0	dsRNA, segmented	Reovirus 1–3, rotaviruses
Adenoviruses	Icosahedral, 70 nm	0	ssDNA	Higher serotypes found mainly in the gut
Parvovirus	Icosahedral, 30 nm	0	ssDNA	Uncertain whether viruses like parvoviruses found in gastroenteritis really belong to the group
Coronaviruses	Helical ?, 80–160 nm	+	ssRNA	Human enteric coronavirus not cultivated or studied in detail

*Electron micrographs of typical virus particles are shown as illustrations to other chapters.

lipid contained in the envelope can be extracted by ether and this leads to an immediate reduction in the infectivity of the virus—thus, enveloped viruses are *ether* and *chloroform labile.*

Viruses which are basically similar are also separated into serotypes if an immune serum raised against one virus has no effect on another; in a typical case the serum inactivates, or neutralizes, the virus against which it was raised but not another otherwise similar virus. There are, however, great differences in the number of serotypes which occur in different viruses. For example, there are only 2 serotypes of herpes simplex virus, whereas there are about 70 serotypes of enteroviruses. The latter are also subdivided to some extent by their pathogenicity for laboratory animals: the polioviruses are often very neuro-tropic for simians, the coxsackieviruses are pathogenic for suckling mice, and the echoviruses grow readily only in tissue cultures. Some serotypes are, how-ever, on the borderland between such groups, which are therefore convenient for practical purposes but of little fundamental taxonomic importance.

Table 1 is a summary of some of the main features of viruses which occur in the alimentary tract, or resemble those that do. Electron micrographs of many of the viruses can be found in the chapters which deal with particular organisms.

Virus Replication

There is an obvious and necessary relationship between the composition of different sorts of virus particle and the way they replicate when they enter cells, but there are also common features which arise from the fact that they are all nonmotile objects which need to come into intimate contact with the internal apparatus of the cell, without which they are unable to use or repli-cate the limited amount of genetic information they contain.

Viruses must first reach the cell surface, and they must be carried most of the way there passively—on air currents, in food, by peristaltic activity, and so on. Thereafter, in the vicinity of the cell, they may travel the last part of the distance by diffusion and become attached to specific receptors of various sorts found on the cell membrane. The method by which viruses enter cells is not well understood, but many seem to trigger a process akin to pinocytosis in which they become enfolded in a vacuole and drawn into the cell that way. They still have to pass the cell membrane, and this also is ill understood, but in every case the particle has to pass this barrier and become "uncoated," that is, lose its protein coat so that the nucleic acid within it is released and able to become metabolically active. The details may be different with various viruses, and are certainly more complicated than this brief description suggests. For example, it is known that some viruses, such as reoviruses, need to be digested by trypsin-like enzymes to become infective, and while enteroviruses become uncoated in the cytoplasm, adenoviruses move to the nucleus.

The replication of viral DNA resembles the processes which take place when cellular DNA replicates. From the viral DNA in the nucleus or the cyto-plasm, an RNA polymerase transcribes a strand of messenger RNA which then becomes attached to polysomes in the cytoplasm and directs the produc-tion of virus peptides, which include more enzymes and the structural peptides needed to form a new virus particles. The DNA is also replicated by a DNA polymerase and incorporated into the particles of which it forms the core. Particles may form in the cytoplasm or nucleus, sometimes in crystalline arrays, and these are then released when the cell breaks down. Viruses which bud through membranes may be released from the cell surface in this process or accumulate in the cisternae of the endoplasmic reticulum.

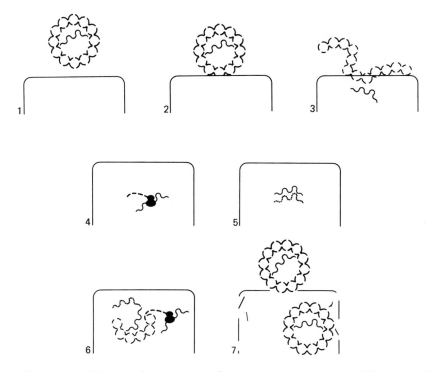

Figure 1   Scheme of replication of a simple positive-strand RNA virus. (1) Virus is adsorbed to the cell. (2) Virus particle attaches to specific receptors. (3) Virus particle becomes uncoated and RNA is released into the cell. (4) RNA attached to a ribosome directs the synthesis of virus peptide. (5) Using the virus-induced enzyme (not shown), a second "negative" strand of RNA is synthesized. (6) Using the negative strand as a template more positive RNA strands are made and incorporated into particles made of subunits. The subunits are formed by folding the peptides translated from a different section of the viral RNA. (7) The cell disintegrates, and virus particles are shed.

Viral RNA may replicate in various ways. In the simplest, the positive-stranded virus enters the cell, and is translated like an ordinary messenger RNA (Fig. 1). The peptides formed include a polymerase which produces a copy of the original RNA-negative virus strand. This in turn is copied again to produce a series of positive strands, each of which can then be inserted into a group of peptides which form a particle around it, or it may become bound to a peptide to form a nucleoprotein and this complex may lie beneath a cell membrane in which other viral proteins are inserted instead of cell proteins. The virus particle is then formed as the surface membrane bulges, then forms a bud which surrounds the nucleocapsid, and is finally nipped off. However, if the virus RNA is negative stranded the virus particle contains an enzyme which produces a positive stranded copy when the virus enters the cell, which can then be translated and carry on the process of replication.

Pathogenicity of Viruses

Viruses do not produce toxins which can act outside the cells they parasitize or in remote parts of the body. They have direct effects on the function and structure of cells they invade, and they also evoke immune responses. These immune responses in many cases have the main effect of terminating the infection by neutralizing virus or by destroying infected cells, but they may also contribute to the disease process. Nevertheless, the first and most important key to the production of disease is that many viruses are able to multiply freely in only a limited range of cells; even though two viruses may seem by electron microscopy or biochemical examination to be very similar they may affect only very different species. Even if they affect the same species they may attack different cells within it. A good example is given by two coronaviruses of pigs. One is transmissible gastroenteritis (TGE), which multiplies only in differentiated enterocytes of the villi of the small intestine. Thus it is very strictly a pathogen of the gastrointestinal tract of the pig, and it multiplies freely in the small intestine until all the enterocytes are destroyed. The disease which follows is a result of the loss of function of these cells, so there is a lack of digestion and adsorption of food. Later, the insusceptible cells of the crypts of Lieberkühn multiply and migrate up the villus and differentiate so that, provided the animal does not die of acute dehydration, all is restored as it was before. However, a closely related virus apparently produces marked gastrointestinal symptoms by quite different mechanisms. This is the virus of vomiting and wasting disease. It infects the upper and lower respiratory tract and also the stomach and jejunum where it invades Auerbach's and Meissner's plexus. From there it spreads via peripheral nerves to the central nervous system (CNS), where it first causes marked involvement of the brain stem, spreading later to the rest of the nervous system. It seems likely that the vomiting is due to involvement of the brain stem, where the "vomiting center" is situated, and that the involvement of the plexus impairs peristalsis and so the absorption of food, giving rise to the typical wasting. It is not surprising either that, as the CNS may be widely involved, a very similar virus has been isolated from the CNS and named the hemagglutinating encephalitis virus.

In these cases the evolution of the disease can be understood as a result of the specific tropism of the viruses for particular cells. These tropisms in turn are the results of the function of the nucleic acid and proteins referred to earlier. However, there are examples showing how particular viral proteins, for instance in reoviruses [4], are involved in the virulence or tropism of the virus; thus it is clear that the pathogenicity of viruses is under genetic control. It is in this sense that we understand the common observation that to pass a virus in an unusual host or by an unusual route will usually decrease its pathogenicity. From this we infer that mutants have been selected which replicate better in the new host system but less well in the original host. It is on this basis that viruses have been attenuated for use as vaccines.

In a number of cases viruses may spread from the gut into the bloodstream, in some cases via the lymphatics, and this viremia may distribute the virus to many other tissues, such as the skin or CNS; this is the mechanism by which enteroviruses, such as polioviruses and coxsackieviruses, produce a generalized disease process.

Immunity and Immunization

The host develops immunity against viruses as it does against other infectious agents, and it is commonly found that on reexposure to an intestinal virus an individual resists infection. This resistance is usually serotype specific. There are also other resistance factors that develop on aging and in other ways. The subject will not be developed here since it is referred to in detail in other chapters, particularly Chaps. 6 and 18.

Virus Cytopathology

When a virus replicates in a cell it may have profound effects on the cell's functioning. In some cases the cell may die; in others the cell may survive and the virus, too, and the cell may undergo malignant transformation though there is no evidence that this happens in the intestinal tract. Cell death is commonly observed in virus diagnostic tests when cells in a tissue culture which form a uniform monolayer are seen to round up and detach from the glass, the so-called cytopathic effect (CPE; Fig. 2). However, this is an end result which may follow a number of different processes inside the cell. In some instances infected cultures disintegrate cell by cell; in others they form syncytia; in some there are marked cytoplasmic changes, such as formation of vacuoles or inclusion bodies; and in others the main effects are in the nucleus. All these are a consequence of various metabolic and biochemical changes which take place in the cells. At present there is no information about the details of these changes in many of the tissues in which cytopathology is observed. However, from in vitro studies we know, for instance, that poliovirus inhibits protein synthesis in the host cell, though some other enteroviruses can replicate in cells and produce no obvious change. An eosinophilic cytoplasmic mass forms, and the nucleus becomes distorted and eventually shrinks (pyknosis) or breaks up (karyorrhexis). The cell suddenly becomes rounded. Adenovirus replication occurs in the nucleus, the normal structure of which is replaced by masses of virus particles.

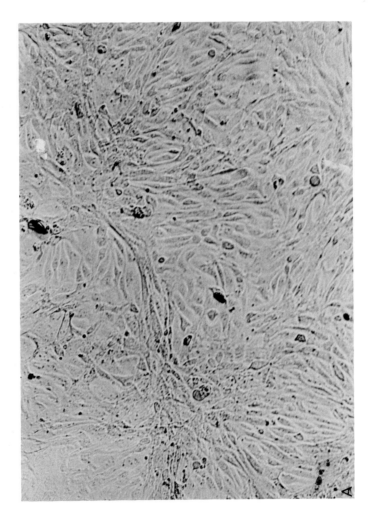

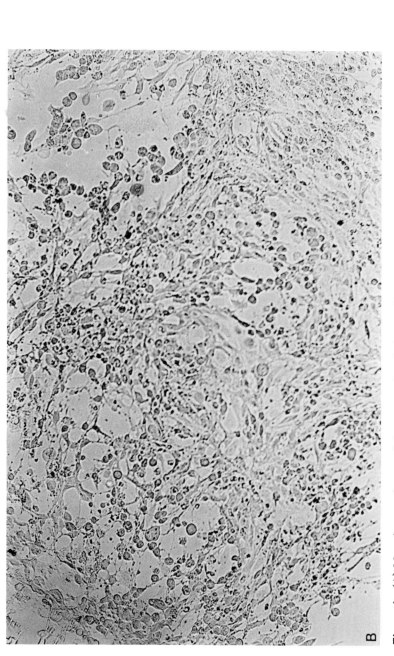
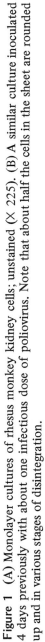

Figure 1 (A) Monolayer cultures of rhesus monkey kidney cells; unstained (X 225). (B) A similar culture inoculated 4 days previously with about one infectious dose of poliovirus. Note that about half the cells in the sheet are rounded up and in various stages of disintegration.

Coronaviruses bud at membrane surfaces, and the cell may become vacuolated or syncytia may form by the fusion of plasma membranes; eventually such cells die also, though there is still much to learn about the biochemical stages in this process.

It is important to remember also that many viruses show remarkable cell specificity. It is commonly found that a virus only infects certain species, and this is often paralleled by the results of tests in vitro. For instance, most strains of poliovirus infect the human and, in the laboratory, the monkey, but not lower animals. Likewise, in the test tube, fibroblasts and kidney cells from human and monkey are susceptible to infection with polioviruses, but cells from rabbits, calves, or chickens are not susceptible. However, within each animal, cells of different tissues may vary enormously in susceptibility. In fact, the pattern of disease often reflects this. Poliovirus multiplies in the pharynx and in Peyer's patches, but may also enter the blood and invade motor cells of the CNS. Rotaviruses, on the other hand, seem rarely to generalize, and usually replicate in the mature enterocytes of the upper intestinal villi. Rotaviruses and many other viruses recently found in the intestine grow in the laboratory only with great difficulty, and this is probably because so far we have no way of culturing cells with the microanatomical and physiological characteristics of enterocytes to which they seem to be so exquisitely and exclusively adapted.

The way in which the replication of viruses finally damages cells has been studied in some detail, and it is clear that very different mechanisms may be found. Poliovirus infection "switches off" the synthesis of host cell proteins, but this may not be immediately responsible for cell death. It has been suggested that the release of lysosomal enzymes into the cytoplasm may be the key role, but it is certainly not a universal cause, though it may well play a role in continuing the process of cell death and autolysis once these have begun. Adenovirus infection makes cells round up, but they continue to metabolize and produce acid. Viruses that bud from cell surfaces may continue to do so for long periods of time, and in some cases the cell may only become embarrassed when it can no longer synthesize further membrane lipid. However, little is known about coronavirus cytopathogenicity—and these are the only viruses that reproduce by budding which are likely to affect the human gut.

Virus Diagnosis

The diagnosis of virus infections follows the general principles and methods used in detecting microbial infections in general [2,3]. The first group of techniques is directed at recognizing the presence of a virus and preferably identifying it in some detail, and the second aims to detect the immune response of the host to the presence of foreign antigens, namely, the various viral peptides.

The most sensitive methods of detecting viruses are those in which infectious virus is propagated in the laboratory, usually in a tissue culture, though it is still necessary to inoculate suckling mice to detect many type A coxsackieviruses. Feces are collected and either stored frozen or processed immediately. The specimen is suspended in buffered saline with added antibiotics, is clarified on a bench centrifuge, and then approximately 0.1 ml volumes are inoculated into tissue cultures of susceptible cells, usually in rolled test tubes. After a few days or weeks many enteroviruses or adenoviruses replicate and kill the cells, and a cytopathic effect is observed. The medium contains virus, the properties of which are tested, for instance for resistance to ether or to estimate the size of the particle by passage through membranes of known porosity. The treated medium is tested in further cultures to determine whether infectious virus is still present. For final identification it is usually necessary to neutralize the virus (i.e., render it noninfectious for tissue culture) by mixing it with specific animal antiserum. In this way it is serotyped. Other tests such as complement fixation, hemagglutination, and hemagglutination inhibition may also be useful.

Virus particles can also be detected with a high degree of probability by other methods. These are basically visualization of the virus by electron microscopy, particularly when large numbers of characteristic particles are shed, or by detecting viral antigens by an immunologic test such as complement fixation, immunofluorescence, or radioimmunoassay. These are described in some detail in Chaps. 3, 4, and 9. It is a striking consequence of the use of some of these techniques in the study of the virology of the gastrointestinal tract that it has been possible to investigate in some detail the nature and role of viruses which still cannot be cultivated in the laboratory: in earlier days we would have been unable to prove that they existed.

It is also possible to diagnose infection by detecting a rising titer of antibodies in sera collected early and late in the course of a disease. This was done first in the case of enteroviruses and adenoviruses, and more recently with others such as rotaviruses. There are numerous possible techniques, but they are not always practical and have different advantages and disadvantages. If there are many serotypes and the test used is type specific, then antibody measurements are useful only to confirm infection in a case from which the virus has already been isolated, e.g., enterovirus infections. In other instances there may be a common antigen found in all viruses of the group, and tests for antibody to this may be useful even though the viruses may be found in many serotypes when examined by neutralization or by other tests that detect antigens at the surface of the virus particle; an example of this situation is the use of complement fixation tests in adenovirus infections.

Etiologic Significance

It is important to remember that even when infection with a virus has been detected by direct or indirect means it is not proved that the virus causes any disease that the patient may have. A classic example of this lies behind the naming of the enteric cytopathic human orphan viruses, the echoviruses, the orphan implying that they were viruses "in search of a disease," either because they had been found only in the feces of healthy children or because they were not regularly associated with disease.

The classic criteria deciding that a virus causes a disease have been modified from the original "Koch's postulates." Such modified criteria might read:

1. The agent must be shown to be present in most cases of a disease.
2. It should be present in a significantly lower proportion of subjects of similar age and other characteristics who are without disease and living in the same epidemiologic environment.
3. The agent should, if possible, be transmitted serially in the laboratory and then shown to cause a disease like that found in the patient on inoculation into a susceptible host. If the virus cannot be passaged it should be tested in a susceptible host and it should be shown again that those hosts that are affected show laboratory evidence of infection.

Thus the organisms can only be shown to be causing disease on a group or statistical basis. In individual cases it may still be impossible to be sure whether any agent detected caused the disease observed.

References

1. C. H. Andrews, and H. G. Pereira, *Viruses of Vertebrates,* Bailliere Tindall, London, 1972.
2. F. Fenner and D. O. White, *Medical Virology,* Academic, New York, (1976).
3. B. N. Fields, in D. A. J. Tyrrell, Mechanisms of viral pathogenesis and virulence, *Nature, 280*:193 (1979).
4. N. R. Grist and E. J. Bell, *Diagnostic Methods in Clinical Virology,* 3rd Ed., Blackwell, Oxford, (1979).
5. A. Z. Kapikian, R. H. Yolken, H. B. Greenberg, R. G. Wyatt, A. R. Kalicia, R. M. Chanock, and H. W. Kim, *Gastroenteritis Viruses in Diagnostic Procedures for Viral, Rickettsial and Chlamydial Infection* (E. H. Lennette and N. J. Schmidt, eds.), American Public Health Association, Washington, D.C., 1979, pp. 927–995.
6. D. A. J. Tyrrell, D. J. Alexander, J. D. Almeida, C. H. Cunningham, B. C. Easterday, D. J. Garwes, J. C. Hierholzer, A. Kapikian, M. R. Macnaughton, and K. McIntosh, Coronaviridae: Second report. *Intervirology, 10*: 321.

— 2

Methods of Gastroenteritis Virus Culture In Vivo and In Vitro

Richard G. Wyatt and Walter D. James National Institute of Allergy and Infectious Diseases, Bethesda, Maryland

Those viruses associated in recent years with acute gastroenteritis in humans have been refractory or relatively resistant to growth in cell and organ culture systems [18,20]. These viruses include rotaviruses, the Norwalk virus group, adenoviruses, coronaviruses, and other small round viruses such as astroviruses and caliciviruses. On the other hand, viruses such as the echoviruses and certain coxsackieviruses, which can be isolated with relative ease from the contents of the enteric tract, have not emerged as major etiologic agents of acute diarrheal disease despite great expectations resulting from early reports on their presence in fecal specimens [20]. Thus, as the study of newer infectious agents causing diarrhea began, in vitro cultivation methods did not play a major role. Examination of specimens by electron microscopy (EM) and the use of animal models, however, have been important tools in the study of rotaviruses [20]. For many of these other agents, which do not replicate efficiently either in tissue culture or in animal model systems, classification and characterization attempts have been based mainly on the morphologic appearance of virus particles by EM [18,20,26,36].

The methods discussed in this chapter represent only a beginning in the cultivation of some of these newly recognized viruses. Since such viruses have in common the environment from which they are recovered, the conditions of growth defined for one virus may be applicable to others. In the sections which follow, rotaviruses will be considered first because of their importance and because more information is available on them than on the other groups.

In Vivo Cultivation Systems

Rotaviruses

Human rotavirus has been shown to replicate and produce diarrhea in a variety of newborn animals, including gnotobiotic calves, piglets, and lambs, as well as conventional piglets and colostrum-deprived rhesus monkeys; human rotavirus has also been shown to induce diarrhea in a small number of susceptible adult volunteers by the oral route [17,20,21,34,35,42,48,53,54,56]. In animal studies, virus is introduced directly into the enteric tract orally, by stomach tube, or by injection into the duodenum at the time of laparotomy as in the case of gnotobiotic calves. In the animal systems, the virus has been demonstrated to replicate only in the small intestine, usually in mature mucosal epithelial cells covering approximately the distal half of villi; immature crypt cells are spared (Fig. 1A) [53,54]. When examined by negative-stain EM, the virus in fecal samples is usually present in both complete and incomplete forms, i.e., with and without the outer capsid. The maximal quantity of virus is shed in diarrheal feces early and usually coincides with onset of diarrhea. Diarrheal or even nondiarrheal feces rich in virus particles can be processed further for use as antigen in complement fixation (CF), immune adherence hemagglutination assay (IAHA), enzyme-linked immunosorbent assay (ELISA), and the fluorescent focus neutralization test; purified virus can also be used to prepare hyperimmune sera in animals [20]. When generating antigen in gnotobiotic animals in this fashion, a useful by-product is infection serum directed against the human rotavirus used as inoculum.

Norwalk Virus

Norwalk virus has been administered to a variety of animals including mice, guinea pigs, rabbits, kittens, calves, baboons, chimpanzees, and rhesus, marmoset, owl, patas, and cebus monkeys, but has failed to produce disease in them [20]. Humans appear to be the only host susceptible to the development of diarrhea with Norwalk virus, although chimpanzees become infected as evidenced by development of a serum antibody response and shedding of viral antigen in feces. The antigen shed in chimpanzee feces has been recovered mainly in a soluble form and thus is of limited usefulness in studies on the biochemical composition of Norwalk virus [17].

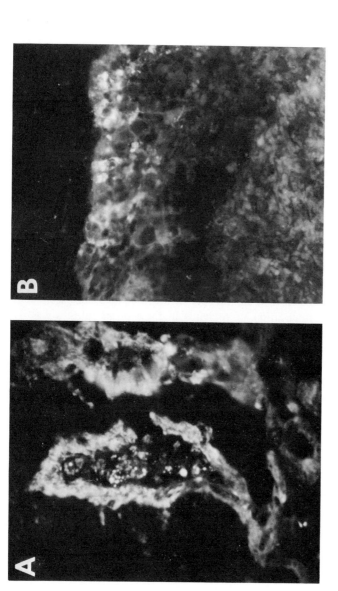

Figure 1   Rotaviral antigens detected by immunofluorescence in differentiated tissues. (A) Lower small intestine of newborn rhesus monkey 24 h after administration of human rotavirus; viral antigens are mainly in villous epithelial cells, and crypts are spared (×250). (B) Human embryonic intestinal organ culture 9 days after inoculation with human rotavirus; scattered epithelial cells contain viral antigens (×160). (A, From Ref. 53; B, from Ref. 55.)

Other Human Enteric Viral Pathogens

No useful in vivo systems have been reported for the study of human adeno-viruses, coronaviruses, or other small round viruses.

Organ Culture Systems

Rotaviruses

The use of organ culture offers the theoretical advantage of supplying differen-tiated cell populations for the cultivation of viruses, such as rotavirus, observed to replicate in mature villous epithelial cells. Epizootic diarrhea of infant mice (EDIM) virus, the first rotavirus to be visualized by ultrathin section EM was sub-sequently cultivated to a limited extent in mouse intestinal organ cultures of ileum, cecum, and colon, but not esophagus or duodenum [39]. The infec-tivity of the culture harvests for mice was used to assess replication in this early study. Later attempts to cultivate EDIM virus efficiently in vitro failed, thus viral antigen was generated by experimentally infecting mice and provided the major source of EDIM virus for study.

Human embryonic intestinal organ culture has been used with limited success in the cultivation of human rotavirus [55]. Of 15 strains derived from different infants and young children, 3 were shown to grow using indirect immunofluorescence (IF) to detect viral antigens; one strain ("D") was pas-saged serially four times in this system [54,55]. Virus replicated in the cyto-plasm of villous epithelial cells (Fig. 1B). After infection was initiated in indi-vidual cells or in small foci, virus did not spread further to involve adjacent cells. Further evidence for replication of rotavirus in these organ cultures was ob-tained using ultrathin section EM; rotavirus particles were seen 15 days follow-ing inoculation (Fig. 2).

The scarcity of suitable human embryonic intestine and the inefficient growth of rotavirus in this system have limited its usefulness. In additional studies, porcine, bovine, and rhesus monkey embryonic intestine of comparable age supported the growth of human rotavirus less well than did human em-bryonic intestine (R. G. Wyatt et al., unpublished).

Specific Methodology

Organ cultures of human embryonic intestine, derived from 9- to 16-week-old fetuses, were established in Petri dish culture maintained with L-15 (Leibovitz) medium without serum. Cultures were incubated on a rocker plat-form at $33°C$ without added CO_2. Under these conditions, cultures could be maintained for up to approximately 3 weeks with recognizable villous archi-tecture [11].

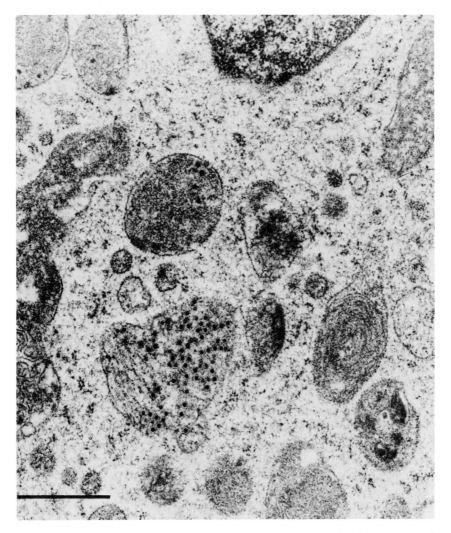

Figure 2 Electron micrograph of rotavirus particles in ultrathin section of human embryonic intestinal organ culture 15 days after inoculation with human rotavirus. Particles have an electron-dense core and are considered to be "full" (bar = 1 μm).

Dishes were inoculated with 0.2 ml of undiluted 2% fecal filtrates per dish. At various intervals following inoculation, explants were removed and frozen sections prepared for IF microscopy to monitor viral growth; ultrathin sections of explants were prepared following fixation in glutaraldehyde. Fluid medium or organ explants in culture medium were frozen and thawed three times for further passage experiments [55].

Norwalk Virus and Other Human Viral Enteric Pathogens

The use of human embryonic intestinal organ culture appears to have failed in the purpose for which the system described above was originally developed, i.e., to cultivate Norwalk virus [5]. However, the successful cultivation of a coronavirus recovered from an outbreak of gastroenteritis in adults has been reported using explants of human embryonic intestine [9,10].

Cell Culture Systems

Rotaviruses

Despite intensive efforts by many investigators around the world, there remained in 1980 relatively few isolates of rotavirus which grew efficiently in cell culture systems. Efficient replication is here defined as the ability of a rotavirus isolate to undergo serial passage with a growth yield sufficient to permit characterization of the strain. Certainly, diagnosis of rotavirus infection by isolating virus from diarrheal feces using routine cell culture methods was not useful.

First Isolations

Successful cultivation of two unidentified viruses, later recognized to be rotaviruses, was reported first by Malherbe and Strickland-Cholmley in South Africa with the isolation in 1958 of Simian Agent (SA)-11 virus from the rectal swab of an asymptomatic vervet monkey and the offal ("O") agent in 1965 from slaughterhouse waste [27]. No special procedures were utilized to propagate these strains in primary vervet monkey kidney cell cultures (Table 1). Neither of these strains was associated with diarrhea, nor were they recognized until much later to resemble reoviruses morphologically.

Later, successful cultivation of rotavirus associated with neonatal diarrhea in calves was first achieved by Mebus and colleagues in 1971 [32]. Two strains of this neonatal calf diarrhea virus (NCDV) were propagated as summarized in Table 1. The cultivation of additional strains of bovine rotavirus, as well as porcine, avian, human, and simian rotavirus, is also outlined [1,2,7,25,30,31,44,46, 51].

In 1980 the cultivation of human rotavirus ("Wa") in primary African green monkey kidney (AGMK) cell cultures was reported (Fig. 3) [51]. The Wa strain was selected from a group of 42 diarrheal stools by examining them for their ability to initiate infection in AGMK cells, using techniques of trypsin treatment and low-speed centrifugation, which are described later. This human

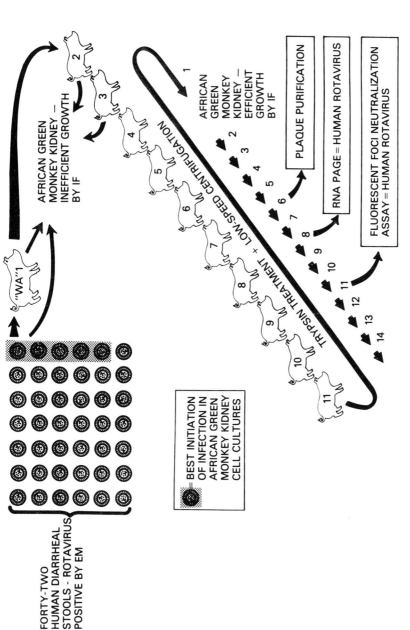
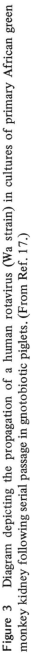

Figure 3 Diagram depicting the propagation of a human rotavirus (Wa strain) in cultures of primary African green monkey kidney following serial passage in gnotobiotic piglets. (From Ref. 17.)

Table 1 Techniques Used for Cell Culture Propagation of Selected Rotaviruses from Animals and Humans

Rotavirus recovered from:	Association with diarrhea	Investigator (year)	Strain designation
Vervet monkey	No	Malherbe and Strickland-Cholmley (1967) [27]	SA-11
Slaughterhouse waste	Unknown	Malherbe and Strickland-Cholmley (1967) [27]	0 agent
Calf	Yes	Mebus et al. (1971) [32]	(a)NCDV-Cody
			(b)NCDV-Lincoln
Calf	Yes	Bridger and Woode (1975) [7]	NCDR (UK, Compton)
Calf	Yes	McNulty et al. (1976) [30]	Northern Ireland
Calf	Yes	L'Haridon and Scherrer (1976) [25]	Thiverval-Grignon
Calf	Yes	Babiuk et al. (1977) [2]	C-486
Calf	Yes	Almeida et al. (1978) [1]	WRV-310
Piglet	Yes	Theil et al. (1977) [46]	(a) OSU
			(b) EE
Chickens, turkeys	Yes	McNulty et al. (1979) [31]	Undesignated
Human infant	Yes	Wyatt et al. (1980) [51]	Wa
Rhesus monkey	Yes	Stuker et al. (1980) [44]	(a) S:USA:78:1 (MMU17959) (b) S:USA:78:2 (MMU18006)

*Continuous cell line.

Cells used in initial isolation	Exogenous enzyme used in initial isolation	Number of passages in experimental animals prior to initial isolation (species)
1° Vervet monkey kidney	None	None
1° Vervet monkey kidney	None	None
1°Fetal bovine choroid plexus, 1° fetal bovine thyroid 1° fetal bovine lung, embryonic bovine trachea*	None	Seven (bovine)
1° Fetal bovine kidney	None	Two (bovine)
1° Calf kidney	None	None
2° Calf kidney	None	None
1° Fetal bovine kidney, 1° fetal sheep kidney	None	None
1° Fetal bovine kidney 1° African green monkey kidney, BSC-1	Trypsin	None
1° Calf kidney	None	None
1° Porcine kidney	Pancreatin	Seven (porcine)
1° Porcine kidney	Pancreatin	Two (porcine)
Chick embryo liver, chick embryo kidney	Trypsin	None
1° African green monkey kidney	Trypsin	Eleven (porcine)
1° Cynomolgus monkey kidney 1° Cynomolgus monkey kidney	None	None

rotavirus strain was subsequently passaged 11 times in gnotobiotic piglets, after which it replicated efficiently in AGMK cultures with a titer of $10^{5.2}$ fluorescent foci per milliliter at passage 14. Wa strain was confirmed to be human rotavirus based on the migration pattern of its RNA segments and by cross-neutralization tests with other rotaviruses using distinguishing sera made against them [19,51].

Very recently two groups of Japanese investigators described the successful isolation of several strains of human rotaviruses (not shown in Table 1) in roller tube cultures of MA104 cells [57,58]. It has also been possible to cultivate human rotaviruses by the use of genetic reassortment with temperature-sensitive mutants of bovine rotavirus [59,60]. Further details on these recent exciting advances appear in Chapter 19.

Cell Types Used

Kidney cells in primary culture from a variety of species were the cell types most frequently used for the initial isolation of rotaviruses listed in Table 1, although currently cell lines such as MDBK, PK-15, IBRS-2, BSC-1, LLC-MK$_2$, Buffalo green monkey kidney, CV-1, and MA-104 are being used successfully [1, 2,4,14,15,25,29,30,37,41,45,50]. These cell lines have the advantage of being less costly than primary cells, but offer the disadvantage that viral strains passaged in them cannot be considered as potential vaccine candidates for human use.

Detection of Viral Growth

Rotaviruses growing in cell cultures have been detected by a variety of methods, including EM, immune EM, CF, IF, radioimmunoassay (RIA), and ELISA, as well as by the development of cytopathic effect (CPE) and plaque formation [20]. Early reports of rotavirus CPE included a description of characteristic "flagging," in which cells remain partially attached to the surface of the culture vessel and wave in the medium [18,49]. CPE can also take the form of nondescript granular degeneration of the cell monolayer; lytic foci may also be observed. Small eosinophilic inclusions have been seen in kidney cell cultures infected with NCDV, SA-11, and O agent [27,49], but the appearance of inclusions has not been used widely to assess viral growth. Cultures can also be infected without obvious CPE, and for this reason, as well as for monitoring early replication, IF is useful. Cultures grown in plastic dishes or on coverslips can be fixed with methanol or acetone, respectively, and examined by direct or indirect immunofluorescence microscopy. Antigens of human rotavirus (Wa), for example, are detected in the cytoplasm of infected cells, beginning with the appearance of finely granular fluorescence as early as 6 h after inoculation and progressing to homogeneous or very coarsely granular fluorescence within 24 h (R. G. Wyatt et al., unpublished). Foci of infected cells are prominent with some rotavirus strains, while with others, scattered single cells are infected with less obvious cell-to-cell spread (Fig. 4).

Plaque assays for rotavirus growth are becoming useful as the necessary techniques are developed [13,29,37,41,50]; these methods will be specifically outlined later.

Use of Proteolytic Enzymes

In recent primary isolations of rotaviruses, treatment with exogenous proteolytic enzymes has been used extensively; the use of trypsin or pancreatin was essential in the cultivation of porcine, avian, and human rotaviruses [2,12, 31,46,51]. Even in the case of some rotaviruses already adapted to grow in cell culture, viral titers increase when virus is incubated with trypsin prior to inoculation [2,4]. In the case of bovine rotaviruses (NCDV-Lincoln, UK, and C-486), an approximate 20- to 100-fold increase in titer is observed when the inoculum is treated with trypsin, compared with untreated viral inoculum [2,4,20]. While trypsin exerts an effect on the virus itself, the mechanism for this action has not been elucidated. By analogy with reovirus and influenza virus, trypsin may act by cleaving surface polypeptide(s) of rotavirus [22,43]. Addition of trypsin to the maintenance medium during viral replication also enhances growth [1,45], perhaps by acting on progeny virus produced during early replication cycles. The enhancement of infectivity to a lesser extent than with trypsin has been demonstrated by incubating bovine rotavirus (NCDV-Lincoln) with protease and lactase prior to inoculation and by adding elastase or α-chymotrypsin to maintenance medium in cultures of porcine rotavirus (OSU) [4,45]. The ability of most rotaviruses to form plaques in monolayer culture is clearly enhanced by the addition to overlays of suitable concentrations of trypsin which permit cells to remain attached, but at the same time act on virus.

The concentrations of trypsin used vary depending on the purity of the preparations. Although it is useful to know the enzymatic activity of each preparation used, an optimal trypsin concentration is usually determined in each laboratory. For example, in the cultivation of human rotavirus (Wa) the virus is incubated with trypsin (Sigma Type IX) at a final concentration of 10 μg/ml prior to inoculation of cultures with serial dilutions of this material [51]. For plaque formation with Wa human rotavirus, 0.5 μg/ml of the same trypsin is added to an agarose overlay; primary AGMK, CV-1, and MA-104 cells usually tolerate this concentration for 5–7 days. Similar concentrations of trypsin have been used for animal rotaviruses.

Use of DEAE-Dextran

DEAE-dextran has been used to enhance rotavirus plaque formation but has a lesser enhancing effect than trypsin and is not essential for plaquing [29, 41].

Animal Passage Prior to Cultivation in Cell Cultures

Among the special procedures used in initial isolation of the rotaviruses listed in Table 1, multiple (2–11) serial passages in experimentally infected

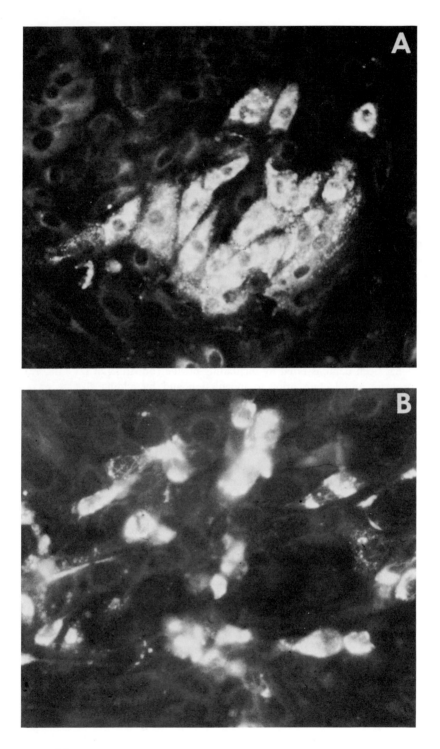

24

piglets or calves were performed prior to the successful cultivation of certain rotaviruses, including two bovine, two porcine, and a single human strain [32, 46,51]. During these passages of virus in animals, the virus may have undergone the process of mutation, which then permitted growth of the strains.

Low-Speed Centrifugation

Low-speed centrifugation of fecal specimens containing rotavirus onto cell monolayers and detection of viral antigens by IF has been described as a method of rotavirus diagnosis. The technique was first described using the IBRS-2 continuous cell line and later, the LLC-MK$_2$ line [3,8]. While it is unlikely that virus particles are deposited directly on the cells at the speeds used, e.g., 1200g or 3000g, heavy viral aggregates may be concentrated on the cell surface [40]. Another possibility is that an alteration of the cell membrane may occur which results in increased numbers of infected cells. By the use of this procedure, various rotaviruses initiate infection in cell cultures more efficiently, although successful serial propagation of rotaviruses has not resulted from its use alone [40,47]. In the adaptation of human rotavirus (Wa) in primary AGMK cells, cultures inoculated with trypsin-treated virus were spun at 1400g at 37°C for 1 h [51]. An approximate 10-fold increase in viral titer was observed as a result of this low-speed centrifugation. This procedure is also a useful step in the fluorescent focus neutralization test because it enhances infectivity [47].

Methods for Plaquing Rotaviruses

The first rotavirus to be plaqued successfully was bovine rotavirus (NCDV-Lincoln); Matsuno and colleagues working in Japan used trypsin and DEAE-dextran to facilitate plaque formation of this virus [29]. Subsequently other bovine, porcine, simian, and human rotaviruses have been plaqued using for the most part techniques similar to those of Matsuno et al. [37,41,51,52]. The development of improved methods in this area is advancing the characterization of rotaviruses as well as their genetic manipulation. Studies by Matsuno and colleagues showing gene reassortment between bovine rotavirus (NCDV-Lincoln) and ultraviolet-treated simian rotavirus (SA-11) and by Greenberg and colleagues demonstrating reassortment between temperature-sensitive bovine rotavirus (UK) and human rotaviruses were made possible by plaquing methods [17,28, 59,60]. Because these methods are similar, some of the techniques used for

---

Figure 4 Rotaviral antigens detected by immunofluorescence in monolayer culture. (A) NCDV-Lincoln in primary bovine embryonic kidney; such focus formation appears when virus spreads from cell to cell (×160). (B) Human rotavirus (Wa) on first passage in primary African green monkey kidney; scattered cells are infected (×312).

plaquing only bovine and human rotaviruses will be described here in order to make comparisons.

Bovine Rotavirus Plaque Assay [29,50]. In an early study by Welch and Twiehaus [49], plaques could not be produced consistently using NCDV (Lincoln and Cody) in bovine embryonic kidney cell monolayers; medium used in those experiments was Hanks' balanced salt solution with 0.5% lactalbumin hydrolysate, 5% fetal calf serum, 0.9% ionagar, and in certain experiments, DEAE-dextran.

Matsuno and colleagues later reported successful plaque formation of NCDV-Lincoln in MA-104 cells [29]. Cell monolayers were grown in 50 mm plastic dishes for 4 days; monolayers were washed with phosphate-buffered saline (PBS) containing 0.2% bovine serum albumin (BSA) and virus dilutions made in PBS with BSA were inoculated (0.1 ml per dish). After adsorption for 1 h at 37°C, an overlay was added consisting of Eagle's Minimum Essential Medium (MEM) with added $NaHCO_3$, 0.8% agarose, 100 μg/ml DEAE-dextran, and 2 μg/ml crystalline trypsin (Sigma). After 3 days incubation, a second overlay containing neutral red was added, and plaques were counted the following day. The results obtained by Matsuno and colleagues are shown in Fig. 5; clearly the best plaque formation was observed when trypsin and dextran were both used in the overlay, when compared with DEAE-dextran alone or no additives. Large plaques formed when trypsin alone was added, but the number increased by about sixfold when DEAE-dextran was added as well [29].

Plaque formation by another bovine rotavirus strain (UK) was reported at the IV International Congress for Virology at The Hague [50]. This virus was plaqued in cell cultures of primary AGMK, primary calf kidney, and two continuous lines, CV-1 and MA-104. The addition of proteolytic enzyme to the overlay is not required for the production of plaques with the UK virus. However, because pretreatment of undiluted virus with trypsin was found to increase the titer by up to 100-fold, UK virus is now routinely incubated with an equal volume of trypsin solution (20 μg/ml) for up to 90 min at 38°C prior to making serial dilutions. Sigma crystalline trypsin, type IX, is dissolved in PBS (pH 7.4) to make a stock solution containing 2 mg/ml which is stored in small aliquots at -20°C; the appropriate dilution is made just before use. Virus dilutions are made in L-15 with 0.5% gelatin, glutamine, and antibiotics (L-15/gel) and inoculated in 1 ml amounts onto monolayers washed three times with L-15/gel. After adsorption for 60–90 min at -38°C, plates are washed once with L-15/gel and overlayed with either (1) L-15 medium containing 0.9% methylcellulose, 5% agamma or fetal calf serum, glutamine, and antibiotics, or (2) Eagle's MEM containing 0.9% agarose, 5% agamma or fetal calf serum, glutamine, and antibiotics. With the use of the L-15/methylcellulose overlay, plates are incubated for 7 days in humidified air without added CO_2 at 38°C, the op-

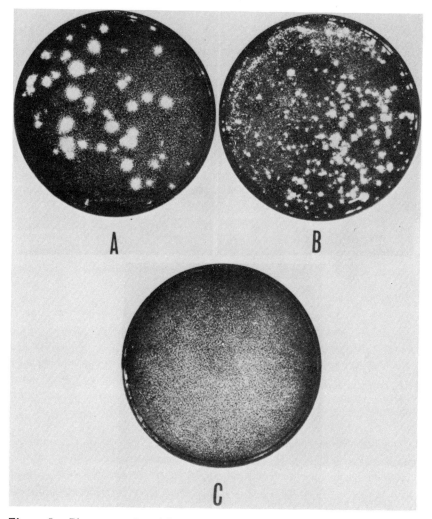

Figure 5 Plaques produced by bovine rotavirus (NCDV-Lincoln) in MA-104 cell monolayers. (A) Agar overlay contains DEAE-dextran and trypsin; 4 days after inoculation. (B) Agar overlay contains only DEAE-dextran; 6 days after inoculation. (C) Agar overlay without DEAE-dextran or trypsin; 6 days after inoculation. (From Ref. 29.)

timal temperature for plaquing UK virus under these conditions. Plates are then fixed with formalin and stained with hematoxylin and eosin or, more easily, with crystal violet prior to counting plaques. Plaques produced optimally by UK virus in this system are illustrated in Fig. 6. With the use of the Eagle's

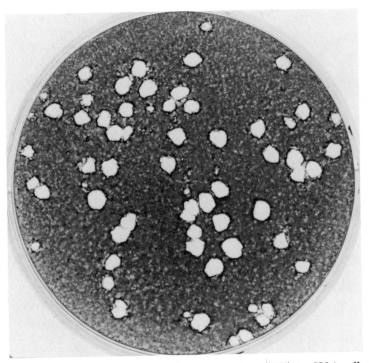

Figure 6 Plaques produced by bovine rotavirus (UK) in CV-1 cell monolayers. Overlay consists of L-15 medium containing 0.9% methylcellulose, 5% agamma calf serum, glutamine, and antibiotics. Plaques vary in size but have a distinct margin.

MEM/agarose overlay, plates are incubated at 38°C in 5% CO_2 humidified atmosphere for 3–7 days, at which time a second overlay containing neutral red is added. Plaques are then counted and picked 1–3 days later.

Human Rotavirus Plaque Assay [52]. Confluent cell monolayers of primary AGMK, CV-1, or MA-104, are grown in six-well plastic dishes. Numerous other cell types have been screened for growth of Wa strain by IF (Table 2); while growth was detected in additional cell types, suitable plaques were only observed in three. In some cases, cells did not tolerate the trypsin necessary for plaque formation. Cells are washed three times with L-15/gel to remove serum used in cell cultivation. Prior to inoculation of virus, it is mixed with an equal volume of trypsin solution (20 μg/ml) as described above for plaquing bovine rotavirus (UK). Virus-trypsin mixture is then incubated for as long as 90 min at 37°C, after which serial 10-fold dilutions are made in L-15/gel. Into a single well of duplicate six-well dishes, 1 ml of each dilution is inoculated.

Table 2 Growth of Human Rotavirus (Wa) in Various Cell Cultures Measured by Immunofluorescence and Plaque Formation[a]

	Cell type (titer of standard Wa pool: PFU/ml or FF/ml)	
Description of growth	Primary cells	Continuous cell lines
A. Plaque formation and development of fluorescent foci	African green monkey kidney (10^5 FF/ml; 2×10^5 PFU/ml)	CV-1 (10^5 FF/ml; 9×10^5 PFU ml) MA-104 (10^5 FF/ml; 6×10^5 PFU/ml)
B. Development of fluorescent foci without efficient plaque formation	Cynomolgus monkey kidney (10^4 FF/ml) Calf kidney (10^4 FF/ml)	LLC-MK$_2$ (10^5 FF/ml) Buffalo green monkey kidney (10^4 FF/ml) HRT-18 (10^3 FF/ml) BSC-1 (10^2 FF/ml)
C. No growth detected at lowest dilution tested (10^{-1} or 10^{-2})	Guinea pig kidney[b] Hamster kidney[b] Rabbit kidney[b] Chick embryo[b] Hamster embryo[b] Rat embryo[b] Swiss mouse embryo[b]	MA383 L929 HeLa[b] HEp-2[b] Vero[b] AV-3[b] MA185[b] FL human amnion[b]

[a]*Note*: All cell cultures were produced by MA Bioproducts; HRT-18 cells were kindly supplied by Dr. W. A. F. Tompkins, Univeristy of Illinois, Urbana, Illinois, and MA104 cells by Dr. E. H. Bohl, Ohio Agricultural Research and Development Center, Wooster, Ohio.
[b]Cells examined only for development of fluorescent foci 24–48 h after inoculation; the monolayers degenerated rapidly under conditions used for plaquing.

Adsorption takes place at $37°C$ without added CO_2 for 1 h, after which the inoculum is removed and cells are washed once with L-15/gel. Overlay is added consisting of Eagle's MEM with Earle's salts, 0.9% agarose, glutamine, gentamicin, amphotericin B, and trypsin (0.5 μg/ml) prepared from the same stock solution described above. After incubation for 4 to 5 days at $37°C$, a second overlay is added consisting of Eagle's MEM with 0.9% agarose and neutral red (0.067 mg/ml of overlay). Plaques are counted 1 and 2 days later; plates may be fixed with formalin and stained with crystal violet after maximal plaque production has been observed. Such a plate is shown in Fig. 7, which represents a titration of a Wa stock suspension containing approximately 10^5 plaque-forming units (PFU)/ml. Plaques can be readily counted but are not uniform in size and have an indistinct margin. At lower dilutions of the virus (10^{-1} and 10^{-2}), the cell sheet is completely destroyed.

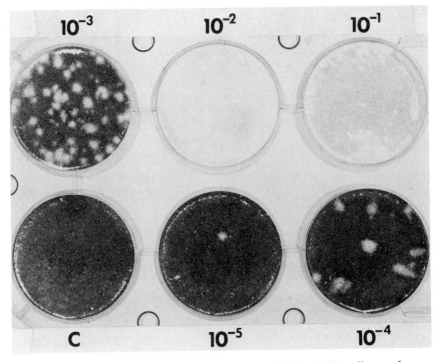

Figure 7 Plaques produced by human rotavirus (Wa) in CV-1 cell monolayers. Virus is diluted 10^{-1} through 10^{-5}. Overlay consists of Eagle's MEM containing 0.9% agarose, trypsin (0.5 μg/ml), glutamine, and antibiotics. Plaques vary in size and have an indistinct margin.

Serum neutralization of virus by the method of plaque reduction can be measured by mixing a standard amount of virus, yielding approximately 30 PFU per well, with test serum dilutions for 1 h at 37°C [52]. The serum-virus mixtures are inoculated into wells, and the test is continued as described above. This and similar procedures are useful in establishing serologic identification of rotaviruses adapted to grow in cell culture [13,52].

Norwalk Virus

No cell culture systems have been identified in which Norwalk or related viruses will grow. The use of a sensitive RIA that is now available should aid in these studies [20].

Adenoviruses

Many of the adenoviruses visualized by EM in stools of pediatric patients with diarrhea cannot be grown in cell culture and are referred to as fastidious or noncultivable enteric adenoviruses [16,20,38]. However, limited replication of these enteric adenoviruses in human amnion cells (HAE-70) has been demonstrated by Retter et al. using IF and by detecting characteristic intranuclear inclusions; spread of virus to adjacent cells was not observed with these fastidious strains. This is in contrast to cultivable adenovirus strains which exhibit spread from cell to cell [38].

Coronaviruses

Few associations of coronaviruses with diarrhea in humans have been made, in spite of the recognition of animal coronaviruses (e.g., transmissible gastroenteritis of pigs and bovine coronavirus) as important animal pathogens. These animal coronaviruses possess the ability to grow in cell cultures [6,33].

Human coronavirus, identified in one gastroenteritis outbreak in adults, was propagated in a limited fashion in cultures of human embryonic kidney cells as well as human embryonic intestinal explants [9,10]. Recently, Chaney and LaPorte reported at the XI Perspectives in Virology Symposium in New York on the detection of coronaviruses in an outbreak of hemorrhagic diarrhea occurring in infants in Paris; these coronaviruses were reported to grow in HRT-18 cells [17,61].

Astroviruses

Limited replication of astroviruses has been observed in cultures of human embryonic kidney using indirect IF to detect replication. Attempts to passage astroviruses in cell cultures and establish productive infection failed [23,24].

Caliciviruses and Other Human Enteric Viral Pathogens

No suitable cell culture systems have been reported for the growth of calicivirus or other small round viruses recovered from human diarrheal stools.

Conclusion

Methods of culture for the viral agents which cause gastroenteritis are beginning to emerge and to be useful with certain of these viruses, especially rotavirus. However, cultivation of rotavirus is still not routine, and only a limited number of strains adapted to grow in cell culture exists. Yet with the current foothold, rapid progress should ensue over the next few years, and the methods developed for rotavirus cultivation should be applied to other fastidious enteric viruses. These techniques include serial propagation in a susceptible host prior to attempted growth in vitro, the use of more sensitive assay systems to detect viral growth, the search for and development of more sensitive cell culture systems (e.g., MA-104 cells) for propagation of virus, and the use of proteolytic enzymes and other potential activators of infectivity to enhance viral replication.

References

1. J. D. Almeida, T. Hall, J. E. Banatvala, B. M. Totterdell, and I. L. Chrystie, The effect of trypsin on the growth of rotavirus, *J. Gen. Virol., 40*:213–218 (1978).

2. L. A. Babiuk, K. Mohammed, L. Spence, M. Fauvel, and R. Petro. Rotavirus isolation and cultivation in the presence of trypsin, *J. Clin. Microbiol. 6*:610–617. (1977).

3. J. E. Banatvala, B. Totterdell, I. L. Chrystie, and G. N. Woode, In vitro detection of human rotaviruses, *Lancet, 2*:821 (1975).

4. B. B. Barnett, R. S. Spendlove, and M. L. Clark, Effect of enzymes on rotavirus infectivity, *J. Clin. Microbiol., 10*:111-113.

5. N. R. Blacklow, R. Dolin, D. S. Fedson, H. DuPont, R. S. Northrup, R. B. Hornick, and R. M. Chanock, Acute infectious nonbacterial gastroenteritis: Etiology and pathogenesis. A Combined Clinical Staff Conference at the National Institutes of Health, *Ann. Intern. Med., 76*:993–1008 (1972).

6. E. H. Bohl, Transmissible gastroenteritis. In *Diseases of Swine,* 4th Ed., (H. W. Dunne and A. D. Leman, eds.), Iowa State University Press, Ames, Iowa, (1975), pp. 168–188.

7. J. C. Bridger and G. N. Woode, Neonatal calf diarrhoea: Identification of a reovirus-like (rotavirus) agent in faeces by immunofluorescence and immune electron microscopy, *Br. Vet. J., 131*:528-535.

8. A. S. Bryden, H. A. Davies, M. E. Thouless, and T. H. Flewett, Diagnosis of rotavirus infection by cell culture. *J. Med. Microbiol., 10*:121-125 (1977).

9. E. O. Caul and S. K. R. Clarke, Coronavirus propagated from patient with non-bacterial gastroenteritis, *Lancet, 2*:953 (1975).

10. E. O. Caul, and S. I. Egglestone, Further studies on human enteric coronaviruses, *Arch. Virol., 54*:107-117 (1977).

11. R. Dolin, N. R. Blacklow, R. A. Malmgren, and R. M. Chanock, Establishment of human fetal intestinal organ cultures for growth of viruses, *J. Infect. Dis., 122*:227-231 (1970).

12. S. G. Drozdov, L. A. Shekoian, M. V. Korolev, and A. G. Andzhaparidze, Human rotavirus in cell culture: Isolation and passage, *Vopr. Virusol., 4*: 389-92 (1979).

13. M. K. Estes, and D. Y. Graham, Identification of rotaviruses of different origins by the plaque reduction test, *Am. J. Vet. Res., 41*:151-152 (1980).

14. M. K. Estes, D. Y. Graham, C. P. Gerba, and E. M. Smith, Simian rotavirus SA-11 replication in cell cultures, *J. Virol., 31*:810-815 (1979).

15. A. L. Fernelius, A. E. Ritchie, L. G. Classick, J. O. Norman, and C. A. Mebus, Cell culture adaptation and propagation of a reovirus-like agent of calf diarrhea from a field outbreak in Nebraska, *Arch. Ges. Virusforsch., 37*:114-130 (1972).

16. G. W. Gary, Jr., J. C. Hierholzer, and R. E. Black, Characteristics of non-cultivatable adenoviruses associated with diarrhea in infants: A new subgroup of human adenoviruses, *J. Clin. Microbiol., 10*:96-103. (1979).

17. H. B. Greenberg, R. G. Wyatt, A. R. Kalica, R. H. Yolken, R. Black, A. Z. Kapikian, and R. M. Chanock, New insights in viral gastroenteritis. In *Perspectives in Virology*, Vol. 11 (M. Pollard, ed.), Raven, New York, 1980, pp. 163-187.

18. I. H. Holmes, Viral gastroenteritis, *Prog. Med. Virol., 25*:1-36 (1979).

19. A. R. Kalica, R. G. Wyatt, and A. Z. Kapikian, Detection of differences among human and animal rotaviruses, using analysis of viral RNA, *J. Am. Vet. Med. Assoc. 173*:531-537 (1978).

20. A. Z. Kapikian, R. H. Yolken, H. B. Greenberg, R. G. Wyatt, A. R. Kalica, R. M. Chanock, and H. W. Kim, Gastroenteritis viruses. In *Diagnostic Procedures for Viral, Rickettsial and Chlamydial Infections* 5th Ed., (E. H. Lennette and N. J. Schmidt, eds.), American Public Health Association, Washington, D.C., 1979, pp. 927-995.

21. A. Z. Kapikian, R. G. Wyatt, M. M. Levine, R. H. Yolken, et al., Oral administration of a human rotavirus to volunteers: Induction of illness and correlates of resistance, (in preparation).

22. H.-D. Klenk, R. Rott, M. Orlich, and J. Blodorn, Activation of influenza A viruses by trypsin treatment, *Virology, 68*:426-439.

23. J. B. Kurtz, T. W. Lee, J. W. Craig, and S. E. Reed, Astrovirus infection in volunteers, *J. Med. Virol., 3*:221-230 (1979).

24. T. W. Lee, and J. B. Kurtz, Astroviruses detected by immunofluorescence, *Lancet, 2*:406 (1977).

25. R. L'Haridon and R. Scherrer, Culture in vitro du rotavirus associe aux diarrhees neonatales du veau, *Ann. Rech. Vet., 7*:373-381 (1976).

26. C. R. Madeley, Comparison of the features of astroviruses and calciviruses seen in samples of feces by electron microscopy, *J. Infect. Dis., 139*: 519-523 (1979).

27. H. H. Malherbe and M. Strickland-Cholmley, Simian virus SA-11 and the related "O" agent, *Arch. Ges. Virusforsch, 22*:235-245 (1967).

28. S. Matsuno, A. Hasegawa, A. R. Kalica, and R. Kono, Isolation of a recombinant between simian and bovine rotaviruses, *J. Gen. Virol., 48*:253-256 (1980).

29. S. Matsuno, S. Inouye, and R. Kono, Plaque assay of neonatal calf diarrhea virus and the neutralizing antibody in human sera, *J. Clin. Microbiol., 5*: 1-4 (1977).

30. M. S. McNulty, G. M. Allan, and J. B. McFerran, Isolation of a cytopathic calf rotavirus, *Res. Vet. Sci., 21*:114-115 (1976).

31. M. S. McNulty, G. M. Allan, D. Todd, and J. B. McFerran, Isolation and cell culture propagation of rotaviruses from turkeys and chickens, *Arch. Virol., 61*:13-21 (1979).

32. C. A. Mebus, M. Kono, N. R. Underdahl, and M. J. Twiehaus, Cell culture propagation of neonatal calf diarrhea (scours) virus, *Can. Vet. J. 12*: 69-72 (1971).

33. C. A. Mebus, E. L. Stair, M. B. Rhodes, and M. J. Twiehaus, Neonatal calf diarrhea: Propagation, attenuation, and characteristics of a coronavirus-like agent, *Am. J. Vet. Res., 34*:145-150 (1973).

34. C. A. Mebus, R. G. Wyatt, R. L. Sharpee, M. M. Sereno, A. R. Kalica, A. Z. Kapikian, and M. J. Twiehaus, Diarrhea in gnotobiotic calves caused by the reovirus-like agent of human infantile gastroenteritis, *Infect. Immun., 14*:471-474. (1976).

35. P. J. Middleton, M. Petric, and M. T. Szymanski, Propagation of infantile gastroenteritis virus (Orbi-group) in conventional and germfree piglets, *Infect. Immun., 12*:1276-1280 (1975).

36. P. J. Middleton, M. T. Szymanski, and M. Petric, Viruses associated with acute gastroenteritis in young children, *Am. J. Dis. Child., 131*:733-737 (1977).

37. S. Ramia and S. A. Sattar, Simian rotavirus SA-11 plaque formation in the presence of trypsin, *J. Clin. Microbiol., 10*:609-614 (1979).

38. M. Retter, P. J. Middleton, J. S. Tam, and M. Petric, Enteric adenoviruses: Detection, replication, and significance, *J. Clin. Microbiol., 10*:574-578 (1979).

39. D. Rubenstein, R. G. Milne, R. Buckland, and D. A. J. Tyrrell, The growth of the virus of epidemic diarrhoea of infant mice (EDIM) in organ cultures of intestinal epithelium, *Br. J. Exp. Pathol., 52*:442-445 (1971).

40. B. D. Schoub, A. R. Kalica, H. B. Greenberg, D. M. Bertran, M. M. Sereno, R. G. Wyatt, R. M. Chanock, and A. Z. Kapikian, Enhancement of antigen incorporation and infectivity of cell cultures by human rotavirus, *J. Clin. Microbiol., 9*:488-492 (1979).

41. E. M. Smith, M. K. Estes, D. Y. Graham, and C. P. Gerba, A plaque assay for the simian rotavirus SA-11, *J. Gen. Virol., 43*:513-519 (1979).

42. D. R. Snodgrass, C. R. Madeley, P. W. Wells, and K. W. Angus, Human rotavirus in lambs: Infection and passive protection, *Infect. Immun., 16*: 268-270 (1977).

43. R. S. Spendlove, M. E. McClain, and E. H. Lennette, Enhancement of reovirus infectivity by extracellular removal or alteration of the virus capsid by proteolytic enzymes, *J. Gen. Virol., 8*:83-94 (1970).

44. G. Stuker, L. S. Oshiro, and N. J. Schmidt, Antigenic comparisons of two new rotaviruses from rhesus monkeys, *J. Clin. Microbiol., 11*:202-203 (1980).

45. K. W. Theil, and E. H. Bohl, Porcine rotaviral infection of cell culture: Effects of certain enzymes, *Am. J. Vet. Res., 41*:140-143 (1980).

46. K. W. Theil, E. H. Bohl, and A. G. Agnes, Cell culture propagation of porcine rotavirus (reovirus-like agent), *Am. J. Vet. Res., 38*:1765-1768 (1977).

47. M. E. Thouless, A. S. Bryden, T. H. Flewett, G. N. Woode, J. C. Bridger, D. R. Snodgrass, and J. A. Herring, Serological relationships between rotaviruses from different species as studied by complement fixation and neutralization, *Arch. Virol., 53*:287-294 (1977).

48. A. Torres-Medina, R. G. Wyatt, C. A. Mebus, N. R. Underdahl, and A. Z. Kapikian, Diarrhea in gnotobiotic piglets caused by the human reovirus-like agent of infantile gastroenteritis, *J. Infect. Dis., 133*:22-27 (1976).

49. A. B. Welch, and M. J. Twiehaus, Cell culture studies of a neonatal calf diarrhea virus, *Can. J. Comp. Med., 37*:287-294 (1973).

50. R. G. Wyatt, R. M. Chanock, and W. D. James, Characterization of rotavirus using plaque assay (Abstract #W35/8). In *Abstracts of the Fourth International Virology Congress,* The Hague, Centre for Agricultural Publishing and Documentation, Wageningen, The Netherlands, p. 461.

51. R. G. Wyatt, W. D. James, E. H. Bohl, K. W. Theil, L. J. Saif, A. R. Kalica, H. B. Greenberg, A. Z. Kapikian, and R. M. Chanock, Human rotavirus type 2: Cultivation in vitro, *Science, 207*:189-191 (1980).

52. R. G. Wyatt, H. B. Greenberg, W. D. James, A. L. Pittman, A. R. Kalica, J. Flores, R. M. Chanock, and A. Z. Kapikian, Definition of human rotavirus serotypes by plaque reduction assay (submitted manuscript).

53. R. G. Wyatt, A. R. Kalica, C. A. Mebus, H. W. Kim, W. T. London, R. M. Chanock, and A. Z. Kapikian, Reovirus-like agents (rotaviruses) associated with diarrheal illness in animals and man. In *Perspectives in Virology,* Vol. 10 (M. Pollard, ed.), Raven, New York, 1978, pp. 121-145.

54. R. G. Wyatt, and A. Z. Kapikian, Viral agents associated with acute gastroenteritis in humans, *Am. J. Clin. Nutr., 30*:1857-1870 (1977).

55. R. G. Wyatt, A. Z. Kapikian, T. S. Thornhill, M. M. Sereno, H. W. Kim, and R. M. Chanock, In vitro cultivation in human fetal intestinal organ culture of a reovirus-like agent associated with nonbacterial gastroenteritis in infants and children, *J. Infect. Dis., 130*:523-528 (1974).

56. R. G. Wyatt, D. L. Sly, W. T. London, A. E. Palmer, A. R. Kalica, D. H. Van Kirk, R. M. Chanock, and A. Z. Kapikian, Induction of diarrhea in colostrum-deprived newborn rhesus monkeys with the human reovirus-like agent of infantile gastroenteritis, *Arch. Virol., 50*:17-27 (1976).

57. K. Sato, Y. Inaba, T. Shinozaki, R. Fujii, and M. Matumoto, Isolation of human rotavirus in cell cultures, *Arch. Virol., 69*:155-160 (1981).

58. T. Urasawa, S. Urasawa, and K. Taniguchi, Sequential passages of human rotavirus in MA104 cells, *Microbiol. Immunol., 25*:1025-1035 (1981).

59. H. B. Greenberg, A. R. Kalica, R. G. Wyatt, R. W. Jones, A. Z. Kapikian, and R. M. Chanock, Rescue of non-cultivatable human rotavirus by gene reassortment during mixed infection with *ts* mutants of a cultivatable bovine rotavirus, *Proc. Natl. Acad. Sci., 78*:420-424 (1981).

60. H. B. Greenberg, R. G. Wyatt, A. Z. Kapikian, A. R. Kalica, J. Flores, and R. Jones, Rescue of thirty-three strains of non-cultivatable human rotavirus by gene reassortment (submitted manuscript).

61. J. Laporte and P. Bobulesco, Growth of human and canine enteric coronaviruses in a highly susceptible cell line: HRT 18. In *Perspectives in Virology,* Vol. 11 (M. Pollard, ed.), Raven, New York, 1980, pp. 189-193.

3

Electron Microscopy and Immune Electron Microscopy for Detection of Gastroenteritis Viruses

Heather A. Davies   Clinical Research Centre,
Harrow, Middlesex, England

Electron Microscopy

The resolving power of the electron microscope enables viruses to be identified on the basis of their characteristic morphology [45]; this may be done rapidly using negative staining [11] of suitable clinical material.

The presence of virus particles in clinical specimens from patients with gastroenteritis may be determined in two ways. First, rapid identification, from a few minutes to several hours, may be made of virus particles recovered directly from feces [21,23,26] using negative staining. The differential diagnosis of smallpox (Variola major and Variola minor) and chickenpox (Herpes zoster) [17,44,48] and the detection of respiratory viruses from nasopharyngeal secretions [22,34], were achieved using negative staining. Second, biopsy or autopsy tissue specimens from areas of the alimentary tract can be examined for the presence of virus particles using the longer (i.e., 1 week) procedure of ultrathin sectioning [31]. This method is usually reserved for tissues of particular interest or research topics; the technique of negative staining is the one of choice for routine rapid diagnosis.

Samples for virus isolation can be obtained at any stage of the illness and prepared using either of the above two methods. However, feces should be collected within 5 days of the onset of symptoms, when maximum excretion of virus occurs; this period may vary according to the virus. Only those of adeno-viruses, enteroviruses, rotaviruses, and caliciviruses have been reported [18,20, 29,39]. The samples should be kept cool and reach the laboratory without any delay.

Since the first report by Flewett et al. [26] of noncultivable rotaviruses in feces, detected by negative staining, many reviews have followed [12,16,24, 49]. Madely [46] suggested that viruses found in feces can be placed into three groups: cultivable, noncultivable, and bacteriophages, all of which are discussed in this book.

Methodology

The negative staining method for rotaviruses was first published by Flewett et al. [26] and has been adopted by many workers in the field. A 10-20% w/v suspension of feces is prepared in phosphate-buffered saline (PBS) and clarified on the bench centrifuge at 1500g for 20 min. Differential centrifugation is performed as in most routine virus diagnostic laboratories; the supernatant is withdrawn and centrifuged at 12,000g for 30 min at 4°C, and the supernatant from this at 100,000g for 1 h at 4°C to pellet the virus. This ultracentrifugation should be performed in a swing-out rotor so that the pellet forms at the bottom of the tube. The g values stated can be converted to revolutions per minute by referring to a nomogram that shows the relationship between revolutions per minute, g value, and radius of rotation; e.g., 1500g is equivalent to 3000 rev/min on a bench centrifuge. The supernatant is tipped off, the tubes left inverted to drain for 5 min, and the inner walls wiped with filter paper to remove all the residual liquid. The pellet is resuspended in 2-3 drops of PBS by placing the tubes in an ultrasonication bath for 30 s.

A drop of the suspension is put on a microscope slide and a parlodion-carbon 400 mesh grid [32] is placed, membrane surface downward, onto the drop for 5 min. The grid is removed using fine curved forceps, the edge blotted, and then touched thrice onto the surface of a drop of distilled water, blotted each time, and finally touched onto the surface of a drop of 2% w/v potassium phosphotungstate at pH 6.5, for 10 s, blotted, and allowed to air-dry. Prepared grids may be stored undesiccated at room temperature before they are examined; the maximum time period of storage is 3-5 years.

An alternative method of grid preparation is to dip the grid into a drop of resuspended pellet and allow the adherent drop to almost dry, while the grid is left at one edge of the slide, before dipping in distilled water and staining as in the first method. Care must be exercised to avoid cross-contamination between samples, and it is advisable to dip the forceps into methylated spirit and flame them between each preparation; the grids are then examined in the electron microscope at a recommended viewing magnification of 28,000X; micrographs are taken at 51,300X.

A third method by Caul et al. [14] involves mixing 4 ml of a 20% clarified fecal suspension with saturated ammonium sulfate solution to give a final concentration of 60%. This is left at 4°C for 1 h and the precipitate ultracentrifuged at 50,000g for 2 h. The pellet is resuspended in 4 drops of distilled water and negatively stained grids prepared. Care must be exercised in the interpretation of micrographs of small (i.e., less than 30 nm) viruses, as the morphology may be obscured by contaminating proteins (Cubitt, personal communication).

The process of ultracentrifugation is time consuming and may not fit in well with routine work in the laboratory. It is, however, possible to routinely examine fecal suspensions by negative staining prior to their inoculation into tissue culture. Also, Middleton et al. [47] used a very rapid technique for electron microscopy (EM) by mixing a small amount of crude feces with 1% ammonium acetate, placing a drop on a membrane-coated grid, blotting, and then negatively staining. Both these methods lack the advantage of concentration that ultracentrifugation affords, but they are rapid. However, either of these can be used as a screening test and any feces or fecal suspensions that are negative can be ultracentrifuged as above and reexamined. Figure 1 shows the various viruses that can be found in feces.

One extra step can be introduced when preparing grids: the virus suspension, either as a resuspended pellet or a routine suspension, has salts in the medium which can be removed by the agar diffusion method of Anderson and Doane [3]. This step effectively concentrates the particles and removes the salts. By applying the grid onto a drop of suspension which is on a small (1 mm^3) block of 1.5% agar in distilled water, the diluent is completely absorbed and the grids can then be negatively stained. An alternative method is to use agar-filled wells of a plastic disposable microtiter plate, containing wells with a diameter of 7 mm.

In the search for unknown viruses in feces, one more method should be emphasized as a research tool. Cesium chloride buoyant density purification was used by Appleton et al. [6] to detect the Ditchling agent, a 28 nm virus particle with a buoyant density of 1.38-1.4 g/cm^3, from an outbreak of winter vomiting. The methodology involves differentially centrifuging 2 ml of fecal suspension to pellet the virus as described above. This is resuspended in 0.5 ml of distilled water and layered onto 5 ml of cesium chloride in distilled water, density 1.39 g/cm^3. This is ultracentrifuged in a swing-out rotor at 100,000g for 18 h at 4°C. Twenty to twenty-five fractions are collected of approximately 0.2 ml each. The fractions in the region of density 1.38-1.4 g/cm^3 are examined using the agar diffusion method of grid preparation [3]. The method is time consuming and thus useful only as a research tool, but it has the advantage of concentrating and purifying small virus particles from the crude fecal suspension, thus increasing the possibility of detection.

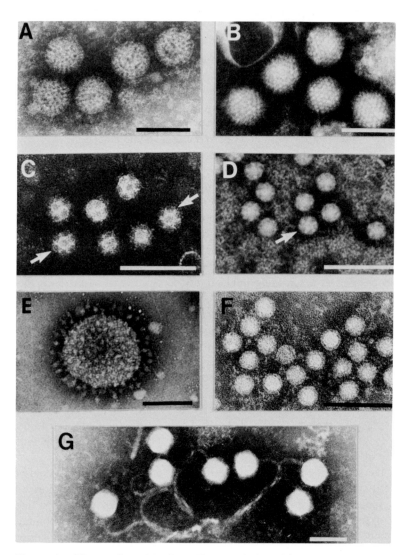

Figure 1 Viruses found in feces from patients with gastroenteritis, negatively stained with 2% potassium phosphotungstate at pH 6.5. Bars present 100 nm. (A) Rotaviruses: "smooth" particles showing the double coat. (B) Adenoviruses: The icosahedral morphology is evident. (C) Calciviruses: Two particles (arrowed) exhibiting the characteristic morphology of a six-pointed star. (D) Astroviruses: Some particles show a five- or six-pointed star on the surface (arrowed). (Courtesy of Dr. C. R. Madeley.) (E) Coronavirus: Pleomorphic particle with surface projections of approximately 20 nm in length [15]. (Courtesy of E. O. Caul.) (F) Small round viruses (SRV): Particles with no obvious morphology and a diameter of 27 to 30 nm. (G) Bacteriophages: These particles have hexagonal heads with long flexible tails all attached to a piece of bacterial debris.

Summary

The electron microscope has been an invaluable diagnostic and research tool. It has the advantage of detecting viruses which cannot be cultivated in tissue culture, and in addition, individual specimens can be examined shortly after reception in the laboratory. Thus, in an emergency situation, the electron microscope can provide a rapid result.

Many artefacts and other constituents are present in negatively stained preparations of fecal extracts, including bacterial cell wall components [19], host cell membranes, and bacteriophages (viruses which parasitize bacteria). The latter group contains a variety of morphologic types; some are hexagonal, with a diameter of 75 nm, and may be confused with adenoviruses. Others, 27–30 nm in diameter, are also hexagonal and may be confused with small round viruses (SRV) [46]. An experienced electron microscopist is able to discriminate between such constituents and enteric virus particles.

The detection of viruses in ultrathin sections of biopsy or autopsy tissues may be equivocal. Their morphology is not as distinct in sections as it is in negatively stained preparations. Viruses must be present as complete particles, and if they are present in large numbers (e.g., after replication) a diagnosis can be made. However, if only a few scattered particles are seen in the section, identification is difficult. Rotaviruses were first detected in ultrathin sections of the jejunum of children with nonbacterial gastroenteritis by Bishop et al. [10]. Adenoviruses were found in the small intestine, taken at autopsy, of a 16-month-old child with gastroenteritis [54]. Many artefacts have been mistaken for viruses, particularly in Crohn's disease, both in ultrathin sections of biopsy material and in tissue culture isolation [30,55].

There are a few disadvantages of EM. First, the sensitivity is not great, as a minimum concentration of 10^6 particles per milliliter is required before they can be observed. Second, the instrument is expensive and may not be available in many small diagnostic laboratories. Third, the number of specimens that can be examined in a working day are fewer than in other tests. EM has largely been superceded by immunofluorescence (IF) [13], radioimmunoassay (RIA) [35] and enzyme-linked immunosorbent assay (ELISA) [57] for rotavirus antigen or antibody detection. A useful comparison of tests by Ellens et al. [25] was made in the detection of calf rotavirus antigens in feces. However, the electron microscope will continue to be used by many laboratories for viruses other than rotaviruses or particles of the Norwalk agent type until other tests are devised that are as reliable and as sensitive as EM.

Immune Electron Microscopy

The term *immune electron microscopy* (IEM) was first used by Almeida and Waterson [2] to describe the observation by negative staining in the electron microscope, of a reaction between virus and specific antibody. This review was preceded by reports of this antigen-antibody reaction in relation to plant virology in 1941 by Anderson and Stanley [4] and by von Ardenne et al. [51]. For animal viruses the first two reports appeared simultaneously and the method was demonstrated by Anderson et al. [5] and Lafferty and Oertelis, in 1961 [41].

The technique involves the interaction of antibody with virus particles; if conditions are optimal, aggregation of the virus particles occurs. As a serologic test, IEM is specific, as was demonstrated first by Hummeler et al. [33] who showed that heat-inactivated poliovirus was antigenically different from fresh virus. This was followed by many reports using a mixture of polyoma- and papillomaviruses [1], influenza virus [7,42], herpesvirus [53], avian infectious bronchitis virus [9], and two serotypes of rhinovirus [36].

IEM was not applied to the problem of noncultivable fecal gastroenteritis viruses of humans until 1972, when Kapikian [38] detected 27 nm virus particles in an outbreak of gastroenteritis in Norwalk, Ohio. In this study, virus particles present in a fecal suspension were aggregated by antibodies present in a volunteer's convalescent serum. Evidence of infection was demonstrated in most volunteers when acute and convalescent sera were tested against the Norwalk agent.

IEM has proved a valuable asset in detecting fecal viruses in patients with gastroenteritis.

Methodology

The original method is described by Almeida and Waterson [2] and has been slightly modified by Kapikian et al. [38] and Flewett et al. [28]. The serum under test is inactivated at 56°C for 30 min and then ultracentrifuged at 100,000g for 60 min to deposit any aggregated protein and other debris. This last step is not essential in a routine assay but a cleaner preparation is obtained.

To 0.5 ml fecal suspension, prepared as previously explained, 0.1 ml of undiluted, 1/10 or 1/100 dilution of serum in PBS is added; these are mixed thoroughly and incubated at a chosen temperature and time, namely, 37°C for 1 or 2 h, 4°C overnight, or 37°C for 1 h and 4°C overnight. The mixture is then made up to 5 ml (the capacity of the ultracentrifuge tube) and centrifuged in a swing-out rotor. The mixture may also be made up to 1.0 ml or even lesser volume when using firm tubes for a Sorvall centrifuge with the SS-34 rotor. The speed used is designed to pellet the virus-antibody aggregates and is lower than that for single particles; 35,000g for 90 min is recommended by Kapikian et al. [38] for smaller fecal viruses, although Almeida and Waterson [2] suggest 27,000g for 30 min for similar sized poliovirus-antibody aggregates.

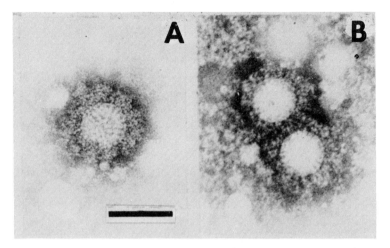

Figure 2   Rotavirus particles observed following incubation of a stool filtrate with homologous human convalescent serum and further preparation for electron microscopy. The antibodies around the particles can be seen as a "fuzz." Bar represents 100 nm. (From Ref. 39.)

The supernatant is poured off, and the pellets are treated in the same manner as those from fecal suspensions. The resultant negatively stained preparation may be obscured by high molecular weight material from either the virus suspension or the serum. This can be reduced if the pellet is resuspended in PBS and ultracentrifuged again. It is possible to omit the ultracentrifugation step if the concentration of virus particles is high, e.g., 10^{10} particles per milliliter. Under such circumstances grids can be prepared directly after the mixture has been incubated [43].

One technique that can also be classified as an IEM technique is the examination of precipitin lines in Ouchterlony gel diffusion plates. Smaller viruses penetrate the pores of the agar gel as do the antibody molecules, and the precipitin line is formed of virus-antibody complexes. These are released from the agar by cutting out the line with a scalpel, freezing it, cutting it into small pieces, and then thawing it. A drop of negative stain is added, and grids prepared. This technique was used by Watson et al. [52] for polyomavirus particles and by Beale and Mason [8] who demonstrated that "full" and "empty" poliovirus particles were antigenically different. This method is a very useful check on the composition of precipitin lines.

IEM can be used in many ways in the diagnostic laboratory. It is useful for the direct detection in patients' stools of noncultivable viruses using the patient's convalescent serum, e.g., Norwalk agent [38]. This enables an epidemiologic relationship to be established. Second, seroconversion can be demonstrated if the patient's acute and convalescent sera are assayed, thus giving evidence of infection. The concentration of antibody around the particles has been graded by assessing the amount of "fuzz" around the particles (Fig. 2) [27,37, 38]. Third, cross-reactions between viruses that are morphologically similar can be studied and antigenic similarities noted. Woode et al. [56] showed that "rough" rotavirus particles from all animal species had group antigens, but antigen(s) conferring type-specificity were found on the double-coated "smooth" particles. Thornhill et al. [50] showed the antigenic relationship of virus particles found in three isolated outbreaks of gastroenteritis in the United States, and Appleton et al. [6] demonstrated that the Ditchling agent from winter vomiting disease was antigenically unlike Norwalk agent. Fourth, serotyping can be carried out using IEM. Luton [43] showed that serotyping of adenoviruses was not only possible but quicker than the routine neutralization test. This was also used by Flewett et al. [27] who serotyped a noncultivable adenovirus 7 directly from a fecal suspension. Zissis and Lambert [58] used IEM to show the existence of two serotypes of human rotavirus and that the type-specific antigens are located on the outside of the virus particle.

Other viruses found in feces of patients with gastroenteritis, apart from those already mentioned, have been aggregated by convalescent sera, though not with acute sera or at a significantly lower dilution. These include astroviruses [40], caliciviruses [18] and minireoviruses [47]. The "parvovirus-like" Ditchling agent demonstrated in an outbreak of winter vomiting by Appleton et al. [6] was aggregated by the patients' convalescent sera only, as no acute sera were available.

There are a few disadvantages of IEM. First, a costly electron microscope is required, although now more and more laboratories are equipped with one. Second, if the concentration of particles in the fecal suspension is low, the few aggregates formed in the reaction may be missed on the grid. However, single particles heavily coated with antibody may be observed. Third, optimum antibody and antigen concentrations must be achieved for aggregation to occur. It should be stressed, however, that aggregation per se does not indicate the presence of antibody since certain viruses or virus-like particles may aggregate nonspecifically. Thus it is essential to evaluate the amount of antibody coating the particles even if they are in a group. The dilutions of particle-containing material or of serum can be varied to help determine the nature of the aggregation observed. This will assist in studying the significance of the particles. However, reaction with the appropriate paired sera and demonstration of a seroresponse to the particle in question is an essential early step in studies aimed at determining the significance of a particle. Fourth, very large aggregates may be formed which completely cover the grid, and are so dense that the image is dark and the grid has to be discarded. These last two, however, can be circumvented by using several dilutions of sera. The fifth disadvantage is that paired sera are not always available, and often convalescent sera are not collected as the patient is discharged within a short time.

Summary

IEM has many advantages and in some cases is more useful than direct electron microscopy. Small noncultivable fecal viruses with no distinct morphology can be detected more easily than by direct EM; however, fine structural detail can be obscured by the attached antibodies. The particles are also concentrated by aggregation, again facilitating their detection. Alternatively, if the number of particles is small, single particles may be heavily coated with antibody, thus facilitating the recognition of even some low-titered preparations. Furthermore, serologic assay can be performed and also the serotyping of viruses. IEM is a very rapid technique when compared with routine virus isolation in tissue culture and subsequent serotyping by neutralization tests.

References

1. J. Almeida, B. Cinader, and A. Howatson, Structure of antigen-antibody complexes, *J. Exp. Med., 118*:327-340 (1963).
2. J. D. Almeida, and A. P. Waterson, The morphology of virus-antibody interactions, *Adv. Virus Res., 15*:307-338 (1969).
3. N. Anderson, and F. W. Doane, Agar diffusion method for negative staining of microbial suspensions in salt solutions, *Appl. Microbiol., 24*:495-496 (1972).
4. T. F. Anderson, and W. M. Stanley, Study by means of electron microscope of reaction between tobacco mosaic virus and its antiserum, *J. Biol. Chem., 139*:339-344 (1941).
5. T. F. Anderson, N. Yamamoto, and K. Hummeler, Specific agglutination of phages and polio virus by antibody molecules as seen in the electron microscope, *J. Appl. Physics, 32*:1639 (1961).
6. H. Appleton, M. Buckley, B. T. Thom, J. L. Cotton, and S. Henderson, Virus-like particles in winter vomiting disease, *Lancet i*:409-411 (1977).
7. M. E. Bayer, and E. Mannweiler, Antigen-antibody reactions of influenza virus as seen in the electron microscope, *Arch. Virusforsch., 13*:541-547 (1963).
8. A. J. Beale, and P. J. Mason, Electron microscopy of poliovirus antigen antibody precipitates extracted from gel diffusion plates, *J. Gen. Virol., 2*: 203-204 (1968).
9. D. M. Berry, and J. D. Almeida, The morphological and biological effects of various antisera on avian infectious bronchitis virus, *J. Gen. Virol., 3*: 97-102 (1968).

10. R. F. Bishop, G. P. Davidson, I. H. Holmes, and B. J. Ruck, Virus particles in epithelial cells of duodenal mucosa from children with acute non-bacterial gastroenteritis, *Lancet, 2*:1281-1283 (1973).

11. S. Brenner, and R. W. Horne, A negative staining method for high resolution electron microscopy of viruses, *Biochim. Biophys. Acta, 34*:103-110 (1959).

12. A. S. Bryden, H. A. Davies, R. E. Hadley, T. H. Flewett, C. A. Morris, and P. Oliver, Rotavirus enteritis in the West Midlands during 1974, *Lancet 2*: 241-243 (1975).

13. A. S. Bryden, H. A. Davies, M. E. Thouless, and T. H. Flewett, Diagnosis of rotavirus infection by cell culture, *J. Med. Microbiol., 10*:121-125 (1977).

14. E. O. Caul, C. R. Ashley, and S. I. Egglestone, An improved method for the routine identification of faecal viruses using ammonium sulphate precipitation, *FEMS Micro. Lett., 4*:1-4 (1978).

15. E. O. Caul, W. K. Paver, and S. K. R. Clarke, Coronavirus particles in faeces from patients with gastroenteritis, *Lancet 1*:1192 (1975).

16. Colloquium on selected diarrhoeal diseases of the young, *J. Am. Vet. Med. Assoc., 173*:511-676 (1978).

17. J. G. Cruickshank, H. S. Bedson, and D. H. Watson, (1966). Electron microscopy in the rapid diagnosis of smallpox, *Lancet 2*:527-530 (1966).

18. W. D. Cubitt, D. A. McSwiggan, and W. Moore, Winter vomiting disease caused by calicivirus, *J. Clin. Pathol., 32*:786-793 (1979).

19. A. Dalen, The presence in faecal extracts of bacterial cell wall components resembling viral structures, *Acta. Pathol. Microbiol. Scand. [B], 86*:249-251 (1978).

20. G. P. Davidson, R. R. W. Townley, R. F. Bishop, I. H. Holmes, and B. J. Ruck, Importance of a new virus in acute sporadic enteritis in children, *Lancet 1*:242-246 (1975).

21. F. W. Doane, and N. Anderson, Electron and immunoelectron microscopic procedures for diagnosis of viral infections. In *Comparative Diagnosis of Viral Diseases,* Vol. II, Chap. 13 (E. Kurstak and C. Kurstak, eds.), 506-539 (1977).

22. F. W. Doane, N. Anderson, K. Chatiyanonda, R. M. Bannatyne, D. M. Mc-Lean, and A. J. Rhodes, Rapid laboratory diagnosis of paramyxovirus infections by electron microscopy, *Lancet 2*:751-753 (1967).

23. F. W. Doane, N. Anderson, A. Zbitnew, and A. J. Rhodes, Application of electron microscopy to the diagnosis of virus infections, *Can. Med. Assoc. J., 100*:1043-1049 (1969).

24. H. L. Du Pont, B. L. Portnoy, and R. H. Conklin, Viral agents and diarrheal illness, *Ann. Rev. Med., 28*:167-177 (1977).

25. D. J. Ellens, P. W. de Leeuw, P. J. Straver, and J. A. van Balken, Comparison of five diagnostic methods for the detection of rotavirus antigens in calf faeces, *Med. Microbiol. Immunol., 166*:157-163 (1978).

26. T. H. Flewett, A. S. Bryden, and H. A. Davies, Virus particles in gastroenteritis, *Lancet 2*:1497 (1973).

27. T. H. Flewett, A. S. Bryden, H. Davies, and C. A. Morris, Epidemic viral enteritis in a long stay children's ward, *Lancet 1*:4 (1975).

28. T. H. Flewett, A. S. Bryden, H. Davies, G. N. Woode, J. C. Bridger, and J. M. Derrick, Relation between viruses from acute gastroenteritis of children and newborn calves, *Lancet 2*:61-63 (1974).

29. J. P. Fox, C. D. Brandt, F. E. Wasserman, C. E. Hall, I. Spigland, A. Kogon, and L. R. Elveback, The Virus Watch Program: A continuing surveillance of virus infections in metropolitan New York families. VI. Observations of adenovirus infections: Virus excretion patterns, antibody response, efficiency of surveillance, patterns of illness and relation to illness, *Am. J. Epidemiol., 89*:25-50 (1969).

30. G. L. Gitnick, M. H. Arthur, and I. Shibata, Cultivation of viral agents from Crohn's disease. A new sensitive system, *Lancet, 2*:215-217 (1976).

31. A. M. Glauert, and N. Reid, In *Practical Methods in Electron Microscopy*, Vol. 3. (A. M. Glaubert, ed.), North-Holland, Amsterdam, 1977, pp. 1–76.

32. M. A. Hayat, Support films. In *Principles and Techniques of Electron Microscopy Biological Applications*, Vol. 1., Chap. 5. Van Nostrand Reinhold, New York, 1970, pp. 323–332.

33. K. Hummeler, T. F. Anderson, and R. A. Brown, Identification of poliovirus particles of different antigenicity by specific agglutination as seen in the electron microscope, *Virology, 16*:84-90 (1962).

34. J. H. Joncas, L. Berthiaume, R. Williams, P. Beaudry, and V. Pavilanis, Diagnosis of viral respiratory infections by electron microscopy, *Lancet, 1*: 956-959 (1969).

35. A. R. Kalica, R. H. Purcell, M. M. Sereno, R. G. Wyatt, H. W. Kim, R. M. Chanock, and A. Z. Kapikian, A microtiter solid phase radioimmunoassay for the detection of the human reovirus-like agent in stools, *J. Immunol., 118*:1275-1279 (1977).

36. A. Z. Kapikian, J. D. Almeida, and E. J. Stott, Immune electron microscopy of rhinoviruses, *J. Virol., 10*:142-146 (1972).

37. A. Z. Kapikian, H. Wha Kim, R. G. Wyatt, W. J. Rodriguez, W. Lee Cline, R. H. Parrott, and R. M. Chanock, Reoviruslike agent in stools: Association with infantile diarrhea and development of serologic tests, *Science, 185*:1049-1053 (1974).

38. A. Z. Kapikian, R. G. Wyatt, R. Dolin, T. S. Thornhill, A. R. Kalica, and R. M. Chanock, Visualisation by immune electron microscopy of a 27 nm particle associated with acute infectious nonbacterial gastroenteritis, *J. Virol., 10*:1075–1081 (1972).

39. A. Kogon, I. Spigland, T. E. Frothingham, L. Elveback, C. Williams, C. E. Hall, and J. P. Fox, The Virus Watch Program: A continuing surveillance of viral infections in metropolitan New York families. VII. Observations on viral excretion, seroimmunity, intra-familial spread and illness association in coxsackie and echovirus infections, *Am. J. Epidemiol., 89*:51-61 (1969).

40. J. B. Kurtz, T. W. Lee, and D. Pickering, Astrovirus associated gastroenteritis in a children's ward, *J. Clin. Pathol.* *30*:948-952 (1977).
41. K. J. Lafferty, and S. J. Oertelis, Attachment of antibody to influenza virus, *Nature, 192*:764 (1961).
42. K. J. Lafferty, and S. J. Oertelis, Interaction between virus and antibody III. Examination of virus-antibody complexes with the electron microscope. *Virology, 21*:91-99 (1963).
43. P. Luton, Rapid adenovirus typing by immunoelectron microscopy. *J. Clin. Pathol. 26*:914-917 (1973).
44. A. D. Macrae, J. R. McDonald, A. M. Field, E. V. Meurisse, and A. A. Porter, Laboratory differential diagnosis of vesicular skin rashes, *Lancet, 2*:313-316 (1969).
45. C. R. Madeley, *Virus Morphology,* Churchill Livingstone, London, 1972.
46. C. R. Madeley, Viruses in the stools, *J. Clin. Pathol., 32*:1-10 (1979).
47. P. J. Middleton, M. T. Szymanski, and M. Petric, Viruses associated with acute gastroenteritis in young children, *Am. J. Dis. Child., 131*:733-737 (1977).
48. J. Nagington, Electron microscopy in differential diagnosis of poxvirus infections, *Br. Med. J., 2*:1499-1500 (1964).
49. D. S. Schreiber, J. S. Trier, and N. R. Blacklow, Recent advances in viral gastroenteritis, *Gastroenterology, 73*:174-183 (1977).
50. T. S. Thornhill, R. G. Wyatt, A. R. Kalica, R. Dolin, R. M. Chanock, and A. Z. Kapikian, Detection by immune electron microscopy of 26- to 27-nm viruslike particles associated with two family outbreaks of gastroenteritis, *J. Infect. Dis., 135*:20-27 (1977).
51. M. von Ardenne, H. Friedrich-Freksa, and G. Schramm, Electronenmikroskopische Untersuchung der Präcipitin reaktion von Tabakmosaikvirus mit Kaninchen antiserum, *Arch. Fürges. Virusforsch., 2*:80-86 (1941).
52. D. H. Watson, G. L. Le Bouvier, J. A. Tomlinson, and D. G. A. Walkey, Electron microscopy of antigen precipitates extracted from gel diffusion plates. *Immunology, 10*:305-308 (1966).
53. D. H. Watson, and P. Wildy, Some serological properties of herpes virus particles studied with the electron microscope, *Virology, 21*:100-111 (1963).
54. A. Whitelaw, H. A. Davies, and J. Parry, Electron microscopy of fatal adenovirus gastroenteritis, *Lancet, 1*:361 (1977).
55. P. J. Whorwell, C. A. Phillips, W. L. Beeken, P. K. Little, and K. D. Roessner, Isolation of reovirus-like agents from patients with Crohn's disease, *Lancet, 1*:1169-1171 (1977).
56. G. N. Woode, J. C. Bridger, J.M. Jones, T. H. Flewett, A. S. Bryden, H. A. Davies, and G. B. B. White, Morphological and antigenic relationships between viruses (Rotaviruses) from acute gastroenteritis of children, calves, piglets, mice and foals, *Infect. Immun., 14*:804-810 (1976).

57. R. H. Yolken, R. G. Wyatt, B. A. Barbour, H. W. Kim, A. Z. Kapikian, and R. M. Chanock, Measurement of rotavirus antibody by an enzyme-linked immunosorbent blocking assay, *J. Clin. Microbiol., 8*:283-287 (1978).

58. G. Zissis, and J. P. Lambert, Different serotypes of human rotaviruses, *Lancet, 1*:38-39 (1978).

__ 4

Enzyme Immunoassays for Detecting Human Rotavirus

Robert H. Yolken The Johns Hopkins University School of Medicine, Baltimore, Maryland

Electron microscopic techniques offer efficient, rapid diagnosis of rotavirus infections. However, such techniques require access to an electron microscope and skilled personnel capable of interpreting electron microscopic studies of specimens. In addition, diagnosis by electron microscopy requires the presence of complete, recognizable viral particles. Because of these limitations, there has been interest in developing techniques for the diagnosis of human rotavirus which do not require an electron microscope. Most of these techniques are immunoassays and have their basis in the fact that specific anti-rotaviral antibodies can be raised in laboratory animals [1]. While immunologic differences between animal rotaviruses and different serotypes of human rotaviruses have been described, the immunologic detection of rotavirus is facilitated by the fact that all known rotaviruses share a common antigen and that antisera prepared to one strain will show cross-reactivity with other strains in most immunoassays [2,5]. Thus, a number of different immunoassays for human rotavirus have been developed. These include counterimmunoelectrophoresis [6], immunofluorescence of tissue culture cells [7], complement fixation (CF) [8], immune adherence [9], free viral immunofluorescent assays (FVIA) [10], solid-phase absorption assays (SPACE) [11], radioimmunoassay [12], and enzyme immunoassay (EIA) [13]. Under optimal conditions, all these assays can provide for the efficient diagnosis of human rotavirus, and the choice of assay can be deter-

51

Table 1 Efficiency and Practicality of Methods Available for Detecting
Human Rotaviruses in Stool Specimens[a]

Method	Efficiency	Practicality[b]
Electron microscopy	4+	1+
Immune electron microscopy	4+	<1+
Complement-fixation (conventional)	1+	4+
Human fetal intestinal organ culture (with FA)	1+	0
Counterimmunoelectro-osmophoresis	3+ to 4+	4+
Fluorescent virus precipitin test	4+	1+
Cell culture (cytopathic effect)	<1+	2+ to 3+
Cell culture (with FA)	1+	<1+
Cell culture (with EM)	<1+	<1+
Centrifugation onto cell culture (with FA)	3+ to 4+	1+
Gel diffusion	1+	4+
Smears (with FA)	1+	4+
Radioimmunoassay	4+	3–4+
Enzyme-linked immunosorbent assay (ELISA)	4+	4+
Immune adherence hemagglutination assay	3+	2–3+
RNA electrophoresis patterns in gels	3+	1+
Modified complement-fixation	3+ to 4+	2–3+

[a]On a scale of 1+ to 4+, where 1+ indicates low degree of efficiency or practicality, and 4+ indicates a high degree of efficiency or practicality.
[b]For large-scale epidemiologic studies, assuming 4+ efficiency.
Source: From Ref. 1.

mined largely on the availability of the necessary reagents and the needs of the laboratory. The relative efficiency and practicality of the rotavirus assays are shown in Table 1.

In our laboratory, enzyme immunoassay has proven to be a versatile technique for the detection of human rotavirus in clinical specimens. Enzyme immunoassays are based on the principle that an antibody molecule can be covalently linked with an enzyme to form a conjugate which retains both immunologic and enzymatic function [14,15]. This antibody-enzyme conjugate can be bound to a virus in a clinical specimen by a variety of steps and allowed to react with substrate to produce a visible color [16]. The sensitivity of enzyme immunoassays is based on the fact that a single molecule of enzyme can react with a large number of molecules of substrate (depending upon the turnover number of the enzyme) without the exhaustion of the enzymatic activity [17]. Since EIA can utilize colorless substrates which yield a visibly colored compound on enzymatic reaction, a great deal of sensitivity can be obtained without the use of sophisticated instrumentation. In fact, in some cases visual readings can be performed with only the naked eye [13]. Points requiring consideration in setting up and evaluating enzyme immunoassays for rotavirus are discussed below.

Reagents

The key to any of the above immunoassays is the use of specific antisera capable of reacting with rotavirus but not with other antigens which might be present in stools. Since human rotavirus grown in tissue culture is not widely available, other sources of antigens must be found for use in producing the specific antibody [1]. Viral particles can be purified from stools by means of a number of physicochemical techniques, including density centrifugation with cesium chloride and zonal centrifugation in sucrose [18,19]. However, it is difficult to obtain pure preparations of rotaviral particles from human stools since the stools contain a large number of extraneous antigens and also because rotavirus present in them might be tightly bound with antibody. When antibody-coated viral particles are used to immunize an animal, antisera to human immunoglobulin are produced as well as antisera to rotavirus [20]. A preferable alternative is to use for immunization human rotavirus that has been grown in germ-free animals such as colostrum-deprived calves and piglets [21]. Rotaviral particles purified from these stools by the abovementioned techniques have been used to immunize laboratory animals such as guinea pigs and goats to produce highly specific antirotaviral antisera [19,22]. However, since reagents obtained from germ-free animals are not widely available, alternate methods of producing antisera to rotavirus have been devised. One of these is to use an animal rotavirus which is capable of growing in tissue culture as a substitute for human antigen. Since animal rotaviruses cross-react with human rotavirus, efficient antisera to human rotavirus can be produced in this way [1,2]. The animal strain which has been most widely used is SA-11, originally isolated from a simian source [25]. This simian rotavirus (SA-11) can be grown in tissue culture cells such as African green monkey kidney, purified by means of genetron extraction and density centrifugation, and used to immunize laboratory animals such as rabbits or guinea pigs. Such antisera have proved to be efficient for use in radioimmunoassay and EIA systems for the detection of human rotavirus [5]. The commercial availability of such antisera would markedly increase the availability of all the rotavirus immunoassays. Recently, the tissue culture cultivation of a strain of human rotavirus has been reported [25]. Antisera from tissue culture grown human rotavirus would be valuable reagents for immunoassays for human rotavirus as well as for the further elucidation of human serotypes.

Solid Phase

All immunoassays which utilize labeled reagents require a step to separate antibody bound to the antigen from antibody which is not bound [16]. Although this separation can be accomplished by means of centrifugation, it is usually simpler to bind one reactant to a solid phase and remove unreacted label by washing the solid phase [24]. A large number of different solid phases have been devised, including plastic test tubes [14], filter papers [26], cyanogen bromide activated disks [27], plastic receptacles [28], protein membranes [29, 30], silicone strings [31], and metal beads [32]. However, the two forms of solid phase which we have found to be most useful are microtitration plates [16] and plastic beads [33]. Plastic microtitration plates and beads have the capability of binding proteins in dilute alkaline solution. While the exact mechanism of this protein binding is not known, it probably occurs by means of hydrogen bonding. This binding is largely irreversible under standard experimental conditions [34]. Nonspecific binding of other reactants is minimized by the saturation of available binding sites by a neutral protein such as fetal calf serum, gelatin, or bovine serum albumin [16,35]. In practice, we have found that a separate saturation step is not needed but that the immunologically neutral protein can be added with the additional reactants. In addition, nonspecific absorption is decreased by the use of a nonionic detergent such as Tween-20 [16,35]. Microtitration plates offer the advantage that each one has 96 wells and thus a large number of tests can be performed in a single test run. However, microtitration plates have the disadvantage that some wells must be wasted if only a small number of samples are assayed in a single test run. In addition, microtitration plates are formed in such a way that is difficult to ensure that the plastic composition of each well is identical. Also, it is difficult to ensure a uniform temperature of all wells during the test procedure. This is especially a problem in the outer wells of the plates, which often give erratic results [36]. These disadvantages are overcome by the use of plastic beads to bind the solid phase. Beads can be formulated with a uniform finish and can be stored in such a way that only the exact number required for the test need be used. In addition, the beads offer a somewhat increased surface area over microtiter wells [33]. Thus, for laboratories running small numbers of assays, beads are preferable to microtitration plates. However, beads do require more manipulation, especially during the washing steps, and are somewhat more expensive. Thus microtitration plates are preferred for use in laboratories which are running large numbers of specimens.

Assay Methods

A number of different types of assay systems can utilize enzyme-linked reactants. However, the two most commonly used for the detection of antigens in clinical specimens are direct assays and indirect assays [37]. Direct EIA, which are analogous to direct immunofluorescence assays [38], utilize an enzyme which is directly linked with the antiviral antibody (Fig. 1). Indirect EIA, like

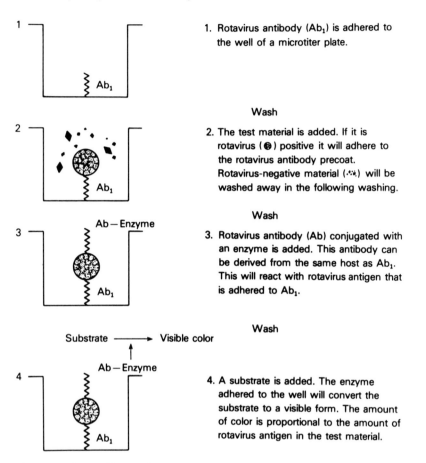

1. Rotavirus antibody (Ab$_1$) is adhered to the well of a microtiter plate.

Wash

2. The test material is added. If it is rotavirus (●) positive it will adhere to the rotavirus antibody precoat. Rotavirus-negative material (⋰) will be washed away in the following washing.

Wash

3. Rotavirus antibody (Ab) conjugated with an enzyme is added. This antibody can be derived from the same host as Ab$_1$. This will react with rotavirus antigen that is adhered to Ab$_1$.

Wash

4. A substrate is added. The enzyme adhered to the well will convert the substrate to a visible form. The amount of color is proportional to the amount of rotavirus antigen in the test material.

Figure 1 Direct ELISA for antigen measurement. (From Ref. 1.)

indirect immunofluorescence assays [39], utilize unlabeled antibody. This unlabeled antibody is measured by the use of an enzyme-labeled antiglobulin which will react with this unlabeled antibody (Fig. 2). Direct EIA offer the advantage that they require one less incubation step. In addition, they can be performed with a single antiviral reagent. However, they suffer from the disadvantage that each antiviral reagent must be linked with an enzyme. This is inconvenient if the laboratory wishes to perform a number of different enzyme immunoassays. Indirect assays, on the other hand, do not require the direct enzyme labeling of the antiviral reagent but rather use enzyme-labeled antiglobulins directed against a species of immunoglobulins. Since enzyme-labeled antiglobulins are available commercially, a laboratory using indirect EIA does not have to perform its own

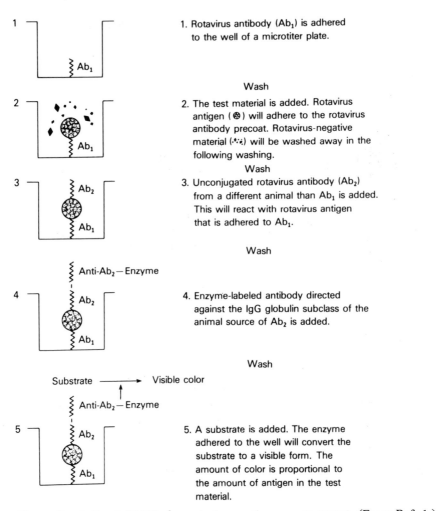

1. Rotavirus antibody (Ab₁) is adhered to the well of a microtiter plate.

Wash

2. The test material is added. Rotavirus antigen (⊕) will adhere to the rotavirus antibody precoat. Rotavirus-negative material (·ⁱ·ⁱ) will be washed away in the following washing.

Wash

3. Unconjugated rotavirus antibody (Ab₂) from a different animal than Ab₁ is added. This will react with rotavirus antigen that is adhered to Ab₁.

Wash

4. Enzyme-labeled antibody directed against the IgG globulin subclass of the animal source of Ab₂ is added.

Wash

5. A substrate is added. The enzyme adhered to the well will convert the substrate to a visible form. The amount of color is proportional to the amount of antigen in the test material.

Figure 2   Indirect ELISA for rotavirus antigen measurement. (From Ref. 1.)

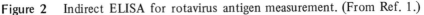

enzyme-labeling procedure. In addition, a single antiglobulin can be used for a number of different enzyme immunoassay systems as long as it is directed to the appropriate animal species [37]. In addition, as in immunofluorescence systems [39], indirect assays are somewhat more sensitive than direct assays, presumably because a single molecule of antiviral antibody can react with a number of molecules of labeled antiglobulin. However, indirect assays do suffer from one major disadvantage. Antibody from two different animal species must be utilized. The use of antibody from two animal species is required to prevent the nonspecific binding of the antiglobulin to the solid phase. Thus the solid-phase antibody must be made in an animal species which will not react with the enzyme-labeled antiglobulin. Fortunately, immunoglobulins from different animal species are sufficiently distinct so that antiglobulins can demonstrate a large degree of specificity, thus allowing for the use of a number of different animal species in indirect immunoassays [37-39].

One form of immunoassay which can utilize a common indicator system but which does not require antibody made in two different animal species is one which makes use of C1q, a fragment of the first component of complement. C1q will bind with antigen-antibody complexes to a much greater extent than it will bind with monomeric immunoglobulin molecules [40]. If C1q is substituted for the labeled second antibody in the direct assay, the amount of C1q bound to the solid phase will be directly proportional to the amount of antigen-antibody complex formed by the binding of antigen to specific antiviral antibody on the solid phase. The amount of binding of C1q can be measured either by utilizing enzyme-labeled C1q or, alternately, by utilizing enzyme-anti-enzyme complexes which will bind to C1q and will subsequently yield colored products by reactions described below [40,41]. Note that preformed antigen-antibody complexes in the specimen will not interfere with the reaction because they will not bind to the solid phase. Experiments in our laboratory have indicated that this assay system can be utilized to detect rotavirus in stool specimens utilizing guinea pig, rabbit, or human rotavirus antibody bound to the solid phase. Analogous C1q systems can also be used to detect other viruses.

Enzyme-Substrate Systems

Although a number of different enzymes can be used in the EIA systems, three enzymes—alkaline phosphatase, peroxidase, and β-galactosidase—have been utilized in most EIA systems (Table 2) [42]. We have generally utilized alkaline phosphatase because of its increased stability under standard laboratory conditions and the fact that preservative solutions such as sodium azide can be used with alkaline phosphatase to prevent microbial contamination [35]. In addition, alkaline phosphatase can utilize a number of different substrates, as described below. However, alkaline phosphatase has the disadvantage that it is relatively expensive. Also, since only mammalian alkaline phosphatase has sufficient specific activity for use in EIA systems [42], the investigator must rely on commercial sources for the enzyme. Thus, many laboratories may choose to use peroxidase or β-galactosidase–conjugated enzymes. EIA for rotavirus utilizing these enzymes will have equivalent sensitivity to the EIA utilizing alkaline phosphatase as long as care is taken to ensure the sterility of the conjugates since preservative solutions such as sodium azide cannot be used with them.

A number of methods of enzyme-antibody conjugation have been developed to link antibody to enzyme [42]. Most of these are based on the binding of the ε-amino groups of proteins by means of a bifunctional cross-linking reagent such as glutaraldehyde. The simplest method is a one-step procedure

Table 2 Comparison of Enzymes Available for EIA*

Enzyme	Source	Uses	Approximate cost per 10,000 tests	Methods of conjugation	Practical substrates available		
					Visual	Fluorescent	Radioactive
Alkaline phosphatase	Calf intestine	EIA,	$80	Glutaraldehyde: 1-step	NP-PO$_4$	MU-PO$_4$ FM-PO$_4$	[^{3}H] AMP
Peroxidase	Horseradish	EIA, HIST	$20	Glutaraldehyde: 1-step Glutaraldehyde: 2-step Sodium M-Periodate	5AS OPD ABTS	NADH	NA
β-Galactosidase	E. coli	EIA, HIST	$20	Glutaraldehyde: P-Benzoquinone N-N′-OPLD	NP-Gal	MU-Gal	NA

*Abbreviations:
ABTS = 2,2-azino-di-(3-ethylbenzothiazolinsulfone-6)diammonium salt.
N-N′-OPLD = N-N′-O-phenylenedimaleimide.
NP-PO$_4$ = Nitrophenyl phosphate.
5AS = 5-Aminosalicylic acid.
OPD = Orthophenylene diamine.
NP-Gal - Nitrophenyl galactose.
MU-PO$_4$ = Methylumbelliferyl phosphate.
FM-PO$_4$ = Fluorescein methylphosphate.
MU-Gal = Methylumbelliferyl galactose.
HIST = Enzyme-mediated histochemical procedure.
NA = Not available.

which consists of mixing antibody, enzyme, and the cross-linking agent glutaraldehyde [14]. Following a suitable reaction interval, the glutaraldehyde is removed by dialysis. This method yields enzyme-antibody conjugates of very high molecular weight. Thus, conjugates prepared in this way should not be used for immunohistology. However, enzyme-antibody conjugates prepared by this method are suitable for EIA. We have found that this method is simple to perform and yields conjugates of reproducible activity.

In the case of peroxidase and β-galactosidase the efficiency of conjugation can somewhat be improved by the use of a two-step procedure. In this procedure [43] the enzyme is first activated with glutaraldehyde. The glutaraldehyde is removed by column chromatography prior to the addition of the immunoglobulin. This method has the advantage of not leading to the cross-linking of antibody molecules to each other with a resulting decrease in the efficiency of the conjugation. However, this method cannot be utilized to conjugate alkaline phosphatase since there are insufficient sites in the enzyme molecule to ensure an adequate activation by this method. In the case of peroxidase, another conjugation method is available which utilizes periodate to link immunoglobulin with the carbohydrate moiety of peroxidase [44]. Since the carbohydrate portion of peroxidase is located far from the active site of the enzyme, this conjugation method does not inhibit the enzymatic activity of peroxidase. However, one disadvantage of this method is that commercial preparations of peroxidase vary in the amount of carbohydrate [42]. It is thus often difficult to obtain conjugates of reproducible activity with this method. Schematic procedures for the above conjugation methods have been previously described [42].

We have found that all these conjugation procedures can be used to produce satisfactory direct and indirect conjugates for the rotavirus EIA systems. Newer methods utilizing benzoquinone [45] and N,N'-O-phenylenedimaleimide [46] have also been described. Further studies will be necessary to ensure the efficiency of conjugates produced by these methods for EIA systems.

Substrates

Most of the substrates utilized in the EIA are colorless compounds which react with enzyme to yield colored compounds. The use of colorigenic substrates has the advantage of utilizing simple instrumentation and offering the option of performing qualitative readings with the naked eye. However, one disadvantage of colorigenic substrates is that a relative large amount of color must be accumulated before they are detectable by a colorimeter. Enzyme assays can thus be made more sensitive by the use of substrates which can be detected in lower concentrations than colorigenic substrates [47]. Thus, a substrate which produces a fluorescent product on reaction with the enzyme can be used. For example, 4-methylumbelliferone (hymecromone) is a fluorescent compound which

Table 3 Comparison of EIA Substrates for Alkaline Phosphatase

Substrate	Type	Concentration used (mol/liter)	Cutoff	Detection limit (moles) (10 min incubation)					
				Substrate	Enzyme theoretical[a]	Enzyme practical	H fl PrP[b]	Rotavirus (Dilution of standard)[c]	CMV (TCID$_{50}$)[d]
P-Nitrophenyl phosphate	Yellow λmax; 405 nm	>10^{-3}	0.01 Optical density unit	$10^{-9.5}$	$10^{-15.5}$	$10^{-15.5}$	10^{-14}	$10^{-2.5}$	1000
4-Methyl umbelliferyl phosphate	Fluorescence λex 330 nm λemit, 450 nm	10^{-4}	1 Fluorescence unit	10^{-12}	10^{-18}	$10^{-17.5}$	$10^{-15.5}$	10^{-4}	30
Methyl fluorescein phosphate	Fluorescence λex, 470 nm λemit, 510 nm	10^{-4}	1 Fluorescence unit	10^{-11}	10^{-17}	$10^{-16.5}$	$10^{-14.5}$	$10^{-3.5}$	100
[^{3}H] adenosine monophosphate	β radiation 10 Ci/mmol	$10^{-5.5}$	500 CPM	$10^{-13.5}$	$10^{-19.5}$	$10^{-18.5}$	10^{-17}	$10^{-4.5}$	3
[^{32}P] adenosine monophosphate	β-radiation 100 Ci/mmol	$10^{-6.5}$	500 CPM	$10^{-14.5}$	$10^{-20.5}$	10^{-19}	NT[e]	NT	NT

[a]Assuming a maximum turnover rate of 10^5 per minute.
[b]Polyribose phosphate of *Hemophilus influenzae* type b.
[c]Dilution of a standard stool suspension from a germ-free calf experimentally infected with human rotavirus.
[d]Cytomegalovirus.
[e]Not tested.

can be detected at an amount ranging up to 10^{-12} mol. However, 4-methyl-umbelliferone is minimally fluorescent when linked with phosphate or galactose molecules [48,49]. Thus, 4-methylumbelliferyl phosphate and 4-methylumbelliferyl galactose can be utilized as substrates for alkaline phosphatase and β-galactosidase, respectively. The use of such substrates allows for the measurement of substantially less enzyme than colorigenic substrates (Table 3). When applied to the measurement of human rotavirus, EIA using fluorescent substrates are more than 10-fold more sensitive than EIA using the same reagents with colorigenic substrates [49]. The potential problem of background fluorescence in clinical specimens is eliminated by the use of the solid-phase assays since interfering material is washed away and only antigen is bound to the solid phase. However, care must be taken to utilize filtered water to minimize the possibility of background fluorescence due to extraneous molecules in the substrate solutins.

Additional sensitivity can be obtained by the use of radioactive substrates for the enzyme-antibody conjugate. One disadvantage of radioactive substrates is that the reaction products must be separated from unreacted substrate. One practical radioactive substrate for alkaline phosphatase is tritium-labeled adenosine monophosophate ($[^3H]$ AMP) [50]. Alkaline phosophatase converts $[^3H]$ AMP into $[^3H]$ adenosine and phosphate. $[^3H]$ Adenosine can be separated from $[^3H]$ AMP by means of ion-exchange chromatography on DEAE-Sephadex since the negatively charged $[^3H]$ AMP will bind strongly to the positively charged ion-exchange resin, while uncharged adenosine will pass through (Fig. 3). The use of a radioactive substrate allows for the detection of between 10^{-19} and 10^{-20} mol of enzyme. EIA using radioactive substrates can be approximately 100-fold more sensitive than the corresponding EIA using colored substrates. It should be noted that while the use of fluorescent and radioactive substrates will allow for the detection of a smaller amount of a standard preparation of rotavirus, the sensitive substrates are not needed in routine clinical use since most patients will shed sufficiently large amounts of antigen in the acute phase of diarrhea to be detected by EIA which use colorigenic substrates. However, the more sensitive substrates are useful in detecting the presence of antigen late in the course of rotavirus diarrhea [49]. They are also useful in experimental studies involving the examination of extraintestinal specimens for rotaviral antigen (Tables 3 and 4) [51].

Nonspecific Reactions

Since enzyme immunoassays offer increased sensitivity over some other immunoassays, they also offer the potential of increased nonspecific reactivity [17]. Generally, three types of nonspecific reactions can occur. One type is caused by the nonspecific binding of enzyme-labeled reactants to the solid-phase

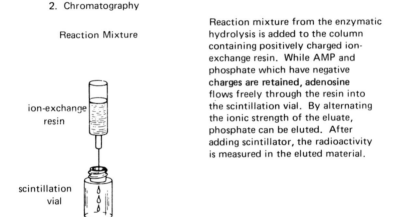

1. Enzymatic Hydrolysis

Adenosine—5'—monophosphate

(H^3 or P^{32} labeled)

Alkaline | Phosphatase

Adenosine (H^3) + Phosphate (P^{32})

2. Chromatography

Reaction Mixture

ion-exchange resin

scintillation vial

Reaction mixture from the enzymatic hydrolysis is added to the column containing positively charged ion-exchange resin. While AMP and phosphate which have negative charges are retained, adenosine flows freely through the resin into the scintillation vial. By alternating the ionic strength of the eluate, phosphate can be eluted. After adding scintillator, the radioactivity is measured in the eluted material.

Figure 3 Chromatographic separation of radioactive products. (From Ref. 50.)

material. We have found that this form of nonspecific binding can be controlled by the dilution of reactants in nonionic detergents such as Tween-20 and non-reactive proteins such as bovine serum albumin, gelatin, or fetal calf serum. The nonreactive reagents should be tested for rotavirus blocking activity prior to use to rule out the possibility of contamination with anti-rotavirus antibody. In addition, the use of reactants at dilute concentrations minimizes nonspecific adherence [35]. For example, we have found that it is seldom necessary to utilize antisera or conjugates at concentrations of greater than 1 μg/ml of immunoglobulin and that nonspecific binding can be kept to a minimum if reactants are used at concentrations in this range. Nonspecific binding can also be minimized by the proper washing of the solid phase with a solution containing a nonionic detergent [16,35]. In the case of microtiter plates, the washing should be perfomred by aspiration. This aspiration procedure can be accomplished by means of a Pasteur pipette attached to a suction apparatus or by means of an aspiration manifold. If beads are used as the solid-phase carriers, the reaction should be

Table 4 Advantages of Types of EIA

Advantage	ELISA	ELFA	USERIA
Substrate	Visible color	Fluorescent	Radioactive (Tritium)
Sensitivity (mol of enzyme)	$10^{-15.5}$	$10^{-17.5}$	$10^{-18.5}$
Cost test	0.05	0.07	0.45
Max. no. tests per day	800	200	100
Separation procedure	Not required	Not required	Column
Biohazard potential	Minimal	Minimal	Moderate
External interference	Minimal	Moderate	Minimal
Instrumentation Availability	Everywhere	Many laboratories	Most laboratories
Cost	0-$10,000	$2,000-15,000	$20,000-30,000
Potential for use in doctors' offices	Good	Slight	None

performed in test tubes which have minimal nonspecific absorption of immunoglobulins or enzymes [33]. We have found that tubes made of borosilicate glass or polycarbonate plastic have the least amount of nonspecific binding. However, the effect of any nonspecific binding to the test tube is minimized if the beads are transferred to a clean test tube at each step in the test procedure.

Nonspecific reactions can also occur in cases in which the antibody recognizes antigens other than the antigen to be tested. This cross-reactivity can be based either on immunologic cross-reactivity due to the nature of the antigen or to contamination of the antigen used to prepare the antibody, thus leading to the elaboration of a nonspecific antibody [17]. This type of nonspecific response can best be avoided by the utilization of antisera prepared with the purest available form of the antigen. When possible, antigens should be purified by means of physicochemical techniques, such as density gradient sedimentation, prior to the immunization of the animals. When this is not possible the antiserum should be absorbed with the appropriate carrier material prior to its use in enzyme immunoassay [52]. From a practical point of view the cross-reactivity potential of antisera should be evaluated by the EIA testing of clinical specimens known to contain irrelevant antigens. This testing should be performed prior to the use of the antiserum for the detection of antigens in clinical specimens. Specificity of actual clinical specimens can be further documented by the use of control reactions, as described below.

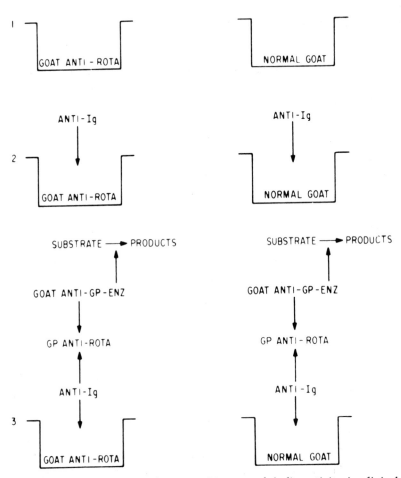

Figure 4 Cross-reactivity due to anti-immunoglobulin activity in clinical specimens. (1) Alternate rows of microtiter plates are coated with goat antirotavirus immunoglobulin and an equal concentration of immunoglobulin from the serum of a goat without demonstrable anti-rotavirus antibody. (2) The specimen is added to both wells. If a nonspecific anti-immunoglobulin is present it will bind to both the goat anti-rotavirus immunoglobulin and the normal goat immunoglobulin. (3) This anti-immunoglobulin will react with the subsequent antisera leading to a reaction in both wells. If rotavirus is also present, there will be an increased reaction in the well coated with the goat anti-rotavirus immunoglobulin. (From Ref. 53.)

A third possible cause of cross-reactivity is due to the nonspecific interaction of material in the test specimen with the immunoglobulin used to coat the plate and used in the further reaction steps. For example, we have found

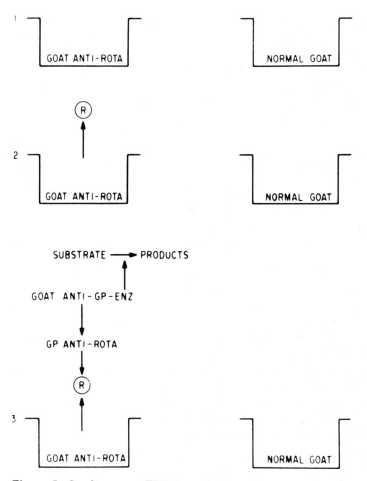

Figure 5 Confirmatory ELISA to distinguish specific rotavirus activity from nonspecific activity due to anti-immunoglobulin activity in the clinical specimens. (1) Alternate rows of microtiter plates are coated with goat anti-rotavirus immunoglobulin and an equal concentration of immunoglobulin from the serum of a goat without demonstrable anti-rotavirus antibody. (2) The specimen is added. If it contains rotavirus it will react with the goat anti-rotavirus immunoglobulin. Nonspecific anti-immunoglobulin will react with both the goat anti-rotavirus immunoglobulin and the normal goat immunoglobulin. (3) Guinea pig anti-rotavirus, enzyme-linked goat anti-guinea pig immunoglobulin, and substrate are sequentially added with washing steps between incubations. Specific rotavirus activity is manifested by a difference in color between the wells coated with goat anti-rotavirus serum and the wells coated with normal goat serum. (From Ref. 53.)

that a number of stools and serum specimens contain an IgM antibody which is capable of reacting with immunoglobulins from a number of different animal species [53]. If these IgM molecules are present in a clinical specimen they will react with the immunoglobulin used to coat the solid phase and also that used for the second antibody and the enzyme-antibody conjugate, thus leading to a nonspecific reaction. The presence of such cross-reacting antiglobulins can be discovered by the use of a control reaction in which preimmunization immunoglobulin at the same concentration as the postimmunization immunoglobulin is used to coat the solid phase. The clinical specimen is tested on separate solid phases coated with both reagents. A specimen containing antigoblulin will react equally to both solid phases, while a specimen containing specific antigen will rect to postimmunization immunoglobulin to a greater extent than the preimmunization immunoglobulin (Figs. 4 and 5). Specific viral reactivity can thus be defined as a difference in the reactivity of the specimen in the two solid phases. The cut-off value for positivity can be determined by the measurement of the mean and standard deviation of the specific reactivity of known negative specimens. Alternately, the specific viral reactivity can be determined for a weakly positive specimen, and this value can be used as the cut off for the positivity of unknown specimens. Since the cross-reactivity is due largely to the IgM class of immunoglobulin molecules, the nonspecific activity can be markedly decreased by the use of a reducing agent such as buffered N-acetyl-L-cysteine (Mucomist) [53]. Reducing agents will inactivate the IgM by the cross-linking of sulfhydryl groups, without affecting the antigenicity of stable viruses such as rotavirus [54]. An additional modification which will reduce this form of nonspecific activity is to utilize a $F(ab')_2$ portion of the immunoglobulin molecule. Since the rheumatoid-like IgM will react predominantly with the Fc portion of the molecule there will be little if any reactivity with the F (ab) $'_2$ portion of the molecule [54,55]. Thus the $F(ab')_2$ fragment of the immunoglobulin molecule, prepared by pepsin hydrolysis of intact IgG [55], should be used in situations in which a great deal of cross-reactivity can occur, such as the use of concentrated crude stool specimens. However, for maximal specificity, control reactions as described above should be performed with each specimen.

Preparation and Use of Substrates

Visible Color

Alkaline Phosphatase
p-nitrophenyl phosphate (Sigma Chemical Company) is prepared at a concentration of 1 mg/ml in 1 M diethanolamine (pH 9.8) containing 0.001 M $MgCl_2 \cdot 6H_2O$. The solution should be used immediately after preparation. After

the development of color, the reaction is stopped by the addition of 25 μl of 3 M NaOH. After the addition of the NaOH, the color will remain unchanged for at least 24 h of storage at 4°C. The color is measured in a colorimeter or microplate reader at a wavelength of 405 nm.

Peroxidase

In 50 ml of 0.01 M citrate-citric acid buffer (pH 5.0) 20 mg of O-phenyl-enediamine is dissolved. Immediately prior to use, 20 μl of 30% H_2O_2 is added. The reaction is stopped by the addition of 25 μl of 2 N H_2SO_4. This will also result in a change of the color from red-brown to dark brown. Since the stoppage of the reaction is incomplete, the reaction should be read immediately at a wavelength of 488 nm.

Fluorescent Substrate (Alkaline Phosphatase)

4-Methylumbelliferyl phosphate is prepared at a concentration of 10^{-4} or 10^{-5} M in 0.01 M diethanolamine buffer (pH 9.8) containing 0.001 $MgCL_2 \cdot 6H_2O$. The substrate should be applied to the wells immediately after preparation. The reaction is measured in a spectrofluorometer at an excitation wavelength of 360 nm (Corning 7-60) and an emission wavelength of 440 nm (Wratten 2A). Because of the possibility of extraneous fluorescent material in ordinary distilled water, filtered water should be used to prepare the substrate solutions. The substrate should be prepared from the crystalline form immediately prior to use.

Tritium-Labeled Substrate (Alkaline Phosphatase)

Tritium-labeled adenosine monophosphate (New England Nuclear), further purified as previously described [50], is diluted to a concentration of 10 μCi/ml in 0.01 M diethanolamine buffer (pH 9.0), containing 0.001 M $MgCl_2 \cdot 6H_2O$ and added to the wells. The amount of tritium-labeled adenosine produced by the hydrolysis of adenosine monophosphate by the bound enzyme is measured by ion-exchange chromatography. In this procedure, the negatively charged, unreacted adenosine monophosphate is bound to positively charged gel, while adenosine passes through the column. The procedure is described as follows:

1. To a small disposable column (Iso-Lab Quik-Sep QS-P) or to a Pasteur pipette plugged with glass wool, 2 ml of DEAE Sephadex A-25 (Pharmacia Fine Chemicals) is added; 2 ml of 0.01 M diethanolamine buffer (pH 9.0) is added on top of the gel.
2. The contents of the wells are added to the column.
3. The adenosine is eluted with 8 ml of 0.01 M diethanolamine (pH 9.0) into a scintillation vial. After the addition of a high-efficiency scintillator (Aquasol II, New England Nuclear) the tritium is counted in a scintillation counter.

The positivity of a specimen is determined by comparison with the appropriate controls as described in the following section, step 9.

Protocols for EIA Assays for Rotavirus

Direct Assay for Antigen

1. Alternate rows of wells of the microtiter plate are coated with a dilution of goat anti-rotavirus serum [or F(ab')₂] and an equal dilution of goat serum [or F (ab) $\frac{1}{2}$] which does not contain measurable antibody to rotavirus.

2. The plate is incubated at least overnight at 4°C. If the plate is not used the next day, it should be covered with parafilm and stored at 4°C until use.

3. The plate is washed five times with PBS-Tween.

4. To the wells of a blank microtiter plate, 50 μl of 20% N-acetyl-1-cysteine (adjusted to pH 7) is added. To four wells containing the N-acetyl-1-cysteine 50 μl of 10% stool suspension or rectal swab is added and incubated for 30 min at -4°C.

5. The contents are transferred to the plate which is coated in step 1, in such a way that each specimen is added to two wells coated with postimmunization sera and two wells coated with preimmunization sera.

6. The plate is incubated for 2 h at 37°C or overnight at 4°C and washed five times with phosphate-buffered saline containing 0.5 ml Tween-20 per liter.

7. Enzyme-labeled anti-rotavirus (either goat or guinea pig) diluted in PBS-Tween containing 2% fetal calf serum (PBST-S) is added to the wells.

8. The plate is incubated for 1 h at 37°C and washed five times with PBS-Tween.

9. The appropriate substrate is added. A rotavirus-specific activity is calculated by subtracting the mean activity of the specimen in the wells coated with the rotavirus-negative serum from the mean activity of the wells coated with the anti-rotavirus serum. The mean and standard deviation of the rotavirus-specific activity of the negative controls is determined. A specimen is considered positive if its mean activity is greater than 2 standard deviations above the mean of the negative controls. Alternately, a specimen can be considered positive if its activity is greater than that of the weakly positive control. This method avoids the need to run a large number of control specimens in each test.

If qualitative visual determinations are used, a specimen is considered positive if its color in the goat anti-rotavirus wells is greater than that of the weakly positive control *and* of the same specimen in the wells coated with normal goat serum.

Indirect Antigen Assay

1. The plate is coated and the specimens are incubated with N-acetyl-l-cysteine and transferred as described in steps 1-6 of the Direct Assay for Antigen.

    2. Unlabeled guinea pig anti-rotavirus diluted in PBST-S is added.

    3. The plate is incubated for 1 h at 37°C and washed five times with PBS-Tween.

    4. Enzyme-labeled anti-guinea pig, prepared in either goat or rabbit, is diluted in PBST-S and added to the wells.

    5. The plate is incubated for 1 h at 37°C and washed five times with PBS-Tween.

    6. Substrate is added, and the results are interpreted as described in steps 10 and 11, Direct Antigen Assay.

Preparation of F(ab')$_2$ Immunoglobulin Fragments [56]

As stated in Nonspecific Reactions, nonspecific reactivity can be minimized by the coating of plates with the F (ab)$_2'$ fragment of immunoglobulin. The F (ab)$_2'$ fractions can be prepared by pepsin hydrolysis of IgG as described below.

Preparation of Globulins

Whole serum is precipitated in saturated ammonium sulfate. The precipitate is spun down at approximately 4000 q, resuspended in 0.01 M phosphate buffer (pH 7.0), and dialyzed overnight against 0.01 M phosphate buffer (pH 7.0).

Isolation of IgG

The above globulin fraction is added to a 10 cm column (Bio-Rad) packed with DEAE-Sephadex equilibrated with 0.01 M phosphate buffer and eluted in 1 ml fractions of 0.01 M phosphate buffer (pH 7.0). The fractions are examined for absorbance at 260 and 280 nm in a spectrophotometer, and the fractions having significant absorbance are pooled and concentrated by vacuum dialysis. The amount of immunoglobulin present is estimated by measuring the absorbance at 260 and 280 nm and by determining the concentration of IgG by means of a standard nomogram [56].

Preparation of F (ab)$_2'$ Fragments

1. The above IgG (2 mg) is dialyzed against three changes of 0.07 M acetate buffer (pH 4.0).

    2. Pepsin is added to a final concentration of 5 mg. The mixture is incubated for 14 h at 37°C.

    3. The mixture is added to a 30 cm column packed with Sephacryl S-200 equilibrated with 0.07 M acetate buffer and eluted in 2 ml fractions with

the same buffer. The first four fractions having a significant absorbance are pooled and concentrated. The amount of $F(ab')_2$ fragments in the resulting solution is measured spectrophotometrically as described above. The solution is stored at $4°C$ with 0.01% sodium azide added as a preservative.

Use of Beads as the Solid Phase

1. Beads are coated by adding 50 beads to 10 ml of antiserum, globulin, or F (ab) $'_2$, at the same concentration used to coat the microtiter plates. The beads are incubated in a shaking water bath for 14 h at $4°C$.

2. The solution is aspirated, and the beads are washed twice with 20 ml of PBS. The beads are air-dried in a $37°C$ incubator. The beads can be stored dry at room temperature until use.

3. The stool specimen or rectal swab is put into a polycarbonate test tube, and an equal volume of 20% buffered N-acetyl-l-cysteine (pH 7.0; Mucomist) is added. Following incubation for 30 min in a shaking waterbath, beads coated with postimmunization and a bead coated with preimmunization antibody are added. (Note that additional beads coated with antibody to other viral agents can be added to the same specimen and processed separately with appropriate reagents.)

4. Following incubation for 2 h at $45°C$ in a shaking waterbath, the beads are removed by aspiration with a Pasteur pipette, dipped in a tube containing 10 ml of PBS-Tween, and transferred to another tube containing a 0.2 ml volume of the next appropriate reagent. The bead is processed utilizing the same order and concentration of reagents as the microtiter wells. Reading is simplified by the placing of substrate and bead in an optically suitable glass test tube and performing the spectrophotometric or fluorometric readings in the same tube.

References

1. A. Z. Kapikian, R. H. Yolken, H. B. Greenberg, R. G. Wyatt, A. R. Kalica, R. M. Chanock, and H. W. Kim, Gastroenteritis viruses. In *Diagnostic Procedures for Viral, Rickettsial and Chlamydial Infections*, 5th Ed., (E.H. Lennette and N. J. Schmidt, eds.), American Public Health Association, Washington, D.C., 1979, pp. 927–995.

2. A. Z. Kapikian, W. L. Cline, H. W. Kim, A. R. Kalica, R. G. Wyatt, D. H. Vankirk, R. M. Chanock, H. D. James, Jr., and A. L. Vaughn, Antigenic relationships among five reovirus-like (RVL) agents by complement-fixation (CF) and development of a new substitute CF antigen for the human RVL agent of infantile gastroenteritis, *Proc. Soc. Exp. Biol. Med., 152*:535–539 (1976).

3. R. H. Yolken, B. Barbour, R. G. Wyatt, A. R. Kalica, A. Z. Kapikian, and R. M. Chanock, Enzyme-linked immunosorbent assay (ELISA) for identification of rotaviruses from different animal species, *Science, 201*:259-262 (1978).

4. R. H. Yolken, R. G. Wyatt, G. P. Zissis, C. D. Brandt, W. J. Rodriguez, H. W. Kim, R. H. Parrott, A. Z. Kapikian, and R. M. Chanock, Epidemiology of human rotavirus types 1 and 2 as studied by enzyme-linked immunosorbent assay, *N. Engl. J. Med., 299*:1156-1161 (1978).

5. G. Cukor, M. K. Berry, and N. R. Blacklow, Simplified radioimmunoassay for detection of human rotavirus in stools, *J. Infect. Dis., 138*:906-910 (1978).

6. P. C. Grauballe, J. Genner, A. Meyling, and A. Hornsleth, Rapid diagnosis of rotavirus infections: Comparison of electron microscopy and immuno-electro-osmophoresis for the detection of rotavirus in human infantile gastroenteritis, *J. Gen. Virol., 35*:203-218 (1977).

7. J. E. Banatvala, B. Totterdell, I. L. Chrystie, and G. N. Woode, In vitro detection of human rotaviruses, *Lancet, 2*:821 (1975).

8. P. J. Middleton, M. T. Szymanski, G. D. Abbott, R. Bortolussi, and J. R. Hamilton, Orbivirus acute gastroenteritis of infancy, *Lancet, 1*:1241-1244 (1974).

9. S. Matsuno and S. Nagayoshi, Quantitative estimation of infantile gastroenteritis virus antigens in stools by immune adherence hemagglutination test, *J. Clin. Microbiol., 7*:310-311 (1978).

10. R. H. Yolken, R. G. Wyatt, A. R. Kalica, H. W. Kim, C. D. Brandt, R. H. Parrott, A. Z. Kapikian, and R. M. Chanock, Use of a free viral immunofluorescence assay to detect human reovirus-like agent in human stools, *Infect. Immun., 16*:467-470 (1977).

11. R. F. Bradburne, J. D. Almeida, P. S. Gardner, R. B. Moosai, A. A. Nash, and R. R. A. Coombs, A solid phase system (SPACE) for the detection and quantification of rotavirus in faeces, *J. Gen. Virol., 44*:615-623 (1979).

12. P. J. Middleton, M. D. Holdaway, M. Petore, M. T. Szymanski, and J. S. Tam, Solid-phase radioimmunoassay for the detection of rotavirus, *Infect. Immun., 16*:439-444 (1977).

13. R. H. Yolken, H. W. Kim, T. Clem, R. G. Wyatt, A. R. Kalica, R. M. Chanock, and A. Z. Kapikian, Enzyme linked immunosorbent assay (ELISA) for detection of human reo-like agent of infantile gastroenteritis, *Lancet, 2*:263-267 (1977).

14. E. Engvall and P. Perlman, Enzyme linked immunosorbent assay (ELISA) III. Quantitation of specific antibodies by enzyme labelled antiglobulin in antigen coated tubes, *J. Immunol., 109*:129-135 (1971).

15. S. Avrameas, Coupling of enzymes to protein with glutaraldehyde. Use of conjugates for the detection of antigens and antibodies. *Immunochemistry, 6*:43 (1969).

16. A. Voller, D. E. Bidwell, and A. Bartlett, Microplate enzyme immunoassays for the immunodiagnosis of virus infections. In *Manual of Clinical Immunoassay* (N. R. Rose and H. Friedman, eds.), American Society of Microbiology, Washington, D.C., 1976, pp. 506-512.

17. A. J. Pesce, D. J. Ford, and M. A. Gaizutus, Qualitiative and quantitative aspects of immunoassays, *Scand. J. Immunol., 8*(Suppl. 7):1-6 (1978).

18. A. Z. Kapikian, A. R. Kalica, J. W. Shih, W. L. Cline, T. S. Thornhill, R. G. Wyatt, R. M. Chanock, H. W. Kim, and J. L. Gerin, Buoyant density in cesium chloride of the human reo-virus like agent of infantile gastroenteritis by ultracentrifugation, electron microscopy, and complement-fixation, *Virology, 70*:564-569 (1976).

19. A. R. Kalica, R. H. Purcell, M. M. Sereno, R. G. Wyatt, H. W. Kim, R. M. Chanock, and A. Z. Kapikian, A microtiter solid phase radioimmunoassay for detection of the human reovirus-like agent in stools, *J. Immunol., 118*: 1275-1279 (1977).

20. H. Wanatabe, I. D. Gust, and I. H. Holmes, Human rotavirus and its antibody: Their coexistence in faeces of infants, *J. Clin. Microbiol., 7*:405-409 (1978).

21. C. A. Mebus, R. G. Wyatt, R. L. Sharpee, M. M. Sereno, A. R. Kalica, A. Z. Kapikian, and M. J. Twiehaus, Diarrhea in gnotobiotic calves caused by the reovirus-like agent of human infantile gastroenteritis, *Infect. Immun., 14*:471-474 (1976).

22. R. H. Yolken, R. G. Wyatt, and A. Z. Kapikian, ELISA for rotavirus, *Lancet, 2*:818 (1977).

23. R. G. Wyatt, A. R. Kalica, C. A. Mebus, H. W. Kim, W. T. London, R. M. Chanock, and A. Z. Kapikian, Reovirus-like agents (rotaviruses) associated with diarrheal illness in animals and man. In *Perspectives in Virology*, Vol. X (M. Pollard, ed.), Raven, New York, 1978, pp. 121-145.

24. B. K. Van Weemen and A. H. Schuurs, Immunoassays using antibody-enzyme conjugates, *FEBS Lett. 43*:215 (1974).

25. R. G. Wyatt, W. D. James, E. H. Bohl, K. W. Theil, L. J. Saif, A. P. Kalica, H. G. Greenberg, A. Z. Kapikian, and R. M. Chanock, Human rotavirus Type 2: Cultivation in vitro, *Science, 207*:189 (1980).

26. H. Wanatabe and I. H. Holmes, Filter paper solid-phase radioimmunoassay for human rotavirus surface immunoglobulins, *J. Clin. Microbiol., 6*:319-324 (1977).

27. M. K. Viljanen, K. Granfors, and J. P. Toivant, Radioimmunoassay of class specific antibodies, *Immunochemistry, 12*:699-705 (1975).

28. H. Park, A new plastic receptacle for solid-phase immunoassays, *J. Immunol. Methods, 20*:349-355 (1978).

29. J. L. Boitieux, G. Desret, and D. Thomas, Immobilization of anti-HB_sAg antibodies on artificial protein membranes, *FEBS Lett., 93*:133-136 (1978).

30. E. P. Halpern and R. W. Bordens, Microencapsulated antibodies in radioimmunoassay, *Clin. Chem., 25*:860-862 (1979).

31. P. Hösli, S. Avrameas, A. Ullman, E. Vogt, and M. Rodrigot, Quantitative ultramicro-scale immunoenzymic method for measuring Ig antigen determinants in single cells, *Clin. Chem., 24*:1325 (1978).

32. K. O. Smith and W. D. Gelle, Magnetic transfer devices for use in solid-phase radioimmunoassays and enzyme-linked immunosorbent assays, *J. Infect. Dis., 136*:5329-332 (1977).

33. B. R. Ziola, M. T. Matikainen, and Salmia, Polystyrene balls as the solif phase of immunoassays, *J. Immunol. Methods, 17*:309-317 (1977).

34. A. Pesce, D. J. Ford, M. Gaizutus, and V. E. Pollak, Binding of protein to polystyrene in solid phase immunoassays, *Biochim. Biophys. Acta, 492*: 399-407 (1977).

35. S. L. Bullock and K. W. Walls, Evaluation of some of the parameters of the enzyme-linked immunosorbent assay, *J. Infect. Dis., 136*:5279-4285 (1977).

36. S. M. Burt, T. Carter, and L. Kricka, Thermal characteristics of microtiter plates used in immunological assays, *J. Immunol. Methods, 31*:231 (1979).

37. R. H. Yolken, Enzyme linked immunosorbent assay (ELISA), *Hosp. Pract., 13*:121 (1978).

38. G. B. Johnson and E. J. Holborow, Immunofluorescence. In *Handbook of Experimental Immunology*, Vol. I (D. M. Weir, ed.), Blackwell, Oxford, 1973, p. 181.

39. E. H. Beutner, E. J. Holborow, and G. D. Johnson, Quantitative studies of immunofluorescent staining, *Immunology, 12*:327 (1967).

40. J. E. Volanakis and R. M. Stroud, Rabbit C_{1q}: Purification, functional, and structural studies, *J. Immunol., Methods, 2*:25 (1972).

41. L. Belanger, Alternative approaches to enzyme immunoassays, *Scand. J. Immunol., 8*:33 (1978).

42. S. Avrameas, T. Ternynck, and J. L. Guesdon, Coupling of enzymes to antibodies and antigens, *Scand. J. Immunol., 8*:7 (1978).

43. S. Avrameas and T. Ternynck, Peroxidase labelled antibody and Fab conjugates with enhanced intracellular penetration, *Immunochemistry, 8* 1175 (1971).

44. P. K. Nakane and A. Kawoi, Peroxidase-labelled antibody. A new method for conjugation, *J. Histochem. Cytochem., 14*:929 (1974).

45. T. Ternynck and S. Avrameas, A new method using P-benzoquinone for coupling antigens and antibodies to marker surfaces, *Ann. Immunol., 127*:197 (1976).

46. K. Kato, K. Y. Hamaguchi, M. Fukui, and E. Ishikaw, Enzyme-linked immunoassay 1. Novel method for synthesis of the insulin-B-D-galactosidase conjugate and its applicability for insulin assay, *J. Biochem., 78*: 235 (1975).

47. K. Kato, Y. Hamaguchi, S. Okawa, E. Ishikawa, K. Kobayashi, and N. Katunuma, Enzyme immunoassay in rapid progress, *Lancet, 1*:40 (1977).

48. E. Ishikawa and K. Kato, Ultrasensitive enzyme immunoassay, *Scand J. Immunol., 8*:43 (1978).

49. R. H. Yolken and P. J. Stopa, Enzyme-linked fluorescence assay (ELFA): An ultrasensitive solid phase assay for the detection of human rotavirus, *J. Clin. Microbiol., 10*:317-321 (1979).

50. C. C. Harris, R. H. Yolken, H. Krokan and I. C. Hsu, Ultrasensitive enzymatic radioimmune assay for detection of cholera toxin and rotavirus, *Proc. Natl. Acad. Sci. USA, 76*:5336-5339 (1979).

51. F. Saulsbury, J. Winkelstein, and R. H. Yolken, Chronic rotavirus infections in immunocompromised children, *J. Pediatr., 97*:61-65 (1980).

52. G. Appleyard and H. T. Zwartouw, Preparation of antigens from animal viruses. In *Handbook of Experimental Immunology*, Vol. I (D. M. Weir, ed.), Blackwell, Oxford, 1973, p. 3.1.

53. R. H. Yolken and P. J. Stopa, Analysis of non-specific reactions in enzyme-linked immunosorbent assay testing for human rotavirus, *J. Clin. Microbiol., 10*:703-707 (1979).

54. J. W. Mehl, W. O'Connell, and J. DeGroot, Macroglobulin from human plasma which forms an enzymatically active compound with trypsin, *Science, 145*:821 (1966).

55. S. Cohen and C. Milstein, Structure and biological properties of immunoglobulins, *Adv. Immunol., 7*:1 (1967).

56. D. R. Stanworth and M. W. Turner, Immunochemical analysis of immunoglobulins and their subunits. In *Handbook of Experimental Immunology*, Vol. I. (D. M. Weir, ed.), Blackwell, Oxford, 1973, p. 101.

5

Viruses and Gastrointestinal Disease

Neil R. Blacklow and George Cukor University of Massachusetts
Medical School, Worcester, Massachusetts

The purpose of this chapter is to review established and postulated relationships of viruses and gastrointestinal tract disease. First, we shall summarize two major types of clinicopathologic events that occur in known acute viral infections of the gut represented by gastroenteritis viruses on the one hand and enteroviruses on the other hand. Occasional secondary infection of the gut is also mentioned. Then, with these well-described events serving as a background, we shall concentrate on a discussion of nondiarrheal diseases of the gastrointestinal tract for which a viral etiology is suggested. These include intussusception, appendicitis, pancreatitis and diabetes mellitus, and inflammatory bowel disease. In each case, we shall critically evaluate the evidence for viral involvement in the disease.

Clinicopathologic Summary of Known Viral Infections of the Gut

Viral infection of the gastrointestinal tract may be expressed in several different clinical forms. The first type of disease is due to direct local damage produced by viral multiplication in the gastrointestinal tract and is clinically manifested as a constellation of acute symptoms including diarrhea, abdominal cramps, nausea, vomitting, and fever. Viral gastroenteritis is the primary subject of this book, and its best documented etiologic agents are the rotaviruses and the

Norwalk-like viruses. The pathology produced by these viruses appears to be confined solely to the gastrointestinal tract without accompanying viremia [2].

A second clinical expression of infection is exemplified by other viruses that replicate for the most part asymptomatically in the gastrointestinal tract but which undergo a viremia, thereby spreading the virus to other target organs where the major syndromes are produced. These viruses are most notably members of the enterovirus group, as well as hepatitis A virus. The syndromes produced by the three groups of enteroviruses (coxsackievirus, echovirus, and poliovirus) are well reviewed elsewhere [3,6], as is the literature on hepatitis A [11]. Enterovirus infection is frequently asymptomatic, and when clinical symptoms develop they are rarely related to the gastrointestinal tract. These viruses do not produce acute diarrheal disease. Target organs that are commonly secondarily infected include the central nervous system (meningitis, poliomyelitis), heart (myopericarditis), muscle (myalgia, pleurodynia), and skin (febrile exanthems). In recent years, chronic neurologic infection in agammaglobulinemic children and a form of acute epidemic hemorrhagic conjunctivitis have also been identified as being produced by infection with enteroviruses [39,57].

A third form of gastrointestinal tract infection is uncommonly recognized clinically and develops when the gut serves as a secondary target of viral infection which is incidentally reached by the hematogenous route. Examples of this mode of infection are hepatitis B and cytomegalovirus [10,15]. Viremic spread to the gut may also account for gastrointestinal symptomatology when it occurs as an incidental part of a generalized viral disease such as influenza B or measles [30].

Thus, the three modes of viral infection of the gastrointestinal tract—primary acute gastroenteritis, other target organ syndromes secondary to viremia, and incidental infection of the gut as a secondary target during viremia emanating from another site—are the result of either a fecal-oral or a systemic viremic mode of viral introduction into the gastrointestinal tract. By far the most common mode of spread is the fecal-oral route through contaminated vehicles such as hands, food, water, and inanimate objects. The major viral agents to be spread in this manner are the enteroviruses, hepatitis A, the gastroenteritis viruses, and occasionally adenoviruses. In order to reach the gut after ingestion, a virus must pass through gastric acid and duodenal bile salts without inactivation. Thus, only nonenveloped, acid-stable viruses may produce direct primary infection of the gut. Labile viruses occasionally reach the gut by the secondary viremic route described above. Some viruses are able to infect both the respiratory and gastrointestinal tracts. Adenoviruses, for example, may be shed asymptomatically in the stool for prolonged periods following acute respiratory tract illness. Many adenoviruses and some enteroviruses may be transmitted by the respiratory route. However, after multiplication in the oropharynx, the virus must be swallowed in order to produce intestinal tract infection and is, of course, subject to inactivation in the stomach and duodenum. For this reason acid-labile viruses such as rhinoviruses do not result in infection of the gut.

Having reviewed the known mechanisms of pathogenesis of virus infections of the gastrointestinal tract, we shall concentrate in the remainder of this chapter on nondiarrheal diseases of the gastrointestinal tract for which a viral etiology has been suggested. Comprehensive reviews of this topic are not readily available in the literature, in contrast to the well-established and well-described forms of infection of the gut described above.

Nondiarrheal Diseases of the Gastrointestinal Tract of Suggested Viral Etiology: General Considerations

A viral etiology has been postulated for several nondiarrheal diseases of the gastrointestinal (GI) tract. These include intussusception, appendicitis, pancreatis and diabetes mellitus, and inflammatory bowel disease (regional enteritis and ulcerative colitis). It may be that viruses are but one of multiple etiologic factors that can produce these diseases. It is possible that for some of these diseases there is a complex pathogenesis having genetic, immunologic, and other environmental factors. It is also possible that rather than being initiators of pathogenesis, viruses may contribute to the exacerbation or remission of certain diseases.

Proving that a nondiarrheal disease of the gastrointestinal tract is caused by a given virus is very difficult. The obvious method is to culture the putative virus from the patient and particularly from the tissues involved. However, live virus may no longer be available for culture by the time operation or autopsy is performed [26]. In addition, no culture systems are available for some viruses infecting the GI tract, such as rotavirus and Norwalk-like viruses. It is possible that some viruses may be present in latent or incomplete forms. Even culture or histologic evidence of infection cannot be considered as conclusive proof of the viral etiology of a disease. This is because virus cultivated from diseased tissue may be an innocent passenger that finds affected cells an appropriate site for replication; in addition, virus recovered from unaffected tissue or secretions may also be an irrelevant innocent bystander. Good epidemiologic studies can be used to establish an association between viral infection and disease but cannot serve as conclusive proof of causation. Properly performed studies require appropriately selected sensitive techniques for detection of virus as well as specific serologic and pathologic data. Prospective studies, in general, are more useful than retrospective studies. Painstakingly selected control populations and appropriately large numbers of patients diagnosed by established clinical criteria are other essential features of a good epidemiologic study. This kind of study is extremely expensive and difficult to perform. The investigations cited below often fall short of at least some of the above criteria. They are, however, useful in indicating the direction that future studies ought to take. Epidemiologic investigations must be relied upon because Koch's postulates are not easily fulfilled for most of these diseases due to difficulties in culturing the virus, lack of a suitable animal model, and inappropriateness of human volunteer studies.

Intussusception

Ileocecal intussusception occurs most commonly in children under the age of 2 years. Enlargement of the mesenteric lymph nodes in the region of the terminal ileum has frequently been observed at laparotomy [26,52]. This finding has led to the suggestion that virus-induced lymphoid hyperplasia may play a causative role in this disease in that a circumferential cuff of intestinal lymphoid tissue may be formed which can conceivably lead to intussusception. In addition, it is possible that viral infection may contribute to the production of intussusception by alteration of intestinal motility [64].

Adenovirus has been frequently isolated from children with intussusception, and high prevalences of serum antibody to adenovirus in such patients have also been reported [19,46,47]. The significance of these findings may be questioned due to the ubiquity of adenovirus, the high prevalence of inapparent infection, and the prolonged fecal excretion of adenovirus following infection. A somewhat stronger suggestion for the pathogenic role of adenovirus in some cases of intussusception comes from the presentation of morphologic evidence of viral replication in appropriate tissue. Yunis et al. [64] have reported that electron microscopic evidence of adenovirus replication was found in the epithelial cells of the appendix or the terminal ileum in one-third of specimens they examined from children undergoing surgery for ileocecal intussusception.

Recent studies by Konno et al. [34] have indicated an association between rotavirus infection and intussusception. Initially, hyperplasia of the intestinal lymphoid tissue including the mesenteric lymph nodes was commonly noted in infants who died with acute rotavirus gastroenteritis [33]. Later, rotavirus was seen by electron microscopy in the stools of 11 of 30 patients with intussusception. This is an extraordinarily high rate of rotavirus excretion in nondiarrheal infants, inasmuch as rotavirus (unlike adenovirus) is rarely seen in such nondiarrheal individuals. Of intussusception patients who shed rotavirus, 70% also experienced a fourfold rise in serum antibody titer to the virus during the course of their illness [34]. Association of rotavirus infection with intussusception also occurred during the cooler months [34], a time when rotavirus infection is commonly seen in temperate climates. Further support for the etiologic role of rotavirus in intussusception is the close correlation in the age distribution of patients with intussusception and patients with acute rotaviral gastroenteritis. In summary, there appears to be an association between rotavirus infection and intussusception; whether the association is etiologic is unknown at present.

Appendicitis

Although plausible mechanisms for the viral induction of appendicitis have been proposed, there is little evidence for the association of the disease with viral infection. It has been suggested that acute viral infection could lead to lymphoid hyperplasia in the appendix, and that this hyperplasia or subsequent healing and scarring might produce acute appendiceal obstruction [28]. It has also been proposed that viruses may infect the appendiceal mucosa and either produce the disease directly or denude the appendix and make it highly susceptible to bacterial infection [26].

It has been reported that appendicitis in childhood tends to occur more frequently during those months in which respiratory infections are most prevalent [36] and that a seemingly large percentage of children in an uncontrolled study experienced upper respiratory tract infection during the 2 weeks prior to or at the time of admission to the hospital for appendicitis [28]. An association between acute appendicitis and lymphoid hyperplasia due to enterovirus infection has been claimed [55]; however, this report has been severely criticized for the inadequacy of controls [27], as well as the small number of patients studied and the specificity of the techniques used [28]. Studies demonstrating virus infection of the appendix during appendicitis, seroconversion during the course of the disease, together with viral study of control subjects have not been reported.

Pancreatitis and Diabetes Mellitus

Infection with mumps virus is among the many recognized causes of pancreatitis [26]. The reported incidence of pancreatitis among patients with parotitis ranges from less than 1% to as high as 25% and occurs more commonly in young adults than in children. Since typical parotitis is not seen in about one-third of mumps cases, it is at least theoretically possible that sporadic episodes of idiopathic pancreatitis in children are caused by mumps virus infection [7]. Acute pancreatitis has on occasion been observed to be the only clinical manifestation of mumps infection [58], and mumps has also been associated with chronic recurring pancreatitis [59].

Cytomegalovirus, like mumps virus, exhibits an affinity for the acinar cells of the salivary gland which share some structural similarities with cells of the pancreas. Typical intranuclear inclusions in the pancreatic cells of infants dying with generalized cytomegalic inclusion disease have often been observed [60,61]. Recipients of renal transplants and immunosuppressive drugs are prone to both pancreatitis [54] and infection with cytomegalovirus [50]. Although a causative relationship between the two entities had been suggested[54], the evidence presented so far is only suggestive. For example, pancreatic homogenates of some renal transplant recipients with generalized cytomegalovirus infection have yielded large amounts of virus even though inclusion-bearing cells were rarely observed during histologic examination of the pancreas [29].

The ability of group B coxsackieviruses to produce necrotizing lesions in the pancreas of infant mice has long been recognized [45]. Lesions of the pancreas have also been found in human infants dying with generalized group B coxsackievirus infections, and types B3 and B4 have been isolated from such cases [31,32]. Coxsackievirus B4 has been recovered from older patients with clinical evidence of pancreatitis [42]. Serologic evidence is also suggestive of an association between group B coxsackievirus infection and acute pancreatitis [1,4].

Damage to the pancreas which results in the destruction of the insulin-secreting β cells of the islets of Langerhans is the cause of insulin-deficiency diabetes mellitus. The hypothesis that certain common human virus infections can occasionally result in such damage was first proposed over 80 years ago [23,24] when an increased prevalence of diabetes following an outbreak of mumps was noted. Several independent lines of evidence have been proposed to show that virus infection plays an etiologic role in the induction of acute onset diabetes mellitus [8,14,43]. The first part of the evidence consists of numerous epidemiologic observations showing an increased prevalence of new cases with onsets in either the winter or early autumn months and a relative paucity of new cases during the spring and early summer [7,37]. It has been suggested that these seasonal trends correspond to the prevalence of certain common virus infections in the community. Further evidence seeks to establish a temporal relationship between certain childhood virus infections and the onset of diabetes. The virus most often implicated has been mumps [23,24,58]. Although most workers report a short interval between parotitis and diabetes, one group noted an increase in the prevalence of new cases of diabetes in New York State several years after community-wide outbreaks of mumps [53]. Pancreatitis infrequently occurs in mumps patients who subsequently develop diabetes mellitus [7]. Rubella virus has also been reported to be diabetogenic based on the increased incidence of this disease in patients with congenital rubella [38].

Strong evidence that viruses have a causative role in diabetes has come from animal studies. Variants of two viruses of human origin, reovirus type 3 and coxsackievirus B4, as well as murine encephalomyocarditis virus, have been shown to infect pancreatic β cells and produce a diabetes-like syndrome in certain in-bred strains of mice [9,43,44,63].

A recent important report [62] fulfills Koch's postulates in associating a variant of coxsackievirus B4 with one human case of acute onset diabetes mellitus. The virus was isolated from the pancreas of a child who died after the onset of diabetic ketoacidosis. Lymphocytic infiltration of the islets of Langerhans and necrosis of β cells were noted. The virus was recovered after inoculation into cell culture. Inoculation of the isolate into genetically susceptible mice resulted in β-cell damage and hyperglycemia. The virus could be recovered from the infected animals. Further documentation included a rise in viral antibody titer in both the patient and infected mice and the finding of viral antigen in the cells of the patient's pancreas. This report is buttressed by an earlier suggestion of serologic association between coxsackievirus B4 infection and acute onset diabetes [16,18]; however, other careful serologic studies have not been confirmatory [13,25].

Finally, it should be noted that the common virus infections may only be a small portion of the etiology of diabetes mellitus and that genetic and immunologic factors appear to play essential roles in determining susceptibility to the disease [8]. Furthermore, it is possible that environmental agents other than viruses (e.g., chemicals) may also be capable of triggering the onset of diabetes. However, further studies are indicated into the viral causation of diabetes. An experimental basis for the viral hypothesis has been established by the demonstration that coxsackieviruses B3 and B4 and mumps virus replicate specifically in insulin-secreting human β cells in culture [48,63].

Inflammatory Bowel Disease

An infectious viral etiology for Crohn's disease (regional enteritis) was first suggested experimentally by the induction in mice of granulomas and chronic intestinal inflammation following inoculation with filtrates of diseased bowel tissue homogenates [5,40,41]. An increased prevalence of lymphocytotoxic antibodies and anti-RNA antibodies in both inflammatory bowel disease patients and their spouses has recently been noted when compared with control groups; these findings are suggestive of a role for environmental agents in inflammatory bowel disease although the interpretation of these data is not clear at present [12,35].

Several laboratories have reported the cultivation of virus-like agents with a greater frequency from involved tissue of inflammatory bowel disease patients than from comparable tissues of control patients. These agents have been described as cytomegalovirus from ulcerative colitis tissue [15], a 30 nm virus-like particle from Crohn's disease [20,21], and a rotavirus-like agent from Crohn's disease [56]. However, when serum antibody prevalences and titers to rotavirus and Norwalk virus were compared in Crohn's disease patients and in matched controls, no significant differences were found [22]. In the cases of rotavirus and cytomegalovirus, it is difficult to present convincing evidence of differing antibody prevalences among groups since the majority of populations possess antibodies to these agents. However, the additional lack of differences in titers makes the association between rotavirus and Crohn's disease unlikely. In addition, the isolation in cell culture of rotavirus-like agents from Crohn's disease tissue could not be confirmed; rather, cell culture contamination with mycoplasma was observed [29a].

Serum antibody to cytomegalovirus has been detected more frequently and at higher mean titer in ulcerative colitis patients compared with matched controls [15]. Biopsies from three of six ulcerative colitis patients yielded cytomegalovirus after culture and serial passage. Important covariables such as the use of steroids and recent history of blood transfusion were controlled for in this study.

An attractive hypothesis involving immune-mediated enterocytolysis [51] has been proposed to explain the possible role of cytomegalovirus in inflammatory bowel disease [49]. The proposed model accounts for many of the clinical aspects of the disease. It is suggested that a viremia occurs during primary cytomegalovirus infection in childhood or early adulthood in some genetically and/or immunologically susceptible individuals so that latent virus infection is established in the epithelial cells of the colon. The virus-specific products, whose synthesis is directed by cytomegalovirus DNA integrated into the host chromosome, cause an antigenic alteration of the cell surface. Immune destruction of these modified host cells results in the patient's disease symptoms. The characteristic exacerbations and remissions of inflammatory bowel disease can be related to the point at which a gradually increasing load of antigenically altered cells reaches the threshold for eliciting episodes of immune-mediated enterocytolysis. The general immunosuppressive effect of steroids could account for the response to these compounds in acute exacerbations of inflammatory bowel disease. The feasibility of this model depends on the demonstration of either virus particle or subviral components in involved inflammatory bowel tissue. Using a hybridization technique, these workers have been able to demonstrate cytomegalovirus DNA in intestinal tissue from only one of four ulcerative colitis patients. However, their procedure was able to detect only one to two genome equivalents of viral DNA per cell, which may not be sufficiently sensitive. It is possible that only a fragment of the viral genome is present in each cell so that final judgment of this intriguing proposed model awaits the development of more sensitive methodology.

Finally, it should be noted that it is possible that viruses may merely be passengers in the denuded gut epithelium of inflammatory bowel disease patients and not etiologic agents. Nonetheless, should this prove to be the case, the presence of these viruses may turn out to have a profound influence on disease progress and exacerbation.

Conclusion

We have summarized clinicopathologic events known to occur in various forms of acute virus infections of the human gastrointestinal tract. These events are well described in the literature and serve as a background for analyzing certain nondiarrheal diseases of the gut for which a viral etiology has been suggested and for which comprehensive reviews are lacking in the literature. A current examination of limited studies on intussusception indicates an association between rotavirus infection and the disease; whether the association is etiologic is not known. There is little evidence at present to support a role for viruses in appendicitis. Viruses are one of the many known, but uncommon causes of acute pancreatitis; more importantly, a recent body of growing persuasive evidence indicates that virus infection (particularly coxsackievirus B4) may be one factor in initiating acute onset diabetes mellitus. Finally, sporadic reports of viral involvement in regional enteritis and ulcerative colitis have yet to be confirmed by controlled, large-scale studies, and any role for virus infection in inflammatory bowel disease is likely to be complex and perhaps intertwined with an immunologic pathogenesis. Our understanding of the role of viruses in various clinical forms of nondiarrheal gastrointestinal disease is clearly limited, although intussusception and some cases of diabetes mellitus seem to be the strongest candidates at present for an etiologic relationship with virus infection.

References

1. B. Arnesjo, T. Eden, I. Ishe, E. Nordenfelt, and B. Ursing, Enterovirus infections in acute pancreatitis; a possible etiological connection, *Scand. J. Gastroenterol., 11*:645-649 (1976).
2. N. R. Blacklow and G. Cukor, Viral gastroenteritis, *N. Engl. J. Med., 304*: 397-406 (1981).
3. E. H. Brown, Enterovirus infections, *Br. Med. J., 1*:169-171 (1973).
4. P. Capner, R. Lendnum, D. J. Jeffries, and G. Walker, Viral antibody studies in pancreatic disease, *Gut, 16*:866-870 (1975).
5. D. R. Cave, S. P. Kane, and D. N. Mitchell, Further animal evidence of a transmissible agent in Crohn's disease, *Lancet, 2*:1122-1124 (1973).
6. J. D. Cherry and D. B. Nelson, Enterovirus infections: Their epidemiology and pathogenesis, *Clin. Pediatr., 5*:659-664 (1966).
7. J. E. Craighead, The role of viruses in the pathogenesis of pancreatic disease and diabetes mellitus, *Prog. Med. Virol., 19*:161-214 (1975).
8. J. E. Craighead, Current views on the etiology of insulin-dependent diabetes mellitus, *N. Engl. J. Med., 299*:1439-1445 (1978).
9. J. E. Craighead and M. F. McLane, Diabetes mellitus; induction in mice by encephalomyocarditis virus, *Science, 162*:913-914 (1968).
10. D. M. Dent, P. J. Days, A. R. Bind, and W. E. Birkenstock, Cytomegalic virus infection of bowel in adults, *S. Afr. Med. J., 49*:669-672 (1975).
11. J. D. Dienstag, W. Szmuness, C. E. Stevens, and R. H. Purcell, Hepatitis A virus infection: New insights from seroepidemiologic studies, *J. Infect. Dis., 137*:328-340 (1978).
12. R. J. DeHoratius, R. G. Strickland, W. C. Miller, N. A. Volpicelli, R. F. Gaecke, J. B. Kirsner, and R. C. Williams, Antibodies to synthetic poly-

ribonucleotides in spouses of patients with inflammatory bowel disease, *Lancet, 1*:1116-1119 (1978).

13. S. E. Dippe, P. H. Bennett, M. Miller, J. E. Maynard, and K. R. Berquist, Lack of causal association between coxsackie B4 virus infection and diabetes, *Lancet, 1*:1314-1317 (1975).

14. A. L. Drash, The etiology of diabetes mellitus, *N. Engl. J. Med., 300*:1211-1213 (1979).

15. G. W. Farmer, M. M. Vincent, L. Fucillo, L. Horta-Barbosa, J. L. Sever, and G. L. Gitnick, Viral investigations in ulcerative colitis and regional enteritis, *Gastroenterology, 65*:8-18 (1973).

16. D. R. Gamble, M. L. Kinsley, M. G. Fitzgerald, R. Bolton, and K. W. Taylor, Viral antibodies in diabetes mellitus, *Br. Med. J., 3*:627-630 (1969).

17. D. R. Gamble and K. W. Taylor, Seasonal incidence of diabetes mellitus, *Br. Med. J., 3*:631-633 (1969).

18. D. R. Gamble, K. W. Taylor, and H. Cumming, Coxsackie viruses and diabetes mellitus, *Br. Med. J., 4*:260-262 (1973).

19. P. S. Gardner, E. G. Knox, S. D. Court, and C. A. Green, Virus infection and intussusception in childhood, *Br. Med. J., 2*:697-700 (1962).

20. G. L. Gitnick, M. H. Arthur, and I. Shibata, Cultivation of viral agents from Crohn's disease: A new sensitive system, *Lancet, 2*:215-217 (1976).

21. G. L. Gitnick and V. J. Rosen, Electron microscopic studies of viral agents in Crohn's disease, *Lancet, 2*:217-219 (1976).

22. H. B. Greenberg, R. L. Gebhard, C. J. McCluin, R. D. Soltis, and A. Z. Kapikian, Antibodies to viral gastroenteritis viruses in Crohn's disease, *Gastroenterology, 76*:349-350 (1979).

23. E. Gundersen, Is diabetes of infectious origin? *J. Infect. Dis., 41*:197-202 (1927).

24. H. F. Harris, A case of diabetes mellitus quickly following mumps, *Boston Med. Surg. J., 140*:465-469 (1899).

25. J. C. Hierholzer and W. A. Farris, Follow-up of children infected in a coxsackie B3 and B4 outbreak: no evidence of diabetes mellitus, *J. Infect. Dis., 129*:741-746 (1974).

26. R. J. Howard, H. H. Balfour, and R. L. Simmons, The surgical significance of viruses. In *Current Problems in Surgery*, Vol. XIV (M. Ravitch, ed.), Yearbook Medical Publishers Inc., Chicago-London, 1977, pp. 1-82.

27. J. G. R. Howie, Virus infection and appendicitis, *Lancet, 2*:182 (1965).

28. R. H. Jackson, P. S. Gardner, J. Kennedy, and J. McQuillin, Viruses in the aetiology of acute appendicitis, *Lancet, 2*:711-715 (1966).

29. R. E. Kanich and J. E. Craighead, Cytomegalovirus infection and cytomegalic inclusion disease in renal homotransplant recipients, *Am. J. Med., 40*:874-882 (1966).

29a. A. Z. Kapikian, M. F. Barile, R. G. Wyatt, R. H. Yolken, J. G. Tully, H. B. Greenberg, A. R. Kalica, and R. M. Chanock. Mycoplasma contamination in cell culture of Crohn's disease material (letter). *Lancet, 2*:466-467 (1979).

30. A. A. Kerr, M. A. P. S. Downham, J. McQuillin, and P. S. Gardner, Gastric flu: Influenza B causing abdominal symptoms in children, *Lancet, 1*:291-295 (1975).

31. S. Kibrick and K. Benirschke, Acute aseptic myocarditis and meningoencephalitis in the newborn child infected with coxsackie virus group B type 3, *N. Engl. J. Med., 255*:883-889 (1956).

32. S. Kibrick and K. Benirschke, Severe generalized disease (encephalohepatomyocarditis) occurring in the new born period and due to infection with coxsackie virus group B. Evidence of intrauterine infection with this agent, *Pediatrics, 22*:857-875 (1958).

33. T. Konno, H. Suzuki, A. Imai, and N. Ishida, Reovirus-like agent in acute epidemic gastroenteritis in Japanese infants; faecal shedding and serologic response, *J. Infect. Dis., 135*:259-266 (1977).

34. T. Konno, H. Suzuki, T. Kutsuzawa, A. Imai, N. Katusushima, M. Sakamoto, S. Kitaoka, R. Tsuboi, and M. Adachi, Human rotavirus infection in infants and young children with intussusception, *J. Med. Virol., 2*:265-269 (1978).

35. S. J. Korsmeyer, R. C. Williams, I. D. Wilson, and R. G. Strickland, Lymphocytotoxic antibody in inflammatory bowel disease: A family study, *N. Engl. J. Med., 293*:1117-1120 (1975).

36. W. E. Ladd and R. E. Gross, *Abdominal Surgery of Infancy and Childhood*, W. B. Saunders, Co., Philadelphia, 1941.

37. D. R. MacMillan, M. Kotoyan, D. Zeidner, and B. Hafezi, Seasonal variation in the onset of diabetes in children, *Pediatrics, 59*:113-115 (1977).

38. M. A. Menser, J. M. Forrest, and R. D. Bransby, Rubella infection and diabetes mellitus, *Lancet, 1*:57-60 (1978).

39. R. R. Mirkovic, N. J. Schmidt, M. Yin-Murphy, and J. L. Melnick, Enterovirus etiology of the 1970 Singapore epidemic of acute conjunctivitis, *Intervirology, 4*:119-127 (1974).

40. D. N. Mitchell and R. J. W. Rees, Agent transmissible from Crohn's disease tissue, *Lancet, 2*:168-171 (1970).

41. D. N. Mitchell and R. J. W. Rees, Further observation on the transmissibility of Crohn's disease, *Ann. N.Y. Acad. Sci., 278*:546-559 (1976).

42. A. M. Murphy and R. Simmul, Coxsackie B4 virus infection in New South Wales during 1962, *Med. J. Aust., 2*:443-445 (1964).

43. A. L. Notkins, Virus-induced diabetes mellitus, *Arch. Virol., 54*:1-17 (1977).

44. T. Onodera, A. B. Jenson, J. W. Yoon, and A. L. Notkins, Virus-induced diabetes mellitus: Reovirus infection of pancreatic B cells in mice, *Science, 201*:529-531 (1978).

45. A. M. Pappenheimer, J. B. Daniels, F. S. Cheever, and T. H. Weller, Lesions caused in suckling mice by certain viruses isolated from cases of so called non-paralytic poliomyelitis and of pleurodynia, *J. Exp. Med., 92*:169-190 (1950).

46. C. S. Potter, Adenovirus infection as an aetiological factor in intussusception of infants and young children, *J. Pathol. Bacteriol., 88*:263-274 (1964).

47. C. W. Potter, W. I. H. Shedden, and R. B. Zachary, A comparative study of the incidence of adenovirus antibodies in children with intussuscep-

tion with that in a control group, *J. Pediatr., 63*:420-427 (1963).

48. G. A. Prince, A. B. Jenson, L. C. Billups, and A. L. Notkins, Infection of pancreatic beta cell cultures with mumps virus, *Nature, 271*:158-163 (1978).

49. J. K. Roche and E. S. Huang, Viral DNA in inflammatory bowel disease. CMV-bearing cells as a target for immune mediated enterocytolysis, *Gastroenterology, 72*:228-233 (1977).

50. R. H. Rubin, B. A. Corsimi, N. E. Tolkoff-Rubin, P. S. Russell, and M. S. Hirsch, Infectious disease syndromes attributable to cytomegalovirus and their significance among renal transplant recipients, *Transplantation, 24*: 458-464 (1977).

51. J. D. Stobo, T. B. Tomasi, K. A. Huizenga, R. J. Spencer, and R. G. Shorter, In vitro studies of inflammatory bowel disease; surface receptors of the mononuclear cell required to lyse allogenic colonic epithelial cells, *Gastroenterology, 70*:171-176 (1976).

52. R. Strang, Intussusception in infancy and childhood: A review of 400 cases, *Br. J. Surg., 46*:484-495 (1959).

53. H. A. Sultz, B. A. Hart, M. Zielezng, and E. R. Schlesinger, Is mumps virus an etiologic factor in juvenile diabetes mellitus? *J. Pediatr., 86*: 654-6 (1975).

54. N. L. Tilney, J. J. Collins, and R. E. Wilson, Hemorrhagic pancreatitis. A fatal complication of renal transplantation, *N. Engl. J. Med., 274*:1051-1057 (1966).

55. T. Tobe, Inapparent virus infection as a trigger of appendicitis, *Lancet, 1*: 1343 (1965).

56. P. J. Whorwell, C. A. Phillips, W. L. Beeken, P. K. Little, and K. D. Roessner, Isolation of reovirus-like agents from patients with Crohn's disease, *Lancet, 1*:1169-1171 (1977).

57. C. M. Wilfert, R. H. Buckley, T. Mohanakumar, J. F. Griffith, S. L. Katz, J. K. Whisnant, P. A. Eggleston, M. Moore, E. Treadwell, M. N. Oxman, and F. S. Rosen, Persistent and fatal central nervous system echovirus infections in patients with agammaglobulinemia, *N. Engl. J. Med., 296*: 1485-1489 (1977).

58. C. L. Witte and B. Schanzer, Pancreatitis due to mumps, *JAMA, 203*: 164-165 (1968).

59. C. B. Wood, R. A. Bradbrook, and L. H. Blumgart, Chronic pancreatitis in childhood associated with mumps virus infection, *Br. J. Clin. Pract. 28*: 67-69 (1974).

60. W. A. Worth and H. L. Howard, New features of inclusion disease of infancy, *Am. J. Pathol., 26*:17-36 (1950).

61. J. P. Wyatt, J. Saxton, R. S. Lee, and H. Pinkerton, Generalized cytomegalic inclusion disease, *J. Pediatr., 36*:271-294 (1950).

62. J. W. Yoon, M. Austin, T. Onodera, and A. L. Notkins, Virus-induced diabetes mellitus: Isolation of a virus from the pancreas of a child with diabetic ketoacidosis, *N. Engl. J. Med., 300*:1173-1179 (1979).

63. J. W. Yoon, T. Onodera, and A. L. Notkins, Virus-induced diabetes mellitus. XV. Beta cell damage and insulin-dependent hyperglycemia in mice infected with coxsackie virus B4, *J. Exp. Med., 148*:1068-1080 (1978).

64. E. J. Yunis, R. W. Atchison, R. H. Michaels, and F. A. DeCicco, Adenovirus and ileocecal intussusception, *Lab. Invest., 33*:347-351 (1975).

6

Immunology of the Gastrointestinal Tract

M. B. Pepys   Royal Postgraduate Medical School,
London, England

The great majority of antigenic materials are derived from the external environment, with which the gastrointestinal tract forms the largest "interface." The gut is unavoidably exposed to food and other components of the diet, and also to the normal commensal flora and their products. There may be exposure to potentially or obligatorily pathogenic microorganisms, parasites, and toxins. The gut is therefore of profound importance in the immunologic organization of the individual and is provided with abundant lymphoid tissue. This gut-associated lymphoid tissue (GALT), which may constitute more than one-third of the total lymphoid mass of the body, has a specific structural and functional organization and characteristic secretory antibody products which are particularly adapted to their local functions. Derangement of immunologic functions of the gut may impair its efficiency as the organ of nutrition and have a permissive role in the pathogenesis of enteric and nonenteric infections. It has also lately been recognized that even slight abnormalities in the handling and response to antigens at mucosal surfaces may be of pathogenetic significance in a number of noninfectious diseases.

It is important to recognize that there are many significant differences between species in the structures and functions subserving immunologic responses in the gastrointestinal tract. There may also be variations with age and intercurrent events, such as common forms of parasite infestation. What follows is largely a synthesis of available clinical and experimental information which may not be applicable generally in every species. For more detailed consideration of individual circumstances reference should be made to the original and review articles which are quoted.

Uptake of Antigen from the Gut

Oral administration of antigen has been known, since the work of Uhlenhuth [1], to be capable of inducing production of circulating antibodies. Subsequent workers have repeatedly demonstrated, in human subjects as well as a variety of experimental animals, that exposure to antigens via the gut can both induce systemic allergic responses and elicit allergic reactions in the gut itself and elsewhere [2-9]. There has thus long been evidence that intact macromolecules or their large fragments which retain immunogenicity and/or immunoreactivity, traverse the mucosa intact. Differing estimates have been reported of the amounts of immunologically intact protein antigens which are absorbed. For example Gurskay and Cooke [10] detected in the circulation 0.02% of a 1 g dose of ovalbumin given intragastrically to fasting infants without gastrointestinal symptoms, whereas 0.1% was absorbed by infants with diarrhea. More recently Hemmings and Williams [11] and Morris and Morris [12] have found that 25 and 15%, respectively, of ingested doses of heterologous radioiodinated IgG reaches the carcass of adult rats in the form of immunoreactive fragments of 20,000-50,000 daltons. Hemmings has extended these observations to other proteins and other animal species and claims that they represent a general phenomenon (see references in Ref. 13).

The following routes have been identified by which macromolecular material from the intestinal lumen traverses the mucosal epithelium and reaches the lamina propria.

1. The enterocytes pinocytose material from the lumen, possibly in some cases as a result of the binding of particular molecules to specific receptors on luminal plasma membrane. This seems to be the case with IgG of maternal origin in the suckling rat and some other mammals [14,15]. Such pinocytosed material may be digested intracellularly following the formation of phagolysosomes, but in some cases it may be protected or only incompletely degraded. Undegraded substances tend to be exocytosed at the lateral basal aspect of the enterocyte and thus reach the lamina propria [16].

2. Under some circumstances molecules from the lumen may also pass through the tight junctions between the enterocytes, but this is probably not an important route in normal conditions.

3. Peyer's patches and other mucosal lymphoid aggregates, including tonsils, appendix, and cecal patches, are covered by a distinctive follicle-associated epithelium [17-20]. This is characterized in the intestine by the lack of goblet

cells or, in the tonsil, of stratified epithelium, and by the presence of specialized epithelial cells, called M cells. These have scattered short protuberances rather than microvilli on their luminal aspect, form cytoplasmic bridges between the usual columnar microvillus-covered epithelial cells, and are intimately related to underlying nests of lymphocytes. The M cells contain a tubulovesicular system, represented by pits on their luminal aspect, which has been shown to mediate the uptake of molecules and particles from the lumen and their transfer to the subjacent lymphoid tissue. The anatomical disposition of the mucosal lymphoid aggregates and the features of the follicle-associated epithelium seem adapted to the trapping of antigens and particulate material from the lumen. Since follicle-associated epithelium and M cells, with their characteristic properties, have been found in association with all the major gut mucosal lymphoid aggregates which have been studied, they must have important functions in the uptake and handling of luminal antigens.

4. Apart from these physiological processes, various degrees of pathological dysfunction of the mucosal epithelium, up to and including frank ulceration, presumably permit abnormal patterns of antigen absorption from the gut lumen to occur.

5. The secretory antibody system plays an important role in regulating the uptake of antigens from the gut [21-23]. The major immunoglobulin class of antibody normally present in the lumen is IgA, predominantly in its secretory form sIgA [22]. This sIgA, the production of which is induced by luminal antigens, is incorporated into the mucus which coats the mucosal epithelium and there it binds specific antigens and so inhibits their systemic uptake [24]. Another process which assists in this so-called immune exclusion function of secretory antibody is the increase in the susceptibility of antigens to digestive enzymolysis when they are complexed with antibody [25]. This is clearly not the only mechanism since IgA also excludes antigens in the respiratory tract [26]. The apparently greater "permeability" of the neonatal compared to the adult gut may be largely a reflection of the immaturity of the secretory antibody system [23]. Similarly, the abnormally high titers of serum antibodies to dietary antigens in individuals with selective IgA deficiency [27,28] may also be in part attributable to impaired exclusion in the gut. Other possible explanations for these phenomena are considered below.

Structure of the Gut-Associated Lymphoid Tissue

Intraepithelial Lymphocytes

Numerous lymphoid cells are present within the mucosal epithelium itself. They lie between the enterocytes and thus in very close relationship to the lumen and its contents. Many, but not all these cells are T lymphocytes, or at least T-cell dependent, while the ultrastructure of a few of them is suggestive of B cells [29-33]. In the follicle-associated epithelium overlying mucosal lymphoid aggregates, such as Peyer's patches or appendix, nests of lymphocytes typically lie enfolded in the cytoplasm of the M cells which provide a thin porous partition from luminal antigens [34]. So-called globule leukocytes may also be present in the epithelium. Elements of their structure and cytochemistry resemble mast cells, and it has been suggested, though not as yet unequivocally established, that T lymphocytes may be capable of transformation into mast cells [35,36].

Lamina Propria Lymphoid Cells

The interstitial tissue of the lamina propria contains abundant lymphoid cells, mostly mature immunoglobulin-secreting plasma cells together with scattered macrophages and occasional lymphocytes. The plasma cells tend to lie in close relationship to the glands of the mucosal epithelium, and the majority of them produce IgA [37,38]. Smaller numbers produce IgM and very few make IgG. Occasional IgE-containing plasma cells may also be found.

Lamina Propria Lymphoid Aggregates

Scattered through the lamina propria are aggregates of lymphoid tissue varying in size from minor cellular foci or nodules to the massive accumulations which surround the appendix in some species (see review in Ref. 39). The most constant feature is the characteristic Peyer's patches, although their site, number, and persistence through adult life vary greatly among the species. Peyer's patches have a follicular structure including both thymus-dependent T lymphocytes and thymus-independent B lymphocytes. There are also abundant macrophages, particularly in the area overlying the lymphoid follicles and immediately beneath the follicle-associated epithelium. The antigen-retaining dendritic reticular cells, which are a notable feature of lymphoid follicles elsewhere in the body, are lacking, but antigens and particles from the lumen clearly have ready access to the patches. Plasma cells are very rarely seen within a Peyer's patch itself, but there may be accumulations of them in the adjacent lamina propria. Lymphoid tissue in the appendix, in those species which possess it, has an overall structure similar to that of the Peyer's patches.

Mesenteric Lymph Nodes

Lymph draining from the gut mucosa, including the Peyer's patches, goes to the mesenteric lymph nodes, which structurally resemble lymph nodes elsewhere. There is, however, morphologic and functional evidence of persistent lymphocyte activation in the mesenteric nodes. Unlike systemic lymphoid tissue, which in good health may have only a minimal antigenic load, the mesenteric nodes are continuously stimulated.

Thoracic Duct

Virtually all the lymph from the gut finally reaches the thoracic duct from which its cellular and other contents enter the systemic circulation. Over half the lymphoid cells in the thoracic duct are T cells, and there is a minor population of activated lymphocytes including both T- and B-cell blasts [31]. The majority of B blast cells are apparently committed to IgA production; they both bear it on their surface and contain it in their cytoplasm [40].

Maturation of the Gut-Associated Lymphoid Tissue

Two major influences contribute to the establishment of the GALT in its normal mature form. These are: (1) the thymus and T cells and (2) the normal microbial flora. In the absence of either of these factors, as in T-cell–deficient [41] or gnotobiotic animals [42], respectively, all components of the GALT which have been enumerated above remain rudimentary, and there is diminished production of secretory antibody. The precise mechanisms for the T-cell dependence of the GALT are not known, but most of the intraepithelial lymphocytes are themselves T cells. Furthermore, it is well recognized that although lymphoid follicles in general are composed largely of B cells, their development and response to antigens require T cells [43]. IgA antibody production, regardless of the route of antigen administration, is also T-cell dependent [44,45]. The role of the microbial flora is less clear. It may provide intense antigenic stimulation, since many microbial products are more potent antigens than, for example, most dietary constituents. There may also be a role for bacterial products, particularly endotoxic lipopolysaccharides as nonspecific mitogens. This latter concept is difficult to generalize because lipopolysaccharides are powerful mitogens only in mice (see discussion in Ref. 39).

Functional Organization of the Gut-Associated Lymphoid Tissue

The GALT is equipped to provide the following functions:

1. Rapid and extensive sampling of antigens from the lumen via the follicle-associated epithelium.
2. Activation of lymphocytes in Peyer's patches by luminal antigens. The blast cells then migrate via the blood and "home back" into the gastrointestinal tract and other mucosal and secretory organs, including the lactating breast.
3. Production by plasma cells in the lamina propria of secretory antibody, chiefly sIgA, with specificity for luminal antigens.

Although the precise mechanisms underlying much of this functional behavior are not yet understood, it is likely that the overall effect is beneficial

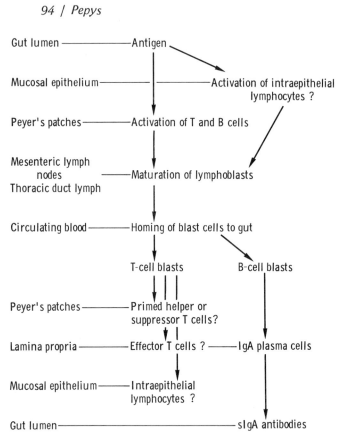

Figure 1 Lymphocyte activation, migration, and function in the gut-associated lymphoid tissue.

to the organism by distributing specific effector cells and antibodies to sites where they can contribute to the exclusion of viable and nonviable antigens (Fig. 1).

Intraepithelial Lymphocytes

The function of the intraepithelial lymphocytes, which are the most "superficial" cells of the GALT, is not known. A significant proportion of them are active blast cells, and while some may be shed, many are engaged in active traffic between the epithelium and deeper tissues [32,33]. They may include "afferent" cells sampling luminal antigen and possibly responding to it before moving elsewhere in the GALT to mature or interact with other cell populations. There may also be "efferent" cells which have already been primed by luminal or other antigens and are serving a local effector function by mediating reactions of delayed hypersensitivity or cellular immunity [46,47].

Handling of Antigen in the Lamina Propria

Soluble or particulate antigens, including microorganisms, which have penetrated the mucosal epithelium, may either be taken up by local macrophages in the lamina propria [48,49] or may travel to and localize in the Peyer's patches [17,50]. The abundant material which readily traverses follicle-associated epithelia tends to be handled by the many macrophages around and within the follicular lymphoid aggregates. The fate of antigens which are not processed locally, or indeed after this has occurred, is not known. The basis for the partition of antigens between blood and lymph is also not known but may be very important. For example, there is evidence that the direct entry of antigen into the portal blood can induce tolerance whereas this does not occur in the presence of a portacaval shunt [51-53].

Peyer's Patches and Lymphoblast Migration

The Peyer's patches, and possibly other follicular lymphoid aggregates in the lamina propria, have a central role in the functioning of the GALT (see review in Ref. 39). There is very active cellular traffic in the patches, particularly of blast cells. Exposure to both viable and nonviable antigens via the intestine, rather than parenterally or by other routes, provokes germinal center formation [54] and activates both T- and B-lymphocyte populations in the Peyer's patches [55-58]. The B blasts are the main source of precursors of the IgA-secreting plasma cells which populate the lamina propria [59-63]. The special features of the microenvironment of the Peyer's patches and/or the properties of the lymphocytes within it which determine this fact are not known. However, there is evidence for a specific population of T cells which regulate IgA synthesis [64], and recently it has been shown that murine Peyer's patches are relatively much richer in helpers and deficient in suppressors for IgA than spleen and peripheral nodes [65]. Having been triggered by antigen under the cooperative influence of T cells and possibly other factors in the patches, the B blasts do not become plasma cells in situ but migrate out via the lymphatics which drain into the mesenteric nodes. From there they finally reach the thoracic duct from which they enter the circulation. Most of these B-cell blasts, originally generated in Peyer's patches, promptly home back into the gut [66]. They extravasate and settle in the lamina propria of the intestine where many then become mature IgA-secreting plasma cells [32,67]. Blast cells taken directly from Peyer's patches do not show gut-homing properties [68]; they apparently acquire this property in the course of their migration out into the mesenteric nodes and thoracic duct. During this process many develop intracellular as well as surface IgA [40,69].

The tendency of B-cell blasts originating from the Peyer's patches and mesenteric nodes to home back into and localize in the gut has both antigen-independent and antigen-dependent components. Such blasts will localize in heterotopic isografts of sterile fetal intestine free of intrinsic antigen [31,70], in the gut of germ-free neonatal rats [71] and in fetal sheep in utero [72]. However, in local segments of intestine containing an extrinsic antigen, there is greater accumulation and enhanced persistence of recirculated B blasts with appropriate specificity [63,73]. There may be some local proliferation of B blasts after recirculation [74], and there is certainly local antibody secretion after segmental exposure to antigen [75]. This double mechanism for gut-homing of the antibody-forming cell precursors is probably advantageous. On the one hand it distributes to the whole gut, and even to other sites such as the respiratory tract and the lactating breast, the specific response to antigens which may only have been locally encountered [76]. It thus enables the mother, for example, to provide the neonate via the colostrum and breast milk with specific passive immunity against those intestinal pathogens to which she has been exposed and is currently responding [77]. On the other hand, the local proliferation or shedding of antigens, for example by enteric microorganisms, can focus the deposition and production of specifically responsive cells and antibodies.

In contrast to the B-cell blasts, the T-cell lymphoblasts generated in Peyer's patches tend, for the most part, to home back into the Peyer's patches [78] and the mucosal epithelium [31]. The function of these recirculated T blasts is not yet clearly defined. They may be the source of a special population of helper cells which have already been primed by luminal antigens and which specifically endow Peyer's patches with their enhanced capacity to generate IgA-forming cell precursors [65]. They may also include the suppressor cells for IgM, IgG, and IgE production which are responsible for orally induced tolerance in some experimental situations (see below).

The mechanisms by which lymphoblasts generated in the gut home back to mucosae are not understood for either T or B cells. Inflammation induced by parasite infestation in the gut is associated with increased nonspecific intestinal homing of T blasts [79]. There is a reasonably clear distinction between the behavior of blast cells generated in the gut and in the spleen or somatic lymph nodes. The latter tend to recirculate and home back into nongut lymphoid tissue as selectively as blasts of enteric origin return to the gastrointestinal tract [80,81]. Small lymphocytes also probably recirculate selectively, at least to some extent, through the enteric or somatic pathway [82].

In addition to their vital role as the source of the precursors of secretory IgA-producing plasma cells, another possible function for Peyer's patches has come to light. It has long been known that the oral administration of antigen can suppress the subsequent response to parenteral immunization [83], and recent evidence suggests that at least one mechanism for this form of tolerance may be the generation in Peyer's patches of suppressor cells which may be in either T- or B-cell populations. These phenomena will be considered below.

Products of the Gut-Associated Lymphoid Tissue

Cells

Exposure to antigens via the gut leading to an allergic response in the GALT generates both T- and B-cell blasts, predominantly in the Peyer's patches as described above. It is not known whether any of these activated cells remain and function in situ, but many undertake the migration and recirculation back into the gut which have been outlined. Most of the B blasts which extravasate into the lamina propria apparently mature into plasma cells and secrete IgA without any further antigen-specific stimulation. It is possible that others persist as B memory cells and may be capable of responding to local antigens by further cell division and direct maturation into plasma cells within the lamina propria [63]. The major target of the gut-homing T-cell blasts is the Peyer's patches, where they may exert regulatory helper and suppressor functions. It is not known to what extent these primed T cells could also function within the lamina propria or the epithelium itself [31], as effector cells with direct cytotoxicity against their specific targets, or as mediators of delayed hypersensitivity or cellular immunity [46,47].

Secretory Antibodies

One of the principal products of the GALT and the one about which most is known is the humoral antibody produced by lamina propria plasma cells and delivered chiefly into the secretions [23,84-86]. The majority of this antibody is in the IgA class. It is secreted by plasma cells in a dimeric form comprising two monomeric IgA molecules linked by a small polypeptide called J chain. In the gut lumen nearly all the IgA molecules are covalently associated with a unique glycoprotein called secretory component which is synthesized by the enterocytes. This secretory form of IgA (sIgA) is largely incorporated into the mucous coat which overlies the epithelium. Some of the IgM which is found in secretions is also associated with secretory component. The secretory forms of immunoglobulin apparently have increased resistance to proteolytic digestion, which may facilitate their functions in the lumen. IgE does not become coupled with secretory component and can be recovered from intestinal secretions only as polypeptide fragments [87,88].

Dimeric IgA has an affinity for secretory component, and it has been suggested, on the basis of immunohistochemical studies in the human, that IgA dimers in the interstitial fluid bind to the plasma membrane of enterocytes via secretory component, which is expressed on their surface. Complexes are then internalized, covalently coupled with secretory component within the cell, and finally secreted onto the luminal aspect [86]. Immune electron microscope studies in pigs have, on the other hand, indicated that IgA and IgM may be transported across the epithelium in membrane-bound vesicles by a process of reverse pinocytosis [89]. Intestinal lymph is rich in IgA [90], and it has recently been shown that once this IgA reaches the circulation it is rapidly and efficiently cleared by the liver and secreted into the bile, whence it reaches the intestinal lumen [91,92]. Although established so far only in rats, this may prove to be an important route for transport of IgA into the gut.

Parenteral immunization may induce some IgA antibody formation systemically as a minor component of the overall response, but there is usually no perceptible secretory antibody formation [93]. In contrast, oral immunization can induce both local, secretory, and systemic responses [5], the former consisting predominantly of IgA [85]. There has been some discussion about whether repeated intestinal exposure to antigen can evoke a secretory antibody response of secondary type, and there are some conflicting data. It seems that with viable, replicating antigens secondary responses may occur but that with nonviable antigens the picture may be obscured by the oral tolerance mechanism (see below). In some experimental systems, parenteral immunization primes for the induction of a secondary intestinal response via the oral route, and may even be more effective than oral priming [73].

Functions of the Gut-Associated Lymphoid Tissue and Secretory Antibody System

Secretory Antibody and Immunity

The most clearly discernible function of immunologic responses in the gut is the protection of the body from enteric pathogens, pathogens which use the gut as their portal of entry, and from toxic nonviable materials. Secretory antibody, particularly IgA, plays a central role in this protective function. Secretory IgA antibody is extremely efficient at binding soluble antigens and agglutinating particulate antigens [22]. It is therefore effective at neutralizing toxins [94,95] and viruses (see Chap. 00), and preventing the adherence of bacteria to epithelia [96], which is a necessary prerequisite for infection or pathogenicity in most cases (see, for example, Ref. 97). The inclusion of secretory IgA in the matrix of mucus which tenaciously coats the epithelial surface seems ideally suited to the exclusion of noxious agents from the epithelium.

Many, but not all, metazoan intestinal parasites induce the production of large amounts of IgE antibody [98]. It is not clear what part, if any, this reaginic antibody plays in eliminating parasites from the gut or preventing reinfestation. It may be involved in the "self-cure" phenomenon which occurs in some infestations. Local immediate hypersensitivity reactions may in general be beneficial by increasing the amount of circulating antibodies and cells which gain access to pathogens localized in or on the mucosa (see discussion in Ref. 99).

Handling of Nonpathogens and Nonviable Antigens

A less clearly defined role of GALT and its products is in the handling and response to nonpathogenic microorganisms and nonviable, intrinsically harmless antigens from the gut lumen. Secretory antibodies play an important part in excluding such materials from the body, but the barrier is not complete since, as mentioned previously, the absorption of a minor proportion of a dietary antigen load is normal. If comparable amounts of antigen were administered parenterally the host would in many cases be sensitized for tissue-damaging hypersensitivity reactions, and yet sensitization by the oral route is relatively rare. This suggests that the gut, the GALT, and its products exert regulatory effects which generally prevent potentially harmful sensitization to antigens from the lumen.

It has long been known that antigen feeding [83] or intragastric instillation of contact-sensitizing chemicals [100] can induce a state of specific immunologic tolerance to subsequent parenteral or dermal sensitization, respectively. These observations have recently been confirmed and extended in several different experimental models, including the antibody response to heterologous erythrocytes in mice [101], the IgG and the IgE responses to heterologous proteins in rats, mice, and guinea pigs [102-105], and contact sensitivity in mice [106]. All the results indicate that primary exposure to antigens via the gut, and hence the GALT, is a potent mechanism for inducing tolerance or at least suppression of those responses which sensitize for hypersensitivity reactions.

A number of possible mechanisms have been proposed on the basis of different experimental results. An IgA antibody response may be induced, leading to circulating antigen-IgA antibody complexes which have immunosuppressive effects [107]. Suppressor T [108,109] or B cells [106] may also be generated in the Peyer's patches. Orally induced tolerance or suppression is, however, neither complete nor a universal phenomenon, since animals and patients can, under some circumstances, be sensitized by the oral route for hypersensitivity reactions elicited either orally or parenterally. Furthermore, normal healthy individuals regularly possess in all immunoglobulin classes serum antibodies directed against their own commensal flora [110,111].

Role of Effector T Cells in the Gut

Delayed hypersensitivity reactions directed against contact-sensitizing chemicals [112,113] and transplantation alloantigens [47] and mediated by T cells can be demonstrated in the gut. There is also evidence that T cells are required to eliminate some parasitic worm infestations from the gut [99], and that the abnormalities of small intestinal mucosal architecture (villous atrophy) seen in such infestations are T-cell dependent [114]. It therefore seems clear that T lymphocytes can exert their usual effector functions in the gastrointestinal tract as in other parts of the body. Their normal role in the regulation of either the commensal flora or pathogenic microorganisms from the lumen is not known. The clinical evidence (see below) from patients with abnormalities of T cells as well as of immunoglobulin production suggests that such a role may exist.

Clinical Abnormalities of Gut Immunologic Function

Immunodeficiency

The clinical consequences of abnormalities in immunologic responses in the gut and the GALT may be seen in patients with various forms of immunodeficiency. Selective IgA deficiency can be completely asymptomatic but is often associated with an increased incidence of autoallergic diseases, gluten-sensitive enteropathy, and malignancy [22]. The increased titers of serum antibodies to dietary antigens in patients with selective IgA deficiency and in patients with gluten-sensitive enteropathy and inflammatory bowel disease may result not only from the failure of IgA and the intact mucosa to exclude antigens, but also from abnormalities of, for example, T-cell regulatory function [64] or other normal mechanisms by which luminal antigens usually induce systemic tolerance. It is interesting that most patients with X-linked hypogammaglobulinemia and some with common variable immunodeficiency, in whom secretory antibodies are virtually absent, have no other clinical, functional, or structural abnormality in the gut. On the other hand, many patients with common variable immunodeficiency, particularly those with abnormalities of T-cell function as well as immunoglobulin deficiency, suffer from a variety of gastrointestinal abnormalities including diarrhea, steatorrhea, intestinal bacterial overgrowth, partial villous atrophy with or without *Giardia lamblia* infestation, nodular lymphoid hyperplasia, gastric atrophy, and an increased incidence of gastrointestinal and other malignancy (see, for example, Refs. 115 and 116). In severe combined immunodeficiency, which without grafting is usually fatal in the first year or so, diarrhea and failure to thrive are often the main complaints and mucosal infection with *Candida albicans* is common.

Inflammatory Disease of the Gut

It is not known to what extent other gastrointestinal diseases which are associated with immunologic abnormalities, such as gluten-sensitive enteropathy, inflammatory bowel disease (Crohn's disease and ulcerative colitis), and pernicious anemia, are a result of underlying abnormalities in the function of GALT,

Gluten-sensitive enteropathy is probably a consequence of hypersensitivity to gluten, manifest as a tissue-damaging reaction in the mucosa of the small intestine [117]. Antibodies to intrinsic factor probably cause vitamin B_{12} deficiency in pernicious anemia, but it is not clear whether these antibodies and the other immunologic abnormalities seen in this condition are primary or secondary [118]. Similarly, in inflammatory bowel disease, there may be a number of immunologic abnormalities, and it is difficult to assess the extent to which these are pathogenetic or are merely epiphenomena. However, antibody and cell-mediated hypersensitivity mechanisms, entirely comparable to those recognized in other parts of the body, can occur in the gastrointestinal tract and lead to local tissue damage. There is evidence for immediate-type hypersensitivity to foods in allergic gastroenteropathy [119], antigen-antibody complex hypersensitivity in gluten-sensitive enteropathy [117], and possibly for delayed hypersensitivity to enterobacterial antigens in Crohn's disease [120,121]. It is conceivable, though not yet firmly established, that hypersensitivity to the products of microorganisms in the gut may contribute to the pathogenesis of enteric infections (see, for example, Ref. 122).

α-Chain Disease

Another aspect of the relationship between enteric infection and gastrointestinal pathology is illustrated by α-chain disease [123]. This condition has been widely reported outside Western Europe and the United States, and is characterized by an abnormal proliferation of intestinal plasmacytoid cells which secrete α-heavy immunoglobulin chains. In its early phase the disorder may respond completely to treatment with broad-spectrum antibiotics and corticosteroids [124], but if left untreated it progresses inexorably to become frankly malignant. Large tumor masses form and can be fatal by causing bowel obstruction, intussusception, or perforation. The etiology of the condition is not known, but the response to treatment suggests that a process leading to malignant transformation of intestinal IgA-secreting plasma cells or their precursors may be initiated by some form(s) of microbial infection.

Atopy

Atopy, which is the inherited predisposition to respond to common environmental antigens by the production of IgE antibodies [125], is apparently associated with the abnormal handling or processing of antigens at mucosal surfaces. Atopic individuals have an increased incidence of transient IgA deficiency in infancy [126]. They tend to respond to experimental [127] or occupational [125] primary exposure to antigens vial mucosal surfaces by producing IgE antibodies, whereas nonatopic individuals do not. It is not clear whether this propensity for IgE production is due to a relative deficit in the "immune exclusion" function of sIgA, abnormalities in the suppressive role of IgA antibody, or suppressor cells, or a combination of factors. In any event atopy is common, involving about 20% of the European and North American populations [125]. There are no reports of investigations looking for altered handling of microorganisms in the gut by atopic subjects, as a result of their mucosal immunologic dysfunction, but it is possible that they exist.

References

1. P. T. Uhlenhuth, NeuerBeitrag zum spezifischem Nachweiss von Eierweiss auf biologischem Wege, *Dtsch. Med. Wochenschr., 26*:734 (1970).

2. J. P. Hettwer and R. A. Kriz, Absorption of undigested protein from the alimentary tract as determined by the direct anaphylaxis test, *Am. J. Physiol., 73*:539 (1925).

3. M. Walzer, Studies in absorption of undigested proteins in human beings. 1. A simple direct method of studying the absorption of undigested protein, *J. Immunol., XIV*:143 (1927).

4. S. J. Wilson and M. Walzer, Absorption of undigested proteins in human beings. IV. Absorption of unaltered egg protein in infants and in children, *Am. J. Dis. Child., 50*:49 (1935).

5. R. M. Rothberg, S. C. Kraft, and R. J. Farr, Similarities between rabbit antibodies produced following ingestion of bovine serum albumin and following parenteral immunization, *J. Immunol., 98*:386 (1967).

6. K. Aas and J. W. Jebsen, Studies of hypersensitivity to fish, *Int. Arch Allergy Appl. Immunol., 32*:1 (1967).

7. I. D. Bernstein and Z. Ovary, Absorption of antigens from the gastrointestinal tract, *Int. Arch. Allergy Appl. Immunol., 33*:521 (1968).

8. P. E. Korenblat, R. M. Rothberg, P. Minden, and R. S. Farr, Immune responses of human adults after oral and parenteral exposure to bovine serum albumin, *J. Allergy, 41*:226 (1968).

9. C. W. Parker, Immune responses to environmental antigens absorbed through the gastrointestinal tract, *Fed. Proc., 36*:1732 (1977).

10. F. L. Gurskay and R. E. Cooke, The gastrointestinal absorption of unaltered protein in normal infants recovering from diarrhea, *Paediatrics, 16*:763 (1955).

11. W. A. Hemmings and E. W. Williams, Transport of large breakdown products of dietary protein through the gut wall, *Gut, 19*:715 (1978).

12. B. Morris and R. Morris, Quantitative assessment of the transmission of labelled protein by the proximal and distal regions of the small intestine of young rats, *J. Physiol. (London), 255*:619 (1976).

13. W. A. Hemmings, The transmission of high molecular weight breakdown products of protein across the gut of suckling and adult rats. In *Antigen Absorption by the Gut* (W. A. Hemmings, ed.), MTP Press Ltd., Lancaster, England, 1978, p. 37.

14. F. W. R. Brambell, The transmission of passive immunity from mother to young. In *Frontiers of Biology*, Vol. 18 (A. Neuberger and E. L. Tatam,

eds.), North Holland Publishing, Amsterdam, 1970.

15. I. G. Morris, The receptor hypothesis of protein ingestion, In *Antigen Absorption by the Gut* (W. A. Hemmings, ed.), MTP Press, Lancaster, England, 1978, p. 3.

16. W. A. Walker and K. J. Isselbacher, Uptake and transport of macromolecular by the intestine. Possible role in clinical disorders, *Gastroenterology, 67*:531 (1974).

17. D. E. Bockman and M. D. Cooper, Pinocytosis by epithelium associated with lymphoid follicles in the bursa of Fabricius, appendix and Peyer's patches. An electron mincroscopic study, *Am. J. Anat., 135*:455 (1973).

18. D. E. Bockman and M. D. Cooper, Early lymphoepithelial relationships in human appendix. A combined light and electronmicroscopic study, *Gastroenterology, 68*:1160 (1975).

19. R. L. Owen and A. L. Jones, Scanning electron microscopic evaluation of Peyer's patches in rats and humans, *Anat. Rec., 175*:404 (1973).

20. R. L. Owen and A. L. Jones, Epithelial cell specialisation within human Peyer's patches: An ultrastructural study of intestinal lymphoid follicles, *Gastroenterology, 66*:189 (1974).

21. J. F. Heremans, *The Secretory Immunologic System*, National Institute of Child Health and Human Development, Bethesda, Maryland, 1969, p. 309.

22. T. B. Tomasi and H. M. Grey, Structure and function of immunoglobulin A, *Progr. Allergy, 16*:81 (1972).

23. W. A. Walker, K. J. Isselbacher, and K. J. Bloch, The role of immunization in controlling antigen uptake from the small intestine, *Adv. Exp. Med. Biol., 45*:295 (1974).

24. C. André, R. Lambert, H. Bazin, and J. F. Heremans, Interference of oral immunization with the intestinal absorption of heterologous albumin, *Eur. J. Immunol., 4*:701 (1974).

25. W. A. Walker, M. Wu, K. J. Isselbacher, and K. J. Bloch, Intestinal uptake of macromolecules. III. Studies on the mechanism by which immunization interferes with antigen uptake, *J. Immunol., 115*:854 (1975).

26. C. R. Stokes, J. F. Soothill, and M. W. Turner, Immune exclusion is a function of IgA, *Nature, 255*:745 (1975).

27. R. M. Buckley and S. C. Dees, Correlation of milk precipitins with IgA deficiency, *N. Engl. J. Med., 281*:465 (1969).

28. T. B. Tomasi and L. Katz, Human antibodies against bovine immunoglobulin M in IgA deficient sera, *Clin. Exp. Immunol., 9*:3 (1971).

29. A. Ferguson and D. M. V. Parrott, The effects of antigen deprivation on thymus-dependent and thymus-independent lymphocytes in the small intestine of the mouse, *Clin. Exp. Immunol., 12*:477 (1972).

30. D. M. V. Parrott and A. Ferguson, Selective migration of lymphocytes within the mouse small intestine, *Immunology, 26*:571 (1974).

31. D. Guy-Grand, C. Griscelli, and P. Vassalli, The gut associated lymphoid system: Nature and properties of the large dividing cells, *Eur. J. Immunol., 4*:435 (1974).

32. M. N. Marsh, Studies of intestinal lymphoid tissue. I. Electron microscopic

evidence of "blast transformation" in epithelial lymphocytes of mouse small intestinal mucosa, *Gut, 16*:665 (1975).

33. M. N. Marsh, Studies of intestinal lymphoid tissue. II. Aspects of proliferation and migration of epithelial lymphocytes in the small intestine of mice, *Gut, 16*:674 (1975).

34. R. L. Owen and P. Nemanic, Antigen processing structures of the mammalian intestinal tract: An SEM study of lymphoepithelial organs, *Scanning Electron Microscopy, II*:367 (1978).

35. H. Ginsberg and L. Sachs, Formation of pure suspensions of mast cells in tissue culture by differentiation lymphoid cells from the mouse thymus, *J. Natl. Cancer Inst. 31*:1 (1963).

36. T. Ishizaka, H. Okudaira, L. E. Mauser, and K. Ishizaka, Development of rat mast cells in-vitro. I. Differentiation of mast cells from thymus cells, *J. Immunol., 116*:747 (1976).

37. P. A. Crabbé and J. F. Heremans, The distribution of immunoglobulin-containing cells along the human gastrointestinal tract, *Gastroenterology, 51*:305 (1966).

38. P. Brandtzaeg, Structure, synthesis and external transfer of mucosal immunoglobulins, *Ann. Immunol. (Inst. Pasteur), 124C*:417 (1973).

39. B. H. Waksman and H. Ozer, Specialized amplification elements in the immune system. The role of nodular lymphoid organs in the mucous membranes, *Prog. Allergy, 21*:1 (1976).

40. A. F. Williams and J. L. Gowans, The presence of IgA on the surface of rat thoracic duct lymphocytes which contain internal IgA, *J. Exp. Med., 141*:335 (1975).

41. D. Guy-Grand, C. Griscelli, and P. Vassalli, Peyer's patches, gut IgA plasma cells and thymic function: Study in nude mice bearing thymic grants, *J. Immunol., 115*:361 (1975).

42. P. A. Crabbé, H. Bazin, H. Eyssen, and J. F. Heremans, The normal microbial flora as a major stimulus for proliferation of plasma cells synthesizing IgA in the gut. The germ free intestinal tract, *Int. Arch. Allergy Appl. Immunol., 34*:362 (1968).

43. G. J. Thorbecke, T. J. Romans, and S. L. Lerman, Regulatory mechanisms in proliferation and differentiation of lymphoid tissue, with particular reference to germinal centre development. In *Progress in Immunology II*, Vol. 3 (L. Brent and E. J. Holbobrow, eds.), North Holland, Amsterdam, 1974, p. 25.

44. J. D. Clough, L. H. Mims, and W. Strober, Deficient IgA antibody responses to arsanilic acid bovine serum albumin in neonatally thymectomised rabbits, *J. Immunol., 106*:1624 (1971).

45. W. B. van Muiswinkel and P. L. van Soest, Thymus dependence of the IgA response to sheep erythrocytes, *Immunology, 28*:287 (1975).

46. A. Ferguson and T. T. MacDonald, Effects of local delayed hypersensitivity on the small intestine, in *Immunology of the Gut*, Ciba Foundation

Symposium 46, new series (R. Porter and J. Knight, eds.), Elsevier/Excerpta Medica/North Holland, Amsterdam, 1977, p. 305.

47. A. Ferguson, Delayed hypersensitivity reactions in the small intestine. In *Antigen Absorption by the Gut* (W. A. Hemmings, ed.); MTP Press Ltd., Lancaster, England, 1978, p. 145.

48. J. Dolezel and J. Bienenstock, Immune response of the hamster to oral and parenteral immunization, *Cell. Immunol., 2*:326 (1971).

49. R. L. Hunter, Antigen trapping in the lamina propria and production of IgA antibody, *J. Reticuloendothelial. Soc., 11*:245 (1972).

50. P. B. Carter and F. M. Collins, The route of enteric infection in normal mice, *J. Exp. Med., 138*:1189 (1974).

51. J. R. Battisto and J. Miller, Immunological unresponsiveness produced in adult guinea pigs by parenteral introductions of minute quantities of hapten or protein antigen, *Proc. Soc. Exp. Biol. Med., 111*:111 (1962).

52. H. M. Cantor and A. E. Dumont, Hepatic suppression of sensitisation to antigen absorbed into the portal system, *Nature, 215*:744 (1967).

53. D. R. Trigor, M. H. Cynamon, and R. Wright, Studies on hepatic uptake of antigen. I. Comparison of inferior vena cava and portel vein routes of immunization, *Immunology, 25*:941 (1973).

54. P. B. Carter and F. M. Collins, Peyer's patches responsiveness to Salmonella in mice, *J. Reticuloendoethel. Soc., 17*:38 (1975).

55. J. W. Muller-Schoop and A. R. Good, Functional studies of Peyer's patches: Evidence for their participation in intestinal immune responses, *J. Immunol., 114*:1757 (1975).

56. M. F. Kagnoff, Functional characteristics of Peyer's patch cells. III. Carrier priming of T cells by antigen feeding, *J. Exp. Med., 142*:1525 (1975).

57. M. F. Kagnoff, Functional characteristics of Peyer's patch lymphoid cells. IV. Effect of antigen feeding on the frequency of antigen-specific B cells, *J. Immunol., 118*:992 (1977).

58. M. K. Wansbrough-Jones, W. J. Doe, and M. B. Pepys, Antigen-binding cells in rabbit Peyer's patches after intestinal immunisation, *Gut, 17s*:400 (1976).

59. S. W. Craig and J. J. Cebra, Peyer's patches: an enriched source of precursors for IgA-producing immunocytes in the rabbit, *J. Exp. Med., 134*: 188 (1971).

60. S. W. Craig and J. J. Cebra, Rabbit Peyer's patches, appendix and popliteal lymph node B lymphocytes: A comparative analysis of their membrane immunoglobulin components and plasma cell precursor potential, *J. Immunol., 114*:492 (1975).

61. J. J. Cebra, R. Kamat, P. Gearhart, S. M. Robertson, and J. Tseng, The secretory IgA system of the gut. In *Immunology of the Gut*, Ciba Foundation Symposium 46, new series (R. Porter and J. Knight, eds.), Elsevier/Excerpta Medica/North Holland, Amsterdam, 1977, p. 5.

62. A. J. Husband, H. J. Monie, and J. L. Gowans. The natural history of the cells producing IgA in the gut. In *Immunology of the Gut*, Ciba Foundation

Symposium 46, new series (R. Porter and J. Knight, eds.) Elsevier/Excerpta Medica/North Holland, Amsterdam, 1977, p. 29.

63. A. J. Husband and J. L. Gowans, The origin and antigen-dependent distribution of IgA-containing cells in the intestine, *J. Exp. Med., 148*:1146 (1978).

64. T. A. Waldmann, S. Broder, R. Krakaver, M. Durm, B. Meade, and C. Goldman, Defect in IgA secretion and in IgA specific suppressor cells in patients with selective IgA deficiency, *Trans. Assoc. Am. Physicians, 89*:215 (1976).

65. C. O. Elson, J. A. Heck, and W. Strober, T-cell regulation of murine IgA synthesis, *J. Exp. Med., 149*:632 (1979).

66. J. L. Gowans and E. J. Knight, The route of recirculation of lymphocytes in the rat, *Proc. R. Soc. Lond. [Biol.], 159*:257 (1964).

67. M. S. C. Birbeck and J. G. Hall, Transformation, in vivo, of basophilic lymph cells into plasma cells. *Nature, 214*:183 (1967).

68. M. McWilliams, J. M. Phillips-Quagliata, and M. E. Lamm, Characteristics of mesenteric lymph node cells homing to gut-associated lymphoid tissue in syngeneic mice, *J. Immunol., 115*:54 (1975).

69. M. McWilliams, M. E. Lamm, and J. M. Phillips-Quagliata, Surface and intracellular markers of mouse mesenteric and peripheral lymph node and Peyer's patch cells, *J. Immunol., 113*:1326 (1974).

70. A. R. Moore and J. G. Hall, Evidence for a primary association between lymphocytes and the small gut, *Nature, 239*:161 (1972).

71. T. E. Halstead and J. G. Hall, The homing of lymph-borne immunoblasts to the small gut of neonatal rats, *Transplantation, 14*:339 (1972).

72. J. G. Hall, J. Hopkins, and E. Orlans, Studies on the lymphocytes of sheep III. Destination of lymph-borne immunoblasts in relation to their tissue of origin, *Eur. J. Immunol., 7*:30 (1977).

73. N. F. Pierce and J. L. Gowans, Cellular kinetics of the intestinal immune response to cholera toxoid in rats, *J. Exp. Med., 142*:1550 (1975).

74. G. Mayrhofer and R. Fisher, IgA-containing plasma cells in the lamina propria of the gut: Failure of a thoracic duct fistula to deplete the numbers in the rat small intestine, *Eur. J. Immunol., 9*:85 (1979).

75. P. L. Ogra and D. T. Karzon, Distribution of poliovirus antibodies in serum, nasopharynx and alimentary tract following segmental immunization of lower alimentary tract with poliovacine, *J. Immunol., 102*:1423 (1969).

76. R. Rundzik, R. L. Clancy, D. Y. E. Percy, R. P. Day, and J. Bienenstock, Repopulation with IgA containing cells of bronchial and intestinal lamina propria after transfer of homologous Peyer's patch and bronchial lymphocytes, *J. Immunol., 114*:1599 (1975).

77. S. Ahlstedt, B. Carlsson, S. P. Fallstrom, L. A. Hanson, J. Holmgren, G. Lidin-Janson, B. S. Lindblad, U. Jodal, B. Kaijser, A. Sohl-Åkerlund, and C. Wadsworth, Antibodies in human serum and milk induced enterobacteria and food proteins. In *Immunology of the Gut*, Ciba Foundation Symposium 46, new series (R. Porter and J. Knight, eds.), Elsevier/Excerpta Medica/North Holland, Amsterdam, 1977, p. 115.

78. J. Sprent, Fate of H_2-activated T lymphocytes in syngeneic hosts, *Cell. Immunol., 21*:278 (1976).

79. M. L. Rose, D. M. V. Parrott, and R. G. Bruce, Migration of lymphoblasts to the small intestine. I. Effect of *Trichinella spiralis* infection on the migration of mesenteric lymphoblasts and mesenteric T lymphoblasts in syngeneic mice. *Immunology, 31*:723 (1976).

80. J. Hopkins and J. G. Hall, Selective entry of immunoblasts into gut from intestin allymph, *Nature, 259*:208 (1976).

81. M. L. Rose, D. M. V. Parrot, and R. G. Bruce, Migration of lymphoblasts to the small intestine. II. Divergent migration of mesenteric and peripheral immunoblasts to sites of inflammation in the mouse, *Cell. Immunol., 27*: 36 (1976).

82. R. G. Scollay, J. Hopkins, and J. G. Hall, Possible role of surface Ig in non-random recirculation of small lymphocytes, *Nature, 260*:528 (1976).

83. H. G. Wells and T. B. Osborne, The biological reactions of the vegetable proteins, I. Anaphylaxis, *J. Infect. Dis., 8*:66 (1911).

84. P. A. Crabbé, A. O. Carbonara, and J. F. Heremans, The normal human intestinal mucosa as a major source of plasma containing γ_A-immuno-globulin, *Lab. Invest., 14*:235 (1965).

85. J. F. Heremans, Immunoglobulin A. In *The Antigens*, Vol. 2, (M. Sela, ed.), Academic, New York, 1974, p. 365.

86. P. Brandtzaeg and K. Baklien, Intestinal secretion of IgA and IgM: A hypothetical model. In *Immunology of the Gut*, Ciba Foundation Symposium 46, new series (R. Porter and J. Knight, eds.), Elsevier/Excerpta Medica/North Holland, Amsterdam, 1977, p. 77.

87. W. R. Brown, B. K. Borthistle, and S. T. Chen, Immunoglobulin E (IgE) and IgE-containing cells in human gastrointestinal fluids and tissues, *Clin. Exp. Immunol., 20*:227 (1975).

88. W. R. Brown and E. A. Lee, Studies on IgE in human intestinal fluids, *Int. Arch. Allergy Appl. Immunol., 50*:87 (1976).

89. W. D. Allen, C. G. Smith, and P. Porter, Localization of intracellular immunoglobulin A in porcine intestinal mucosa using enzyme-labeled antibody, *Immunology, 25*:55 (1973).

90. J. P. Vaerman, C. Andre, H. Bazin, and J. F. Heremans, Mesenteric lymph as a major source of serum IgA in guinea pigs and rats, *Eur. J. Immunol., 3*:580 (1973).

91. I. LeMaitre-Coelho, G. D. F. Jackson, and Vaerman, Rat bile as a convenient source of secretory IgA and free secretory component, *Eur. J. Immunol., 8*:588 (1977).

92. E. Orlans, J. Peppard, J. Reynolds, and J. Hall, Rapid active transport of immunoglobulin A from blood to bile, *J. Exp. Med., 147*:588 (1978).

93. P. L. Ogra, D. T. Karzon, F. Righthand, and M. MacGillivray, Immunoglobulin response in serum and secretions after immunization with live and inactivated poliovaccine and natural infection, *N. Engl. J. Med., 279*: 89 (1968).

94. W. Burrows, J. Kaur, and L. Cercavski, Discussion: The cholera entero-toxin and local immunity, *Ann. N.Y. Acad. Sci., 176*:323 (1971).

95. R. W. Newcomb, K. Ishizaka, and B. C. De Vald, Human IgG and IgA diphtheria antitoxins in serum, nasal fluids and saliva, *J. Immunol., 103*: 215 (1969).

96. R. C. Williams and R. J. Gibbons, Inhibition of bacterial adherence by secretory immunoglobulin A: A mechanism of antigen disposal, *Science, 177*:697 (1972).

97. R. Freter, Mechanism of action of intestinal antibody in experimental cholera. II. Antibody–mediated antibacterial reaction at the mucosal surface, *Infect. Immun. 2*:556 (1970).

98. S. G. O. Johansson, H. Bennich, and T. Berg, The clinical significance of IgE, *Prog. Clin. Immunol., 1*:157 (1972).

99. B. M. Ogilvie and D. M. V. Parrott, The immunological consequences of nematode infection. In *Immunology of the Gut*, Ciba Foundation Symposium 46, new series. (R. Porter and J. Knight, eds.), Elsevier/Excerpta Medica/North Holland, Amsterdam, 1977, p. 183.

100. M. W. Chase, Inhibition of experimental drug allergy by prior feeding of the sensitising agent, *Proc. Soc. Exp. Biol. Med., 61*:257 (1946).

101. C. André, H. Bazin, and J. F. Heremans, Influence of repeated administration of antigen by the oral route on specific antibody-producing cells in the mouse spleen, *Digestion, 9*:166 (1973).

102. H. C. Thomas and D. M. V. Parrott, The induction of tolerance to soluble protein antigen by oral administration, *Immunology, 27*:631 (1974).

103. M. F. David, Prevention of homocytotropic antibody formation and anaphylaxis in rats by prefeeding antigen, *J. Allergy Clin. Immunol., 55*: 135 (1975).

104. J. Quetsch, V. K. Zirkovich, and H. B. Richerson, Tolerogenesis following antigen inhalation and feeding in the mature guinea pig, *Ann. Allergy, 38*: 386 (1977).

105. N. M. Vaz, L. C. S. Maia, D. G. Hanson, and J. M. Lynch, Inhibition of homocytrotropic antibody responses in adult inbred mice by previous feeding of the specific antigen, *J. Allergy Clin. Immunol., 60*:110 (1977).

106. G. L. Asherson, M. Zembala, M. C. C. C. Perera, B. Mayhew, and W. R. Thomas, Production of immunity and unresponsiveness in the mouse by feeding contact sensitising agents and the role of suppressor cells in the Peyer's patches, mesenteric lymph nodes and other lymphoid tissues, *Cell. Immunol., 33*:145 (1977).

107. C. André, J. F. Heremans, J. P. Vaerman, and C. L. Cambiaso, A mechanism for the induction of immunological tolerance by antigen feeding: Antigen-antibody complexes, *J. Exp. Med., 142*:1509 (1975).

108. J. Ngan and L. S. Kind, Suppressor T cells for IgE and IgG in Peyer's patches of mice made tolerant by oral administration of ovalbumin, *J. Immunol., 120*:861 (1978).

109. L. K. Richman, J. M. Chiller, W. R. Brown, D. G. Hanson, and N. M. Vaz, Cellular mechanisms in immunologic tolerance induced by enterically administered soluble protein, *Gastroenterology, 74*:1084 (1978).

110. W. R. Brown and E. Lee, Radioimmunologic measurements of naturally occurring bacterial antibodies. I. Human serum antibodies reactive with *Escherichia coli* in gastrointestinal and immunologic disorders, *J. Lab. Clin. Med., 82*:125 (1973).

110. W. R. Brown and E. Lee, Radioimmunological measurements of bacterial antibodies. II. Human serum antibodies reactive with *Bacteroides fragilis* and *Enterococcus* in gastrointestinal and immunological disorders, *Gastroenterology, 66*:1145 (1974).

112. R. A. Bicks, M. M. Azar, E. Rosenberg, W. G. Dunham, and J. Luther, Delayed hypersensitivity reactions in the intestinal tract. I. Studies of 2,4-dinitrochlorobenzene-caused guinea pig and swine colon lesions, *Gastroenterology, 53*:422 (1967).

113. R. O. Bicks, M. M. Azar, and E. W. Rosenberg, Delayed hypersensitivity reactions in the intestinal tract. II. Small intestinal lesions associated with xylose malabsorption, *Gastroenterology, 53*:437 (1967).

114. A. Ferguson and E. E. E. Jarrett, Hypersensitivity reactions in the small intestine. I. Thymus dependence of experimental "partial villous atrophy," *Gut, 16*:114 (1975).

115. W. R. Brown, D. Butterfield, D. Savage, and T. Tada, Clinical, microbiological and immunological studies in patients with immunoglobulin deficiencies and gastrointestinal disorders, *Gut, 13*:441 (1972).

116. P. E. Hermans and K. A. Huizenga, Association of gastric carcinoma with idiopathic late-onset immunoglobulin deficiency, *Ann. Intern. Med., 76*: 605 (1972).

117. C. C. Booth, T. J. Peters, and W. F. Doe, Immunopathology of coeliac disease. In *Immunology of the Gut*, Ciba Foundation Symposium 46, new series (R. Porter and J. Knight, eds.), Elsevier/Excerpta Medica/ North Holland, Amsterdam, 1977, p. 329.

118. I. Chanarin, The stomach in allergic diseases. In *Clinical Aspects of Immunology*, (P. G. H. Gell, R. R. A. Coombs, and P. J. Lachmann, eds.), Blackwell Scientific, Oxford, 1975, p. 1429.

119. T. A. Waldman, R. D. Wochner, L. Laster, and R. S. Gordon, Allergic gastroenteropathy, *N. Engl. J. Med., 276*:761 (1967).

120. D. M. Bull and T. F. Ignaczak, Enterobacterial common antigen-induced lymphocyte reactivity in inflammatory bowel disease, *Gastroenterology, 64*:43 (1973).

121. W. Bartnik, E. T. Swarbrick, and C. B. Williams, A study of peripheral leucocyte migration in agarose medium in inflammatory bowel disease, *Gut, 15*:294 (1974).

122. T. Matsumura, Studies on bacterial cross allergic reaction on the basis of natural sensitisation by intestinal flora, *Gunma J. Med. Sci., xi*:4 (1962).

123. M. Seligmann, Immunobiology and pathogenesis of alpha chain disease. In *Immunology of the Gut*, Ciba Foundation Symposium 46, new series (R. Porter and J. Knight, eds.), Elsevier/Excerpta Medica/North Holland, Amsterdam, 1977, p. 263.

124. O. N. Manousos, J. C. Economidou, D. E. Georgiadou, K. G. Pratsika-Ougourloglou, S. J. Hadziyannis, G. E. Merikas, K. Henry, and W. F. Doe, Alpha-chain disease with clinical, immunological, and histological recovery, *Br. Med. J., 2*:409 (1974).

125. J. Pepys, Atopy. In *Clinical Aspects of Immunology* (P. G. N. Gell, R. R. A. Coombs, and P. J. Lachmann, eds.), Blackwell Scientific, Oxford, 1975, p. 877

126. J. F. Soothill, C. R. Stokes, M. W. Turner, A. P. Norman, and B. Taylor, Predisposing factors and the development of reaginic allergy in infancy, *Clin. Allergy, 6*:305 (1976).

127. S. Leskowitz, J. E. Salvaggio, and H. E. Schwartz, An hypothesis for the development of atopic allergy in man, *Clin. Allergy, 2*:237 (1972).

7

Basic Rotavirus Virology in Humans

Ian H. Holmes University of Melbourne,
Parkville, Victoria, Australia

On the bases of morphology, chemical composition, and mode of replication, rotaviruses are classified with reoviruses and orbiviruses among the animal virus genera within the family Reoviridae [48]. Rotaviruses generally cause diarrheal disease (enteritis) in infant animals or humans, and asymptomatic or very mild infections in older hosts are also believed to be very common. Rotaviruses have been found infecting a very wide range of animals, and even birds [24,26,38, 41]. Antibodies to rotavirus are so widespread that no isolated human population has ever been found free of them, and one must watch out for their unadvertised presence in commercial antisera, e.g., antiimmunoglobulin sera [26, 41].

Although they grow extremely well in their natural habitat, the intestinal tract, rotaviruses have been very difficult to adapt to cell culture [24,26,38, 88]. This is apparently because they have a high degree of specificity for mature (i.e., differentiated) enterocytes, but infectivity for continuous lines of bovine or monkey kidney cells is enhanced by treatment of the virus inoculum with trypsin [2,5,46,69]. The incorporation of low levels of trypsin in the cell culture medium improves the growth and plaquing ability of even the previously adapted bovine and simian rotaviruses (R. Scherrer, personal communication; S. Sonza, personal communication), and was essential for the cell culture adaptation of avian, porcine, and human strains [41,69,87].

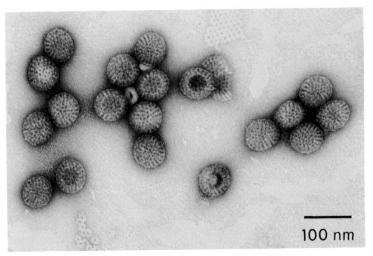

Figure 1 Complete (double-shelled) particles of human rotavirus, negatively stained with potassium phosphotungstate. (Courtesy of J. Esparza and F. Gil, IVIC, Caracas.)

Rotaviruses of calves and piglets are recognized as an important cause of economic loss, and even in the developed countries infections of young children are often serious and can be fatal [15,52]. There are not yet any accurate estimates of morbidity or mortality due to human rotaviruses in the Third World, but the World Health Organization has recognized diarrheal disease as a major public health problem, and wherever surveys have been carried out, the prevalence of rotavirus infections has been considerable [18,24,26,27,32,86,90]. Thus the impetus behind the basic studies to be described is the need for a better understanding of the antigenic variation and growth of rotaviruses, since control has not been achieved by improvements in hygiene and the only hope for prevention seems to be in vaccine development.

Morphology and Morphogenesis

Complete rotavirus particles have a sharply defined circular outline and consist of an outer and an inner capsid surrounding a central core containing the nucleic acid. Whereas the inner capsids of reoviruses are seen only when intact particles have been heat shocked or treated with chymotrypsin, most rotavirus preparations contain a proportion of single-shelled particles [24,26]. The diameter of the central core is about 40 nm, that of the inner capsid is 60 nm, and the outer capsid measures about 70 nm [24,26]. Both single- and double-shelled particles have an obvious subunit structure when negatively stained (Fig. 1), but no agreement has been reached on the number of subunits in the icosahedral shell [16, 45,68].

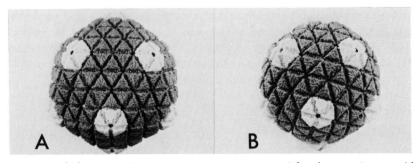

Figure 2 (A) Model of the T = 16 structure proposed for the rotavirus capsid by Esparza and Gil [16], viewed down a threefold axis of symmetry. The model contains 60 "penton" trimers and 260 "hexon" trimers. (B) Model of the T = 13 structure of the rotavirus inner capsid proposed by Roseto et al. [60]. It contains 60 "penton" trimers but only 200 "hexon" trimers. Note that neither structure can be defined in terms of nonoverlapping hexons.

Esparza and Gil [16] illustrated not only particles but also tubules and planar lattices produced by disintegrating virions which show very clearly the trimeric subunits making up the inner capsid shell. Their model had a triangulation number (T) of 16 and consisted of 320 trimers, of which 60 are grouped around the areas of five-fold symmetry (Fig. 2A). More recently, however, undisputable single-sided images of freeze-dried rotavirus particles have been obtaned and it seems more probable that the inner capsid has a skewed, T = 13 lattice [60]. The corresponding model is shown in Fig. 2B; it consists of a total of 260 trimers, i.e., 200 instead of 260 in addition to the 60 around five-fold axes. Neither of these models can be described in terms of nonoverlapping hexon capsomers. In the freeze-dried preparations, symmetrically arranged small holes could be seen in the outer capsid, and it is assumed that these coincide with the more pronounced hollows in the surface of the inner capsid [60].

In thin sections of infected cells rotavirus particles have an electron-dense core 33-35 nm in diameter, then a moderately dense capsid layer to a diameter of 60-70 nm. Virus particles first appear in and around finely granular cytoplasmic areas of "viroplasm," then appear to bud into cisternae of rough endoplasmic reticulum. Later in infection, the main feature of infected cells is the presence of large numbers of virus particles, about 10% retaining a membrane "envelope" but the rest without, in distended cisternae of the endoplasmic reticulum [1,29,43,61]. Masses of convoluted smooth membrane are often situated near the areas where particles enter the cisternae [29,61], and tubules 50-70 nm in diameter are sometimes seen in the cytoplasm or even in the nuclei of infected cells [3,38,61]. On the whole the morphogenesis of rotaviruses and that of orbiviruses appear very similar [54].

Surprisingly, in view of the amount of interest in cell culture propagation of rotaviruses, only one study comparing the morphogenesis of nonadapted rotaviruses in cell cultures with their development in vivo has appeared. McNulty et al. [42] found that during a single passage of nonadapted pig and lamb rotavirus in PK-15 cells, large numbers of particles lacking the normal electron-dense core were produced. The observations await a biochemical follow-up.

Physicochemical Properties

It is now generally agreed that the rotavirus genome consists of 11 segments of double-stranded (ds) RNA [4,17,33,35,55,57,58,62,73,74,75,79]. The pattern of bands seen after gel electrophoresis of the dsRNA varies in detail from strain to strain but is characteristic of all rotaviruses studied (Fig. 3A) and readily distinguishable from the patterns produced by other genera of the Reoviridae. The segments range in molecular weight from about 0.2 to 2.2×10^6 daltons, and the total is $10\text{-}12 \times 10^6$ daltons [4,24,74,75,79].

Estimates of the number and molecular weights of rotavirus polypeptides have been even more varied. There are obvious strain differences, but as in the case of the RNA, there is a clearly recognizable pattern in the bands obtained following electrophoresis in polyacrylamide gels in the presence of sodium lauryl sulfate. The inner capsid is composed of five polypeptides with molecular weights approximately 130, 93, 88, and 42×10^3 daltons, while the outer shell contains three or four of molecular weights 60, 36, and 25×10^3 daltons, and there are probably three nonstructural polypeptides found only in infected cells with molecular weights, 33, 31, and about 17×10^3 daltons [64,70]. In Fig. 3 a typical gel pattern of the polypeptides of the simian rotavirus SA-11 is shown, and the genome coding assignments recently established by Smith et al. [64] are indicated by dotted lines. The polypeptide nomenclature given is that of Thouless [70] as modified by Smith et al. [64], where I indicates an inner capsid polypeptide, O an outer capsid, and NS a nonstructural polypeptide. The polypeptide O_2 (VP-7 of Matsuno and Mukoyama [47] is glycosylated [13,47, 59], and possible one or other of $O_{3/4}$ is also (I. Lazdins, personal communication). Possible due to a strain difference, two distinct bands in the O_2 region are evident in a French strain of bovine rotavirus [13]. Since Fig. 3 was prepared, R. Espejo (personal communication) has shown that O_1 arises by cleavage of I_4 and the segment 5 product may thus be nonstructural.

Cohen et al. [13] have shown that the outer capsid of bovine rotavirus is stabilized by Ca^{2+} ions, and that treatment of complete virions with chelating agents such as ethylenediaminetetraacetic acid (EDTA) or the more specific ethyleneglycolbis(β-aminoethyl ether) – N,N'-tetraacetic acid (EGTA) results in solubilization of the outer shell polypeptides and activation of RNA-dependent RNA polymerase in the single-shelled particles. The single-stranded messenger

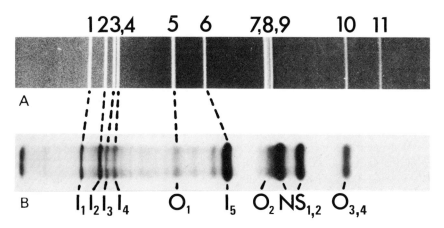

Figure 3 (A) Segments of the genome dsRNA of simian rotavirus (SA-11) separated by electrophoresis in a polyacrylamide gel with discontinuous buffer system, as described by Rodger et al. [57]. The origin of the gel is at the left. (B) Fluorograph showing ^{35}S-labeled polypeptides from an SA-11-infected cell culture, separated by disk electrophoresis in the presence of sodium lauryl sulfate according to Smith et al. The origin is at the left. I denotes a polypeptide of the inner capsid, O means outer capsid, and NS means nonstructural. The cell protein actin (MW 42,000 daltons) is visible just to the left of I_5. The coding assignments by Smith et al. [64] are indicated by dotted lines.

RNA produced in vitro will hybridize with genome dsRNA and is capable of directing synthesis of rotavirus polypeptides in a cell-free translation system [12]. These observations have been confirmed with other rotaviruses, including SA-11 and human strains (S. Rodger, J. Breschkin, and M. Smith, personal communication).

Complete rotavirions have a buoyant density of 1.36 g/cm^3 in cesium chloride (CsCl) and are the infectious form, whereas single-shelled particles band at a density of 1.38 g/cm^3 and appear to be noninfectious [24,26].

Bovine rotavirus has been reported to be slowly inactivated when heated at 60°C, but infectivity was retained for several months at room temperature [84]. Infectivity was not stabilized by molar MgCl$_2$ at 50°C, in contrast to reovirus [81]. Bovine rotavirus is stable at pH 3, but the simian rotavirus SA-11 is unstable below pH 4 [20,44,56,81]. Rotaviruses are stable to ether but readily inactivated by alcohols (R. Schnagl and J. Basthardo, personal communication). The most effective disinfectants for inactivation of rotaviruses appear to be phenolics and iodine-based compounds (R. Schnagl, personal communication) [65,83].

Various procedures have been described for purification of rotaviruses [8, 10,11,58,74]. Needless to say, the use of chelating agents in buffers must be avoided if the aim is intact rotavirus particles. Even so, procedures which yield mainly double-shelled particles of SA-11 virus from cell culture harvests produce mainly single-shelled particles of bovine rotavirus. Recently it has been found that addition of 10 mM $CaCl_2$ to all buffers used during extraction and purification of the Northern Ireland strain of bovine rotavirus greatly increases the yield of double-shelled particles, and other strains may also require extra calcium for stability (J. Basthardo and S. Sonza, personal communication).

Hemagglutination of human, sheep, or guinea pig erythrocytes is a property of double-shelled particles of bovine and simian rotaviruses [31,34,67]. The U.K. strain of bovine rotavirus is said not to hemagglutinate, but the problem may be simply a lack of sufficient double-shelled particles, since the Northern Ireland strain also failed to hamagglutinate until preparations were purified in the presence of added calcium (J. Basthardo, personal communication) [67].

Replication

Very little is known about the cell-surface receptors for rotaviruses, although on the basis of their high degree of specificity for differentiated enterocytes it has been suggested that lactase might be the receptor [28]. This idea has been neither substantiated nor disproven, but the suggestion that lactase was also involved in uncoating of the particles now seems very unlikely. As Cohen et al. [13] have pointed out, the low intracellular Ca^{2+} concentration would ensure uncoating of rotavirus particles as soon as they passed through the plasma membrane of a host cell and entered the cytoplasm.

As in the case of reoviruses, polymerases in the inner capsid synthesize messenger RNA when the outer capsid layer is removed and nucleoside triphosphates are available [11,30]. mRNA molecules corresponding to genome segments 5-11 are detectable in cells infected with the simian rotavirus SA-11, but the transcripts corresponding to the largest four genome segments are difficult to demonstrate (J. Breschkin, personal communication). There also appears to be a lack of these transcripts among the products of in vitro transcription of bovine rotavirus single-shelled particles [12]. It is assumed that rotavirus transcription, like that of reovirus dsRNA, is a conservative process, and that uncoating beyond the single-shelled particle stage does not occur.

At least 12 polypeptides have been detected in rotavirus-infected cells, but pulse-chase experiments have so far failed to detect any cleavage of primary gene products, such as has been found in reovirus-infected cells (M. Smith and I. Lazdins, personal communication) [6,47,70]. Resolution of this dilemma will have to await analysis of tryptic peptides of these polypeptides. The main suggestion of posttranslational processing is found in the case of polypeptide O_1, which is derived from the polypeptide previously designated I_4 by tryptic cleavage after the particle has been released from the cell (R. Espejo, personal communication). Nothing is yet known about control of transcription or translation of rotaviruses in their host cells, but the studies on intracellular proteins clearly show that some control must operate. The polypeptides I_5 and I_2 are the major products both in infected cells and in purified virions, whereas I_3, O_1, and $O_{3/4}$ are quite difficult to detect (Fig. 3B). No functions of the three nonstructural proteins have yet been discovered.

It seems probable, but has not yet been proven, that synthesis of rotavirus dsRNA occurs within precursor particles on ssRNA templates, as has been demonstrated in reovirus multiplication [53]. Rotaviruses also resemble reoviruses in that newly synthesized virions are not rapidly released from infected cells but tend to remain cell associated [19,40,82]. Growth curves for bovine, ovine, and simian rotaviruses have been published, and all have shown that progeny virions are detectable after about 6 h, and reach maximal titers about 18–24 h after inoculation [19,40,42,47,82].

Strains and Antigenic Properties

It has been said that the specificity of rotaviruses is directed to a particular type of cell rather than to a particular animal (or bird) species, and in support of this idea various cross-species transmissions have been documented. Piglets can be infected by bovine, equine, or simian strains as well as by those of porcine origin [25,78,84,85]. Rotaviruses of human origin have been grown in calves, piglets, monkeys, lambs, and dogs, but there does seem to be some degree of host preference and not all transmission attempts succeed [9,37,50,51,66,76, 77,89].

Rotaviruses adapted to growth in cell culture include several bovine strains, simian rotavirus SA-11, and the "O" agent which might be either bovine or ovine; more recently, with the assistance of trypsin treatment of inocula, porcine and human strains have been added to the range [2,8,39,44,49,69,87].

By immune electron microscopy, Flewett et al. [22] first obtained evidence that type-specific antigenic determinants of rotaviruses were located on the outer capsid shell, whereas the inner shell bore common antigens, and subsequent studies using other serologic techniques confirmed this [63,85]. Since infectivity and hemagglutination are both properties of double-shelled rotavirus particles, type specificity is shown by neutralization and hemagglutination-inhibition tests [21,71,72,85]. Zissis and Lambert [92] were able to distinguish two serotypes of human rotavirus by complement fixation (CF), but the main antigens reactive in CF tests are on the inner capsid shell [21,36]. Some common antigen is detectable by CF on the outer capsids of SA-11 and bovine rotavirus, but does not show up by immune electron microscopy (J. Basthardo, personal communication). Rotaviruses are completely cross-reactive when tested by immunofluorescence of infected cells [41,72].

Enzyme-linked immunosorbent assays (ELISA) can distinguish rotaviruses of different animal origins, and in the only intensively studied area, provide evidence of two serotypes of human rotavirus [7,91]. Although they are technically more difficult with human rotavirus, neutralization tests have provided evidence of three or even four serotypes [23,71].

For epidemiologic purposes, the finest discrimination between rotavirus strains is obtained by polyacrylamide gel electrophoresis of their genomes. Differences in migration of any of the 11 dsRNA segments are sufficient to distinguish between isolates [17,18,26,35,57]. Few of the differences between "electropherotypes" are likely to be significant serologically, but rotaviruses appear to breed true both in the laboratory and in the community. A recent electrophoretic study of more than 200 human rotavirus samples collected in Melbourne between 1973 and 1979 has shown that during this period there was a succession of electropherotypes present, some persisting for up to 2 years, and others appearing only briefly (S. Rodger, personal communication).

Future objectives must include the further characterization of the type-specific antigens of rotaviruses: it remains necessary to identify the polypeptides carrying these antigens and the genome segments coding for them. Electropherotyping has so far produced evidence of a multitide of varieties of rotavirus, but in future it is hoped that it will assist studies of the genetic interactions which may give rise to the variety. It seems likely that new rotavirus strains might originate by reassortment of genome segments in doubly infected cells, as has been shown to occur with reoviruses and influenza viruses [14,80]. If so, as a background for possible vaccine development, it will be necessary to establish whether such interactions give rise to antigenic shifts analogous to those affecting immunity to influenza and to see whether "new" genome segments in rotaviruses infecting humans have their origins in other animals or birds. The techniques are now available, but the size of the undertaking should not be underestimated!

References

1. W. R. Adams and L. M. Kraft, Electron microscopic study of the intestinal epithelium of mice infected with the agent of epizootic diarrhea of infant mice (EDIM virus), *Am. J. Pathol., 51*:39-44 (1967).

2. L. A. Babiuk, K. Mohammed, L. Spence, M. Fauvel, and R. Petro, Rotavirus isolation and cultivation in the presence of trypsin, *J. Clin. Microbiol., 6*:610-617 (1977).

3. W. G. Banfield, G. Kasnic, and J. H. Blackwell, Further observations on the virus of epizootic diarrhea of infant mice—an electron microscopic study, *Virology, 36*:411-421 (1968).

4. B. B. Barnett, L. N. Egbert, and R. S. Spendlove, Characteristics of neo-natal calf diarrhea virus ribonucleic acid, *Can. J. Comp. Med., 42*:46-53 (1978).

5. B. B. Barnett, R. S. Spendlove, and M. L. Clark, Effect of enzymes on rotavirus infectivity, *J. Clin. Microbiol., 10*:111-113 (1979).

6. G. W. Both, S. Lavi, and A. J. Shatkin, Synthesis of all the gene products of the reovirus genome in vivo and in vitro, *Cell, 4*:173-180 (1975).

7. C. D. Brandt, H. W. Kim, R. H. Yolken, A. Z. Kapikian, J. O. Arrobio, W. J. Rodriguez, R. J. Wyatt, R. M. Chanock, and R. H. Parrott, Comparative epidemiology of two rotavirus serotypes and other viral agents associated with pediatric gastroenteritis, *Am. J. Epidemiol., 110*:243-254 (1979).

8. J. C. Bridger and G. N. Woode, Characterization of two particle types of calf rotavirus, *J. Gen. Virol., 31*:245-250 (1976).

9. J. C. Bridger, G. M. Woode, J. M. Jones, T. H. Flewett, A. S. Bryden, and H. Davies, Transmission of human rotavirus to gnotobiotic piglets, *J. Med. Microbiol., 8*:565-569 (1975).

10. E. O. Caul, C. R. Ashley, and S. I. Egglestone, An improved method for the routine identification of faecal viruses using ammonium sulphate precipitation, *FEMS Microbiol. Lett., 4*:1-4 (1978).

11. J. Cohen, Ribonucleic acid polymerase activity associated with purified calf rotavirus, *J. Gen. Virol., 36*:395-402 (1977).

12. J. Cohen and P. Dobos, Cell free transcription and translation of rotavirus RNA, *Biochem. Biophys. Res. Commun., 88*:791-796 (1979).

13. J. Cohen, J. Laporte, A. Charpilienne, and R. Scherrer, Activation of rota-virus RNA polymerase by calcium chelation, *Arch. Virol., 60*:177-186 (1979).

14. R. K. Cross and B. N. Fields, Genetics of reoviruses. In *Comprehensive Virology*, Vol. 9 (H. Frankel-Conrat and R. R. Wagner, eds.), Plenum, New York and London, 1977, pp. 291-340.

15. G. P. Davidson, R. F. Bishop, R. R. W. Townley, I. H. Holmes, and B. J. Buck, Importance of a new virus in acute sporadic enteritis in children, *Lancet, 1*:242-245 (1975).

16. J. Esparza and F. Gil, A study on the ultrastructure of human rotavirus, *Virology, 91*:141-150 (1978).

17. R. T. Espejo, E. Calderon, and N. Gonzalez, Distinct reovirus-like agents associated with acute infantile gastroenteritis, *J. Clin. Microbiol., 6*:502-506 (1977).

18. R. T. Espejo, E. Calderon, N. Gonzalez, A. Salomon, A. Martuscelli, and P. Romero, Presence of two distinct types of rotavirus in infants and young children hospitalized with acute gastroenteritis in Mexico City, 1977, *J. Infect. Dis., 139*:474-477 (1979).

19. M. K. Estes, D. Y. Graham, C. P. Gerba, and E. M. Smith, Simian rotavirus SA 11 replication in cell cultures, *J. Virol., 31*:810-815 (1979).

20. M. K. Estes, D. Y. Graham, E. M. Smith, and C. P. Gerba, Rotavirus stability and inactivation, *J. Gen. Virol., 43*:403-409 (1979).

21. M. Fauvel, L. Spence, L. A. Babiuk, R. Petro, and S. Bloch, Hemagglutination and hemagglutination-inhibition studies with a strain of Nebraska calf diarrhea virus (bovine rotavirus), *Intervirology, 9*:95–105 (1978).

22. T. H. Flewett, A. S. Bryden, H. Davies, G. N. Woode, J. C. Bridger, and J. M. Derrick, Relation between viruses from acute gastroenteritis of children and newborn calves, *Lancet, 2*:61-63 (1974).

23. T. H. Flewett, M. E. Thouless, J. N. Pilfold, A. S. Bryden, and J. A. N. Candeias, More serotypes of human rotavirus, *Lancet, 2*:632 (1978).

24. T. H. Flewett and G. N. Woode, The rotaviruses, *Arch. Virol., 57*:1-23 (1978).

25. G. A. Hall, J. C. Bridger, R. L. Chandler, and G. N. Woode, Gnotobiotic piglets experimentally inoculated with neonatal calf diarrhea reoviruslike agent (rotavirus), *Vet. Pathol., 13*:197–210 (1976).

26. I. H. Holmes, Viral gastroenteritis, *Prog. Med. Virol., 25*:1-36 (1979).

27. I. H. Holmes, M. Mathan, P. Bhat, M. J. Albert, S. P. Swaminathan, P. P. Maiya, S. M. Pereira, and S. J. Baker, Orbiviruses and gastroenteritis, *Lancet, 2*:658-659 (1974).

28. I. H. Holmes, S. M. Rodger, R. D. Schnagl, B. J. Ruck, I. D. Gust, R. F. Bishop, and G. L. Barnes, Is lactase the receptor and uncoating enzyme for infantile enteritis (rota) viruses? *Lancet, 1*:1387-1388 (1976).

29. I. H. Holmes, B. J. Ruck, R. F. Bishop, and G. P. Davidson, Infantile enteritis viruses: Morphogenesis and morphology, *J. Virol., 16*:937-943 (1975).

30. J. F. Hruska, M. F. D. Notter, M. A. Menegus, and M. C. Steinhoff, RNA polymerase associated with human rotaviruses in diarrhea stools, *J. Virol., 26*:544-546 (1978).

31. Y. Inaba, K. Sato, E. Takahashi, H. Kurogi, K. Satoda, T. Omori, and M. Matumoto, Hemagglutination with Nebraska calf diarrhea virus, *Microbiol. Immunol., 21*:531-534 (1977).

32. E. S. Jesudoss, T. J. John, M. Mathan, and L. Spence, Prevalence of rotavirus antibody in infants and children, *Indian J. Med. Res., 68*:383-386 (1978).

33. A. R. Kalica, C. F. Garon, R. G. Wyatt, C. A. Mebus, D. H. Van Kirk, R.M. Chanock, and A. Z. Kapikian, Differentiation of human and calf reoviruslike agents associated with diarrhea using polyacrylamide gel electrophoresis of RNA, *Virology, 74*:86-92 (1976).

34. A. R. Kalica, H. D. James, Jr., and A. Z. Kapikian, Hemagglutination by simian rotavirus, *J. Clin. Microbiol., 7*:314-315 (1978).

35. A. R. Kalica, M. M. Sereno, R. G. Wyatt, C. A. Mebus, R. M. Chanock, and A. Z. Kapikian, Comparison of human and animal rotavirus strains by gel electrophoresis of viral RNA, *Virology, 87*:247-255 (1978).

36. A. Z. Kapikian, A. R. Kalica, J. W. Shih, W. L. Cline, T. S. Thornhill, R. G. Wyatt, R. M. Chanock, H. W. Kim, and J. L. Gerin, Buoyant density in cesium chloride of the human reovirus-like agent of infantile gastroenteritis by ultracentrifugation electron microscopy and complement fixation, *Virology, 70*:564-569 (1976).

37. J. S. Light and H. L. Hodes, Studies on epidemic diarrhea of the newborn: Isolation of a filtrable agent causing diarrhea in calves, *Am. J. Public Health, 33*:1451-1454 (1943).

38. M. S. McNulty, Rotaviruses, *J. Gen. Virol., 40*:1-18 (1978).

39. M. S. McNulty, G. M. Allan, and J. B. McFerran, Isolation of a cytopathic calf rotavirus, *Res. Vet. Sci., 21*:114-115 (1976).

40. M. S. McNulty, G. M. Allan, and J. B. McFerran, Cell culture studies with a cytopathic bovine rotavirus, *Arch. Virol., 54*:201-209 (1977).

41. M. S. McNulty, G. M. Allan, D. Todd, and J. B. McFerran, Isolation and cell culture propagation of rotaviruses from turkeys and chickens, *Arch. Virol., 61*:13-21 (1979).

42. M. S. McNulty, W. L. Curran, G. M. Allan, and J. B. McFerran, Synthesis of coreless, probably defective virus particles in cell cultures infected with rotaviruses, *Arch. Virol., 58*:193-202 (1978).

43. M. S. McNulty, W. L. Curran, and J. B. McFerran, The morphogenesis of a cytopathic bovine rotavirus in Madin-Darby bovine kidney cells, *J. Gen. Virol., 33*:503-508 (1976).

44. H. H. Malherbe, and M. Strickland-Cholmley, Simian virus SA11 and the related O agent, *Arch. Ges. Virusforsch, 22*:235-245 (1967).

45. M. L. Martin, E. L. Palmer, and P. J. Middleton, Ultrastructure of infantile gastroenteritis virus, *Virology, 68*:146-153 (1975).

46. S. Matsuno, S. Inouye, and R. Kono, Plaque assay of neonatal calf diarrhea virus and the neutralizing antibody in human sera, *J. Clin. Microbiol., 5*:1-4 (1977).

47. S. Matsuno and A. Mukoyama, Polypeptides of bovine rotavirus, *J. Gen. Virol., 43*:309-316 (1979).

48. R. E. F. Matthews, The classification and nomenclature of viruses, *Intervirology, 11*:133-135 (1979).

49. C. A. Mebus, M. Kono, N. R. Underdahl, and M. J. Twiehaus, Cell culture propagation of neonatal calf diarrhea (scours) virus, *Can. Vet. J., 12*:69-72 (1971).

50. C. A. Mebus, R. G. Wyatt, R. L. Sharpee, M. M. Sereno, A. R. Kalica, A. Z. Kapikian, and M. J. Twiehaus, Diarrhea in gnotobiotic calves caused by the reovirus-like agent of human infantile gastroenteritis, *Infect. Immun., 14*:471-474 (1976).

51. P. J. Middleton, M. Petric, and M. T. Szymanski, Propagation of infantile gastroenteritis virus (Orbi-group) in conventional and germfree piglets, *Infect. Immun. 12*:1276-1280 (1975).

52. P. J. Middleton, M. T. Szymanski, G. D. Abott, R. Bortolussi, and J. R. Hamilton, Orbivirus acute gastroenteritis of infancy, *Lancet, 1*:1241-1244 (1974).

53. E. M. Morgan and H. J. Zweerink, Characterization of transcriptase and replicase particles isolated from reovirus-infected cells, *Virology, 68*:455-466 (1975).

54. F. A. Murphy, E. C. Borden, R. E. Shope, and A. K. Harrison, Physico-

chemical and morphological relationships of some arthropod-borne viruses to bluetongue virus—a new taxonomic group. Electron microscopic studies, *J. Gen. Virol., 13*:273-288 (1971).

55. J. F. F. Newman, F. Brown, J. C. Bridger, and G. N. Woode, Characterization of a rotavirus, *Nature, 258*:631-633 (1975).

56. E. L. Palmer, M. L. Martin, and F. A. Murphy, Morphology and stability of infantile gastroenteritis virus: Comparison with reovirus and bluetongue virus, *J. Gen. Virol., 35*:403-414 (1977).

57. S. M. Rodger and I. H. Holmes. Comparison of the genomes of simian, bovine and human rotaviruses by gel electrophoresis and detection of genomic variation among bovine isolates, *J. Virol., 30*:839-846 (1979).

58. S. M. Rodger, R. D. Schnagl, and I. H. Holmes, Biochemical and biophysical characteristics of diarrhea viruses of human and calf origin, *J. Virol., 16*:1229-1235 (1975).

59. S. M. Rodger, R. D. Schnagl, and I. H. Holmes, Further biochemical characterization, including the detection of surface glycoproteins, of human, calf and simian rotaviruses, *J. Virol., 24*:91-98 (1977).

60. A. Roseto, J. Escaig, E. Delain, J. Cohen, and R. Scherrer, Structure of rotaviruses as studied by the freeze-drying technique, *Virology, 98*:471-475 (1979).

61. L. J. Saif, K. W. Theil, and E. H. Bohl, Morphogenesis of porcine rotavirus in porcine kidney cell cultures and intestinal epithelial cells, *J. Gen. Virol., 39*:205-217 (1978).

62. R. D. Schnagl and I. H. Holmes, Characteristics of the genome of human infantile enteritis virus (rotavirus), *J. Virol., 19*:267-270 (1976).

63. B. D. Schoub, G. Lecatsas, and D. W. Prozesky, Antigenic relationship between human and simian rotaviruses, *J. Med. Microbiol., 10*:1-6 (1977).

64. M. L. Smith, I. Lazdins, and I. H. Holmes, Coding assignments of ds RNA segments of SA 11 rotavirus established by in vitro translation. *J. Virol., 33*:976–982.

65. D. R. Snodgrass and J. A. Herring, The action of disinfectants on lamb rotavirus, *Vet. Rec., 101*:81 (1977).

66. D. R. Snodgrass, C. R. Madeley, P. W. Wells, and K. W. Angus, Human rotavirus in lambs: Infection and passive protection, *Infect. Immun., 16*: 268-270 (1977).

67. L. Spence, M. Fauvel, R. Petro, and L. A. Babiuk, Comparison of rotavirus strains by hemagglutination inhibition, *Can. J. Microbiol., 24*:353-356 (1978).

68. L. M. Stannard and B. D. Schoub, Observations on the morphology of two rotaviruses, *J. Gen. Virol., 37*:435-439 (1977).

69. K. W. Theil, E. H. Bohl, and A. G. Agnes, Cell culture propagation of porcine rotavirus (reovirus-like agent), *Am. J. Vet. Res., 38*:1765-1768 (1977).

70. M. E. Thouless, Rotavirus polypeptides, *J. Gen. Virol., 44*:187-198 (1979).

71. M. E. Thouless, A. S. Bryden, and T. H. Flewett, Serotypes of human rotavirus, *Lancet, 1*:39 (1978).
72. M. E. Thouless, A. S. Bryden, T. H. Flewett, G. N. Woode, J. C. Bridger, D. R. Snodgrass, and J. A. Herring, Serological relationships between rotaviruses from different species as studied by complement fixation and neutralization, *Arch. Virol., 53*:287-294 (1977).
73. D. Todd and M. S. McNulty, Characterization of pig rotavirus RNA, *J. Gen. Virol., 33*:147-150 (1976).
74. D. Todd and M. S. McNulty, Biochemical studies on a reovirus-like agent (rotavirus) from lambs, *Virology, 21*:1215-1218 (1977).
75. D. Todd, M. S. McNulty, and G. M. Allan, Polyacrylamide gel electrophoresis of avian rotavirus RNA, *Arch. Virol., 63*:87-98 (1980).
76. A. Torres-Medina, R. G. Wyatt, C. A. Mebus, N. R. Underdahl, and A. Z. Kapikian, Diarrhea caused in gnotobiotic piglets by the reovirus-like agent of human infantile gastroenteritis, *J. Infect. Dis., 133*:22-27 (1976).
77. S. Tzipori, Human rotaviruses in young dogs, *Med. J. Aust., 2*:922-923 (1976).
78. S. Tzipori and I. H. Williams, Diarrhea in piglets inoculated with rotavirus, *Aust. Vet. J., 54*:188-192 (1978).
79. E. Verly and J. Cohen. Demonstration of size variation of RNA segments between different isolates of calf rotavirus, *J. Gen. Virol., 35*:583-586 (1977).
80. R. G. Webster and W. G. Laver, Antigenic variation in influenza viruses. In *The Influenza Viruses and Influenza* (E. D. Kilbourne, ed.), Academic, New York, 1975, pp. 269-314.
81. A. B. Welch and T. L. Thompson, Physicochemical characterization of a neonatal calf diarrhea virus, *Can. J. Comp. Med., 37*:295-301 (1973).
82. A. B. Welch and M. J. Twiehaus, Cell culture studies of a neonatal calf diarrhea virus, *Can. J. Comp. Med., 37*:287-294 (1973).
83. G. N. Woode, Studies on viral enteritis of calves and pigs. D. Vet. Med. Thesis, University of London, 1978, pp. 41-43.
84. G. N. Woode and J. C. Bridger, Viral enteritis of calves, *Vet. Rec., 96*: 85-88 (1975).
85. G. N. Woode, J. C. Bridger, J. M. Jones, T. H. Flewett, A. S. Bryden, H. A. Davies, and G. B. B. White, Morphological and antigenic relationships between viruses (rotaviruses) from acute gastroenteritis of children, calves, piglets, mice and foals, *Infect. Immun., 14*:804-810 (1976).
86. World Health Organization, The WHO diarrheal diseases control program. *WHO Wkly. Epidemiol. Rec., 16*:121-123 (1979).
87. R. G. Wyatt, W. D. James, E. H. Bohl, K. W. Theil, L. J. Saif, A. R. Kalica, H. B. Greenberg, A. Z. Kapikian, and R. M. Chanock, Human rotavirus type 2: Cultivation in vitro, *Science, 207*:189-191 (1980).
88. R. G. Wyatt, A. R. Kalica, C. A. Mebus, H. W. Kim, W. T.London, R. M. Chanock, and A. Z. Kapikian, Reovirus-like agents (rotaviruses) associated

with diarrheal illness in animals and man. In *Perspectives in Virology*, Vol. 10 (M. Pollard, ed.), Raven, New York, 1978, pp. 121-143.

89. R. G. Wyatt, D. L. Sly, W. T. London, A. E. Palmer, A. R. Kalica, D. H. Van Kirk, R. M. Chanock, and A. Z. Kapikian, Induction of diarrhea in colostrum-deprived newborn Rhesus monkeys with the human reovirus-like agent of infantile gastroenteritis, *Arch. Virol.*, *50*:17-27 (1976).

90. R. G. Wyatt, R. H. Yolken, J. J. Urrutia, L. Mata, H. B. Greenberg, R. M. Chanock, and A. Z. Kapikian, Diarrhea associated with rotavirus in rural Guatemala: A longitudinal study of 24 infants and young children, *Am. J. Trop. Med. Hyg.*, *28*:325-328 (1979).

91. R. H. Yolken, B. Barbour, R. G. Wyatt, A. R. Kalica, A. Z. Kapikian, and R. M. Chanock, Enzyme-linked immunosorbent assay for identification of rotaviruses from different animal species, *Science, 201*: 259-262 (1978).

92. G. Zissis and J. P. Lambert, Different serotypes of human rotavirus, *Lancet, 1*:38-39 (1978).

8

Clinical Features of Rotavirus Infections

T. H. Flewett   East Birmingham Hospital,
Birmingham, England

It has sometimes in the past been the case that after a particular pathogen has been isolated and characterized, cases of infection caused by it have fallen into a pattern not previously recognized. Examples have been benign meningitis with rash associated with coxsackie virus A9 (echovirus 9), hand-foot-and-mouth disease associated mainly with coxsackie virus A16 disease, and the urethritis of kidney graft recipients associated with the BK papovavirus. Isolation of coxsackie B viruses allowed the full extent of what might be called the "expanded Bornholm disease syndrome" to become apparent. But acute infectious diarrhea is such a common disease, so familiar to all clinicians, that few clinical studies of diarrhea known to be caused by viruses have been published, in comparison with acute infective diarrhea caused by other agents. Nevertheless, some differences between virus and bacterial diarrhea have become apparent from studies published in recent years.

Age Distribution

Infections by rotaviruses have been recorded at all ages, from 2 or 3 days after birth to old age; our oldest patient was aged 94 years. Most cases of acute infectious diarrhea associated with rotaviruses have been found between the ages of

125

1 and 6 years, with a peak between 1 and 3 years [4,5,11,26,35,36,46,47,87,88, 98,99]. Konno et al. [48] published a long-term study of over 500 children between December 1974 and March 1977, admitted to the hospital with acute gastroenteritis, finding rotaviruses in 322 (64%) of them. In this series the highest incidence was in children aged between 6 and 11 months—the age when maternal antibody has just been lost and "welcome" is written on the child's tongue for any passing virus. Of the 185 children in this series, fourfold or greater rises in titer were discovered in 130 when acute-phase sera and sera taken in convalescence were compared by the complement fixation test. A very similar age distribution was observed [36] in a pediatric clinic in Brussels, when 148 children presenting with acute gastroenteritis in the course of a year were analyzed. In their series, 74% of the children were less than 2 years of age and 20 had rotavirus infections. They found only one case of diarrhea of bacterial etiology among their patients during the winter months when rotavirus infection was prevalent, but 21 cases in summer months. The average age of the children was 15 months, but in only 23% of patients less than 6 months old were rotaviruses found. (This series is of interest as it relates to children seen as outpatients, very few of whom required admission to a hospital, in a major European city; almost all the published information relates to children who had to be admitted to a hospital, a small and unknown fraction of the total of virus diarrheas of children.) Australian and British age distributions appear to be similar, at least in the big cities. Davidson et al. [26] found the greatest number (115 of 378) between the ages of 1 and 2 years, but 77 aged between 6 months and 1 year. Birch et al. [4], in a study of 400 hospitalized infants and young children, found rotaviruses in 167; the greatest numbers were between the ages of birth and 1 year, declining steadily thereafter, with very few rotavirus cases more than 5 years old. Their youngest patient was 7 days old; their eldest, 10 years. Rotaviruses were found in 31% of children under 6 months, in 50% between 6 months and 3 years, and in 12.5% of those aged 4 years or over. Australian aboriginal children appear to acquire their rotavirus infections slightly earlier in life [79]; in a comparative study of aboriginal and white children admitted to the hospital in Western Australia, rotaviruses were most commonly detected in aboriginal children less than 6 months of age, and in nonaboriginal children between 6 months and 1 year. The proportion of aboriginal patients above 1 year old excreting rotaviruses was much lower than in nonaboriginal patients.

In the city hospitals of North America the age groups attacked have been similar to Europoean and Australian experience. The first study of age distribution by Middleton et al. [63] found that most patients with rotavirus diarrhea were less than 1 year old; the proportion of patients aged 1-2 years, 2-3 years, and over 3 years diminished rapidly with increasing age. Middleton et al. also noted that the virus could infect an adult volunteer. Kapikian et al. [46] found that the mean and median ages of their rotavirus-infected patients were 17.8 and 10 months, respectively. Outbreaks in children of school age must be very rare; however, at least one has been reported [41].

Adults may also be infected, with or without symptoms, [8,9,40,44,46,47, 62,66,96,105]. As well as the volunteer case described by Middleton et al. [63], Flewett et al. [35] mentioned a man aged 20 years whose illness was severe enough for him to be admitted to the hospital. Two adult cases among parents who presumably became infected from their children have been described [66]. von Bonsdorff et al. [9] described two cases of severe acute gastroenteritis in nurses attending sick children, and later in 11 of 42 members of the hospital staff who presented with acute diarrhea. Kapikian et al. [46] also had evidence of 2 clinical and 12 subclinical infections in 14 of 40 adult contacts of sick children. Zissis et al. [105] described cases similar to those reported by Ørstavik et al. [66]. Bolivar et al. [8] have implicated rotaviruses as a cause of "traveller's diarrhea" among adult students from the United States when visiting Mexico. Holzel et al. [44] described 14 cases, aged 24 to 83 years, in an outbreak in a cardiology ward of a hospital. Outbreaks of gastroenteritis among inmates of residential homes for the aged have been investigated by Halvorsrud and Ørstavik [40] and by Flewett (unpublished). Our own oldest patient was aged 94 years. Elias [29] found that the median levels of rotavirus antibody diminished gradually in a hospital population in Birmingham as age increased. Patients whose ages exceeded 80 years possessed little or no neutralizing antibody in their sera. (This study was done using virus from a single sample of feces from one patient as the test reagent, so that it was essentially a study using one serotype of rotavirus only.)

Rotavirus Infection of Neonates

A number of authors have described outbreaks of rotavirus infection in infants a few days old in hospital nurseries [3,6,12-14,65,94]. These outbreaks differed in that they were confined to children in the first few days of life, and that the infection sometimes became endemic in the institution for up to several months. The remarkably mild clinical features will be described below. (One paper [12] referred to rotavirus infection of the placenta, but this has not been confirmed.)

Sex Ratio

Few authors have recorded the sex ratio of their patients, but all of these have noted that males were more numerous than females; Konno et al. [48] found 55% males of 506 children; Shepherd et al. [85] found 63% males among 32 confirmed rotavirus infections; Carr et al. [16] had 60 males in 100 cases, and Davidson et al. [26], 209 in 378 patients (55%). Bearing in mind the excess of male births over females, the greater general resistance of the female, and the tendency in some communities to lavish more care and attention on males than females, it does not seem likely that these figures reflect any genuine difference between the susceptibility of the two sexes. Lewis et al. [55] found no significant difference.

Mechanisms of Infection

Rotaviruses, astroviruses, coronaviruses, and parvoviruses are excreted in enormous numbers in the feces. We have ourselves counted 10^{11} particles per milliliter of feces; samples with such numbers are not uncommon, although among adult contacts [46] and breast-fed neonates [20,94] particles were considerably less plentiful. Particle counts of astroviruses and coronaviruses in feces have not been published. But on the basis of numbers of particles per grid square astroviruses must sometimes be present in numbers as great as rotaviruses, and coronaviruses, in the richest specimens, must be almost as numerous. We have counted parvoviruses in children's feces, finding the almost unbelievable figure of 10^{13} per milliliter of feces—almost unbelievable until one examines electron microscope grids on which there is an almost continuous carpet of these very small viruses. Adenoviruses in feces—when they cause diarrhea, not the adenoviruses of recognized serotypes which can be isolated—are present in enormous numbers. I do not know of anyone who has made precise counts, but comparing electron microscope grids from adenovirus cases with grids from rotavirus cases, up to 10^{10} per gram is a reasonable estimate.

Routes of Infection

Rotaviruses are known to be stable in feces, at least at room temperature in England. Samples of feces sent to Birmingham by air from various parts of the world have often (though not always) contained plenty of viable virus. The infectivity titer of a pot of feces from a calf with diarrhea, left upon the laboratory bench, remained high for a year (Woode, personal communication). It would not, therefore, be surprising if infection were readily carried upon the hands of nurses and other ward staff, or upon hospital ward hardware. If feces are spilt on the floor from a dripping napkin, or if a bedpan is contaminated, or if splashes fall in a sluice, very large numbers of viruses will be deposited even by a very small or inapparent splash, and perhaps be more widely spread as an aerosol. If good ward practice is followed, contaminated surfaces will, of course, be wiped with disinfectant. Surface disinfection which reduces infectivity by a millionfold is doing very well, but if 1000 million viruses are in the contamination, even surface disinfection may not eliminate infectivity.

The way in which coliforms from children with diarrhea can contaminate just about everything in the ward environment was described by Rogers [73] and Hutchinson [45]. Enteric viruses are probably spread around to a similar extent. The particle-infectivity ratio is not reliably known for any of the diarrhea viruses. Infectivity of over 10^6 rotavirus infective units per milliliter of patients' feces has sometimes been determined by counting fluorescent foci in LLC MK$_2$ tissue cultures inoculated by the centrifugation method described by Bryden et al. [10]. Woode found that pig feces containing rotaviruses caused a lethal infection of experimental piglets at a dilution of 10^{-7}. It is reasonable to suppose that infectivity titers in human feces for children may be at least as high. *The Lancet* [53], reviewing viral cross-infection in children's wards, quoted Dr. P. Middleton as saying that the surgical wards in Toronto were the richest source of rotavirus cross-infection. Chrystie et al. [20] and Totterdell et al. [94] had evidence that rotavirus infection in hospital nurseries was being transferred by nurses, and this is in a hospital famous for the standard of its nursing. Control of infection in the average household must be more difficult than in the hospital ward, so it is not surprising that numerous examples of rotavirus infection of adults from children have been reported [47,66,96,105]. Adult infections are often asymptomatic [47]; Kapikian et al. [46] found evidence of infection in 35% of adult contacts in their survey of diarrhea in Washington. (Inapparent infections also occur in adult cows). Although the numbers of viruses found in the feces of subclinical cases are not usually as great as in feces of cases with frank diarrhea, they are large enough to be detected by electron microscopy—at least 10^5, probably 10^6 particles per gram feces, or even more. A mother who does not know she is infected will take less care than one who knows she is.

Can viruses be spread by aerosols? These are no doubt formed in the disposal of feces, when the lavatory is flushed, or in many hospital sluices of the more old-fashioned kind, which remain in many parts of the world, including Great Britain. Dust from dried feces is likely to remain infectious. Mouse rotavirus infection was found to spread from a cage of infected mice to a control cage on the other side of the room unless an air filter barrier was interposed [50,74].

Aerosols and dust might cause infection (1) by contaminating food; (2) by being inhaled and causing local respiratory tract infection, which later spreads to the gastrointestinal tract by the swallowing of virus dripping down from the nasopharynx or coughed up in sputum; (3) by being inhaled and then brought up from the air passages by ciliary action and then swallowed; or (4) by contaminating hands which in turn contaminate food. But although several authors have referred to respiratory tract symptoms and otitis media (see below), there is no evidence that rotaviruses multiply other than in the enterocytes of the small intestine. Tallett et al. [90] could not detect rotavirus in tissue cultures of respiratory tract cells. Lewis et al. [55] were unable to find rotaviruses in throat swabs and nasopharyngeal secretions by electron microscopy. A few attempts to isolate rotaviruses from throat swabs in LLC MK$_2$ cells have failed in our own laboratory. Dr. Kunie Coelho (personal communication) cut frozen sections of rotavirus-infected baby mice and could find no evidence of infection by immunofluorescent staining, except in the small bowel.

Rotavirus Infection in Neonates

Infection of the newborn by rotaviruses has been described by several authors [3,6,12-14,20,65,89,94,103]. The symptoms in these outbreaks have been much milder than those described in older children. The reports of "severity" have varied considerably between different authors. But Totterdell et al. [94] took the view that "loose stools" among neonates are to be expected anyway, and are frequently caused by variations in feeding. They required at least five liquid or semiliquid stools per day before they diagnosed loose stools as "diarrhea" or "gastroenteritis." Other authors who were not so rigorous in their criteria found that most of their excreters of rotaviruses had gastroenteritis. Breast-fed infants were significantly less liable to infection than bottle-fed [20,86,94]. Zissis [103] devised a useful numerical coding for severity of infection; the degree of diarrhea, fever, and vomiting were each coded 0-3. Upon this basis the rotavirus-infected neonates had a much lower score than older children. Totterdell et al. [94] found that only 7 of 76 infected infants had symptomatic gastroenteritis. Murphy et al. [65] found that 84 of 304 (28%) babies excreting rotavirus had diarrhea. They found that five of six metropolitan hospitals in Sydney were affected. Buffet-Janvresse et al. [12] reported that, clinically, rotavirus infections among neonates in a premature baby unit were very mild; though the diarrhea was sometimes profuse it was of short duration and sometimes preceded by a rhinopharyngeal episode. These authors also described rotavirus infection of a placenta in a case of spontaneous abortion. Zissis [103] also reported abortion as a complication of rotavirus enteritis in a pregnant woman. One awaits with interest a second report of rotavirus infection of a placenta. These nursery infections appear to have persisted, in their various centers, for several months.

Other Viruses in Neonates

Murphy et al. [65] found coronavirus-like particles in 2 of 628 stool specimens from neonates in Sydney. Bishop et al. [6] reported that echovirus 22 appeared to be endemic in the nursery of the Royal Children's Hospital, Melbourne, to the extent that it was regarded as "normal flora" and appeared to do no harm. Zissis [103] found that *Escherichia coli* types 055 and 0126 were present in some stools in a nursery outbreak of rotavirus diarrhea in Brussels; the Melbourne infants also had "enteropathic serotypes" of *E. coli* circulating among them, but the presence of these organisms did not appear to be related to symptoms.

In young animals of other species in which antibodies are not transmitted across the placenta, the rule is that the younger the animal the more severe the diarrhea, particularly if it has not been protected by antibody or other antiviral substances [61,93] in mothers' milk. (Crouch and Woode [23] reported that newborn piglets all died in 3 days.) It has been believed until recently that serum IgG antibodies were much less likely to protect than intestinal IgA, but it may not be so.

All the authors who have analyzed the effects of breastfeeding agree that it appears to be beneficial. Welsh and May [100] have contributed a useful review on the antiinfective properties of breast milk. (Among patients in our own hospital exact information about breast feeding has been difficult to compile: breast feeding is so frequently supplemented by the bottle. However, even mixed breast and bottle feeding is probably better than bottle alone.)

Incubation Period

The incubation period in experimental animals can be as short as 19 h [23]. Murphy et al. [65] found 3 of 35 infants infected when only 1 day old. In older children, Flewett et al. [33] reported that secondary cases appeared to follow 2 days after the introduction into a hospital ward of the child who was believed to have been the source of the infection. No doubt the incubation period is influenced to some extent by the dose of virus and perhaps by the age of the infant. The functional reserve in the newborn is not large, and many cells may not need to be destroyed before diarrhea supervenes. The duration of virus excretion in neonates varied from 1 to 9 days [13,14]. Virus excretion occasionally persists longer; in a hospital ward outbreak, one child with congenital dislocation of the hips continued to excrete rotavirus for 29 days [22]. Age at onset varied from 2 to 13 days. In some, excretion of rotavirus preceded the development of diarrhea by 12-72 h [14,43].

Rotavirus infections in temperate climates occur mainly in the winter months: in England, December to the end of March; in Australia, June to September. But nursery infections have shown no such seasonal incidence [12,14, 20,94]; the outbreak described by Bishop et al. [6] took place in December, quite the "wrong" time of year for rotavirus infection in Australia.

Gastroenteritis in Postneonatal Children

The literature describing clinical features of outbreaks of acute rotavirus gastroenteritis in young children is almost entirely based upon studies of children admitted to the hospital. General practitioners in Birmingham say that those sent to the hospital are a small minority of the cases they see, and mothers do not ask the doctor to see every child with diarrhea. We know from numerous antibody studies that almost every child by the age of 7 or 8 years has had a rotavirus infection, and only a very small proportion of these will have been admitted to the hospital. Only, therefore, from observations on outpatients in a pediatric clinic in a not very prosperous area of a large city [36] ; an outbreak in children already in the hospital for some other reason [33] ; a residential nursery [103] ; or from sequential studies of the viral fecal flora in children in a Glasgow slum [83] do we know what the "average" rotavirus gastroenteritis is like. And even these outbreaks among children in the hospital may not have been average because if the infections had been more trivial or subclinical the nurses would not have brought them to our notice.

In the Belgian nursery study [103] diarrhea, vomiting, and fever were assessed and given a code from 0 to 3, in order of severity—frequency of diar-rheic stools (D)' frequency of vomiting (V), and height of fever (F). Assessed thus, 10 children 2-9 months old scored D 11, V 7, and F 4; 11 children 10-24 months old scored D 21, V 12, and F 11; 4 contacts aged 6-39 years returned proportionately higher scores, but the numbers are too small for the difference to be significant. The results do, however, suggest that the younger children were less severely affected. The incubation period and possible routes of infection wee not explored.

In the small series reported by Flewett et al. [33] , three out of six child-ren vomited on the first day of illness. A recent review of the records of these children shows that in three of them vomiting preceded diarrhea by 1-3 days; the diarrhea was very slight for the first 2 days and then became profuse. Fever was absent except on one day in one child. The sequence of illnesses among these children and in other studies of ward cross-infection [22,76] suggested an incubation period of 2-4 days. An adult volunteer suffered nausea on the day 2 and abdominal pains on day 3 [63]. Tufvesson et al. [96], in their study of 31 families infected with rotaviruses, found only one child aged 10 years with a subclinical infection, of a total of 43 infected children, 31 of whom had been admitted to the hospital.

Studies on Hospitalized Children

The clinical pattern of outbreaks of acute gastroenteritis in infants and young children appears to have changed considerably in the last 30 years, at least in Britain. This writer well remembers the shattering outbreaks of vomiting and diarrhea before 1950 which killed young children in large numbers. But the hypernatremic child—with tissues doughy to the touch, neck stiff and limbs rigid, irritable, febrile, convulsing, and usually dying—is rarely seen in our hos-pitals today. Another picture was the limp and drowsy child with lax, nonelastic skin, indrawn cheeks, sunken eyes and depressed fontanelle; febrile; with ex-treme tachycardia; and often dying. The biochemical control of salt and water balance is certainly much better understood nowadays. But one wonders whether the change in severity and mortality is only because of better treatment and better social conditions. Has an important pathogen disappeared, or gone into some unexplained recession, like the powerfully toxigenic, hemolytic streptococcus type 10?

Pullan et al. [69] and Sinha and Tyrrell [87] pointed out that even in the last 10 years, covering a time when the treatment of electrolyte disturbance was already well understood by pediatricians, the pattern has been changing. Nonbacterial enteritis now has a more marked winter prevalence than in earlier years, and the severity of the illnesses has diminished. In the Newcastle-upon-Tyne study [69] of 674 cases, from 1971 to 1975, the percentage with severe dehydration fell from 31% in 1971 to 6% in 1975, and the percentage with serum sodium levels over 150 mEq/L from 27 to 7%. There was a corresponding rise in the proportion of patients with little or no dehydration and with normal serum sodium levels.

The clinical picture of modern gastroenteritis in hospitalized children has been described in detail by comparatively few authors [16,27,39,43,55,71,85, 90]. Hieber et al. [43] compared rotavirus infections in temperate and tropical climates. Abraham and Dammin [1], Lewis et al. [55], and Rodriguez et al. [71] have compared and contrasted the clinical signs and symptoms of rotavirus and bacterial diarrhea, and Ryder et al. [76] and Maiya et al. [58] have done so for these infections in the tropical settings of rural Bangladesh and South India.

Vomiting was the initial symptom of rotavirus diarrhea in 14 of 30 children [85], preceding the diarrhea by 2-36 h; in 69 of 74 [55]; in 58 of 100 with fever [16]; and in half of 27 patients [90]. Rodriguez et al. [71] did not record the timing of the vomiting, which occurred in 96% of their patients, though they observed, as did Lewis et al. [55] and others [31,75], that vomiting occurred more frequently, and lasted longer (mean, 2-6 days) in patients with rotavirus infections than in those whose diarrhea was caused by enterotoxigenic coliforms, or some cause other than rotavirus infection (mean, 0.9 days). On the other hand, Maiya et al. [58] and Abraham and Dammin [1] found no clinical difference between bacterial and nonbacterial enteritis. Perhaps both groups of authors are right; it may all depend on the strains of pathogens causing the diseases studied.

Onset

All authors are agreed that onset is sudden. (It is also often sudden in diarrhea caused by toxigenic *E. coli*, but not always; in the 1968 outbreak in Manchester and Birmingham caused by the serotype O114 the onset was often slow and insidious, with diarrhea persisting and getting worse for day after day.)

Diarrhea

Diarrhea is usually most profuse on the second or third day of disease, and diminishes fairly quickly thereafter, although a few children may continue to excrete rotavirus and have mild diarrhea for longer periods (1-9 days [71], 2-10 days [43], up to 7 days [90]). The median total duration was 4-5 days [55].

Appearance of Feces

In most countries the feces of infants with rotavirus diarrhea vary in shade from yellow to green, but in Japan rotavirus causes a syndrome of "cholera infantum" or, in Japanese, *hakuri*. In this the feces are milky white [48]. We have not seen this in England in children, but I have had a sample of feces from a thoroughbred foal which had the color and consistency of dirty milk, and was teeming with rotaviruses. Dr. David Low (personal communication, 1980) says he has sometimes seen similar feces from Nigerian infants with rotavirus diarrhea. Bloody diarrhea usually indicates a bacterial infection, but may indicate intussusception or the hemolytic-uremic syndrome rather than rotavirus infection [99].

Chronic Diarrhea

Rotaviruses have been found in the feces of five children whose diarrhea persisted from 1 to 6 months [42]. Whether the rotavirus infection came after the original cause of the diarrhea was not established; however, two of the children were IgA deficient and four of them had monosaccharide intolerance. A second wave of replication has been found in experimentally infected piglets; the same may sometimes happen in children, but be missed because the patients have recovered from the first wave of virus replication and gone home. Recently, patients with combined immunodeficiency and X-linked agammaglobulinemia have been found to suffer chronic rotavirus infection; one patient excreted rotavirus for 50 days and another for 80 days. Excretion of virus coincided with diarrhea [78].

Dehydration was found in 83% of rotavirus patients against 40% of others with enteritis [71] and in 13 of 27 in another series [90]. Of all rotavirus patients, 39% required intravenous rehydration (but 75% in the group aged 12-18 months) in the Lewis et al. [55] series; the proportion of children with diarrhea of other causes requiring intravenous treatment was significantly less (see also Ref. 39). (These proportions, of course, relate to the prevalence of nonrotaviral pathogens only over the years of the studies listed; if more virulent strains of bacterial or other nonrotavirus viruses should appear, the findings in future years may well become different.)

Irritability and *lethargy* occurred in one-third to one-half of patients in both rotavirus and nonrotavirus groups [71].

Biochemical Disturbances

Blood urea was elevated in 13% [85] or 50% [71]. Blood pH, bicarbonate, and potassium levels were all significantly reduced in most patients [90], and chloride was significantly increased in nearly all. Hypernatremic (or hypertonic) dehydration (>150 mEq/l) was found only in about 5% of patients [55,71,90]. The incidence of hypernatremia has declined (certainly in England) in recent years, probably as a result of a change to low-solute milks for artificial feeding [59].

Respiratory Symptoms

Earlier authors referred to rhinitis and middle ear and pharyngeal inflammation as being more common in rotavirus than nonrotavirus diarrhea [51,71]; Tallett et al. [90] found (unspecified) respiratory infection in 9 of 27 patients; Hieber et al. [43] found respiratory symptoms in 12 of 16 rotavirus-positive patients in Dallas and in 20 of 41 rotavirus-negative patients in the same series. Lewis et al. [55] found statistically significant differences in clinical features between patients with rotavirus diarrhea and others: patients with rotavirus infection had a history of cough, nasal discharge, or otitis before admission much more frequently than patients with other causes of diarrhea. In Goldwater's [39] series, pharyngitis was much more frequent, especially in children aged 2-5 years.

These results could be explained in one of three ways. (1) rotaviruses multiply even more rapidly in the respiratory tract than in the small bowel. (2) The vomiting which so often precedes diarrhea, and admission to the hospital, causes these changes in the respiratory tract. (The vomiting is often profuse and violent at the beginning, although in the seriously ill child in the later stages it may be no more than a dribble from the mouth.) Vomit in young children could get up the Eustachian tube and set up otitis media. (3) Rotavirus-infected cells rapidly elaborate a toxin which causes these respiratory symptoms. The second explanation at present seems the most likely. A search for rotaviruses in the respiratory tract failed [55], and in my laboratory a search for rotaviruses in a few throat swabs by a tissue culture technique [10] also failed to isolate rotavirus. There is so far no evidence at all to support the third hypothesis.

Second Attacks of Rotavirus Infection

These have been reported by several authors [19,26,37,72]. Fonteyne et al. [37] described a 3-month-old child who had mild symptoms with the first attack and more severe symptoms with the second. The opposite pattern of clinical severity was seen in an older child. These were among five children in a crèche in Brussels, all of whom had rotavirus infection in two successive years: infection in the first year was caused by Zissis and Lambert serotype 1 [104] rotavirus; in the second year by Zissis type 2.

Rodriguez et al. [71] also described a child who had two consecutive rotavirus infections with different serotypes of rotavirus; the first infection was more severe than the second, but even this meager clinical evidence, and also a preliminary experiment in piglets [103], suggests that infection by one serotype may not confer immunity against infection by another. The evidence available so far is quite insufficient to say whether one serotype causes more severe symptoms than another. Differences in severity observed by Yolken et al. [102] suggest that Zissis serotype 2 might be more virulent than serotype 1; however, the differences were not statistically significant.

Complications

Intestinal Hemorrhage

Intestinal hemorrhage has not been noted by most authors, although Delage et al. [27] noted 6 cases of rectal bleeding among 60 patients, and a rash resembling that of Henoch-Schönlein purpura in 2; 1 patient had hematuria. However, in a series of 232 cases in Bangladesh, Taylor et al. [91] recorded bloody diarrhea in only 1 patient.

Intussusception

Occasionally, a child who has had rotavirus gastroenteritis has been discharged from the hospital in Birmingham and shortly afterward readmitted with intussusception, but such cases have been rare (Tarlow, personal communication). But in Japan, Konno et al. [49] found that rotaviruses could be found in 11 of 30 infants with intussusception; adenoviruses were detected in the stools of 8 others of the same 30 patients. Adenovirus infection, of course, has for long been postulated as a cause of intussusception [38,68]. Perhaps like hakuri, Japanese infants are especially liable to rotavirus intussusception.

Encephalitis, Reye's Syndrome

It is always difficult to assess the significance of very rare complications of very common infections. I recall one patient with encephalitis and influenza who would certainly have been added to a series of cases of influenza encephalitis, had his encephalitis only started 3 days after, rather than 3 days before, his influenza. Perhaps any acute infection may very occasionally cause a secondary encephalitis; Salmi et al. [77] described two cases of undoubted encephalitis, with pleocytosis and raised protein levels in the cerebrospinal fluid, associated with rotavirus diarrhea. One child died; at autopsy some cellular infiltration of the brain was found and also the histologic changes of Reye's syndrome in the liver. The other child made a slow recovery.

Because rotavirus infections, and especially nosocomial infections, are so common [33,53,75], we may expect reports that rotaviruses have been detected in all kinds of pediatric syndromes. Before deciding that the rotavirus (or other enteric virus) is even a contributory cause of the syndrome in question, we must carefully assess the evidence [32].

Diffuse intravascular coagulation can be a feature of any massive biochemical disturbance in infants, and may occur with severe hypernatremic dehydration.

Fatal Rotavirus Gastroenteritis

Our pediatricians say that if a child is admitted to the hospital in good time, no matter how severe the infection, they ought not to lose that child. Nevertheless, deaths do occur. Over the last 3 years three deaths have occurred in the East Birmingham Hospital: two were admitted moribund with irreversible electrolyte disturbance; the third died from inhaling vomit.

In small countries where the population is dense, lines of communications are short, and pediatricians expert, as in Holland or Belgium, the mortality rate is very low [95]. In Canada it may take much longer to get a sick child to the hospital. Carlson et al. [15] reviewed 21 fatal cases. Of these, 2 already had another illness, but the remainder had previously appeared healthy. Death in most appeared to have resulted from rapid and severe dehydration, leading to cardiac arrest; 3 had aspirated vomit, and 2 had had seizures.

The Postgastroenteritis Syndrome

"The post-gastroenteritis syndrome is the clinical syndrome when a child who has had an attack of acute gastroenteritis subsequently has intermittant or chronic diarrhoea with or without failure to gain weight following the return to a normal diet" [99]. Authors who have written about this syndrome have not in general distinguished between diarrhea caused by rotavirus and other viruses or bacteria. But it certainly can follow rotavirus infection. The main feature is intolerance to milk when full feeding (especially artificial feeding) is started again. In some patients, biopsy reveals partial villous atrophy, but in others, little obvious histologic change is detectable.

Most of the children are less than 9 months old (below the age when rotavirus disease is most prevalent), and the syndrome is most serious and difficult to manage below the age of 6 months. When the corrected weight of children on admission was below the 3rd percentile the incidence of delayed recovery was more than doubled. Infants from the Indian subcontinent had the highest incidence of delayed recovery [99].

The mechanisms are uncertain and probably manifold. Food allergy, especially cow's milk allergy, has been blamed; some cases have had IgA deficiency [42].

Rotavirus Infection in Adults

Subclinical infections have been described by a number of authors, but clinical infections, sometimes quite severe, also occur [35]. Ørstavik et al. [66], Holzel et al. [44], and von Bonsdorff et al. [9] all described fairly severe attacks, with fever above 39°C, lasting for 2-9 days, in adults. Adults in closed communities seem especially vulnerable. Holzel et al. [44] had a patient of 83 years; we have had one of 94 years in an old people's home (see also Ref. 30). A recent outbreak of rotavirus gastroenteritis in a nursing home for the elderly claimed one death, and several patients, aged between 70 and 90 years, were severely ill [40].

Traveller's diarrhea in the tropics, a syndrome which is endowed with various colorful names, such as "Montezuma's revenge," usually appears to be caused by toxigenic *E. coli* [76], but some cases are caused by rotaviruses [8,97]. Echevarria et al. [28] found that such infections occurred among the natives of the Phillipines, who took them as part of the nature of things, as well as among American visitors.

Astroviruses have been found in the feces of infants both with and without apparent disease [57,67], but do appear to have caused an outbreak of gastroenteritis in children in Oxford [52,54]. The infection has been transmitted to adult volunteers, causing symptoms in some.

Caliciviruses often cause no symptoms at all, but were recovered from an outbreak of winter vomiting disease in a school in London [25] and from the small bowel of a child who died of gastroenteritis [34], where they appeared to be the only pathogen.

Coronaviruses have been found in outbreaks of acute diarrhea and vomiting in teenagers and young adults in England and elsewhere [17,56,67]. Fever and pharyngitis were a feature in some. But in some studies [60,80] they were frequently found in asymptomatic persons, especially among young Indian villagers and Australian aboriginals.

Uncultivable *adenoviruses* were first described as a cause of acute enteritis in 1975 and have since been reported from many countries [21,27,33,48,79, 81,88]. Richmond et al. [70] have recently described an outbreak involving 17 children and 2 adults. Histories of contact suggested an incubation period of about 8-10 days. Diarrhea was severe; most children also vomited. The infection appears to have been more severe than in the small outbreak in a children's ward [33] when vomiting was not a feature. In the interesting case reported by Chiba et al. [19], whose 14-month-old patient had three episodes of diarrhea, caused first by rotavirus, then adenovirus, and again rotavirus, the rotavirus illnesses were associated with vomiting and were more severe than the adenovirus infection in which there was no vomiting.

Two fatal cases are known (see Ref. 101 and Homola, personal communication, 1977).

The *Norwalk agent* will be described in detail elsewhere (Chap. 9). It is of interest here because histologic observation of biopsies from infected adult volunteers [2,82] showed that like rotaviruses, this virus attacks the enterocytes of the tips and sides of villi of the small bowel. Volunteers developed diarrhea; some also had vomiting and abdominal cramps. Respiratory symptoms were not reported.

References

1. A. A. Abraham and G. J. Dammin, Virus isolation studies in infantile diarrhea, *Environ. Child Health,* August:206–211 (1977).
2. S. G. Agus, R. Dolin, R. G. Wyatt, A. J. Tousimis, and R. S. Northrup, Acute infectious nonbacterial gastroenteritis: Intestinal histopathology. Histologic and enzymatic alterations during illness produced by the Norwalk agent in man, *Ann. Intern. Med., 79*:18–25.(1973).
3. M. B. Albrey and A. M. Murphy, Rotaviruses and acute gastroenteritis of infants and children, *Med. J. Aust. 1*(4):82–85 (1976).
4. C. J. Birch, F. A. Lewis, M. L. Kennett, M. Homola, H. Pritchard, and I. D. Gust, A study of the prevalence of rotavirus infection in children with gastroenteritis admitted to an infectious disease hospital, *J. Med. Virol., 1*:69–77 (1977).
5. R. F. Bishop, G. P. Davidson, I. H. Holmes, and B. J. Ruck, Detection of a new virus by electron microscopy of faecal extracts from children with acute gastroenteritis, *Lancet, 1*:149–151 (1974).
6. R. T. Bishop, A. S. Hewstone, G. P. Davidson, R. R. W. Townley, I. H. Holmes, and B. J. Ruck, An epidemic of diarrhoea in human neonates involving a reovirus-like agent and "enteropathic" serotypes of *Escherichia coli, J. Clin. Pathol., 29*:46–49 (1976).
7. N. R. Blacklow, R. Dolin, D. S. Fedson, H. DuPont, R. S. Northrup, R. B. Hornick, and R. M. Chanock, Acute infectious nonbacterial gastroenteritis. Etiology and pathogenesis, *Ann. Intern. Med., 76*:993–1008 (1972).
8. R. Bolivar, R. H. Conklin, J. T. Vollet, L. K. Pickering, H. L. DuPont, D. L. Walters, and S. Kohl, Rotavirus in Travellers' diarrhoea. Study of an adult student population in Mexico, *J. Infect. Dis. 137*:324–327 (1978).
9. C. H. von Bonsdorff, T. Hovi, P. Makela, L. Hovi, and M. Tevalvoto-Aarnio, Rotavirus associated with acute gastroenteritis in adults, *Lancet, 2*:423 (1976).
10. A. S. Bryden, H. Davies, M. E. Thouless, and T. H. Flewett, Diagnosis of rotavirus by cell culture, *J. Med. Microbiol. 10*:121–125 (1977).

11. A. S. Bryden, R. H. Hadley, H. A. Davies, T. H. Flewett, C. A. Morris, and P. Oliver, Rotavirus enteritis in the West Midlands during 1974, *Lancet*, 2:241-243 (1975).

12. C. Buffet-Janvresse, E. Berhard, and H. Magard, Responsabilité des rotavirus dans les diarrhées du nourisson, *Nouv. Presse Méd.*, 5:1249-1251 (1976).

13. D. J. S. Cameron, R. F. Bishop, G. P. Davidson, R. R. W. Townley, I. H. Holmes, and B. J. Ruck, New virus associated with diarrhoea in neonates, *Med. J. Aust.* 1(4):85-86 (1976).

14. D. J. S. Cameron, R. F. Bishop, A. A. Veenstra, G. L. Barnes, I. H. Holmes, and B. J. Ruck. Pattern of shedding of two non-cultivable viruses in stools of newborn babies, *Lancet*, 2:7-13 (1978).

15. J. A. K. Carlsson, P. J. Middleton, M. T. Szymanski, J. Huber, and M. Petric, Fatal rotavirus gastroenteritis. An analysis of 21 cases, *Am. J. Dis. Child.*, 132:477-479 (1978).

16. M. E. Carr, G. D. W. McKendrick, and T. Spyridakis, The clinical features of infantile gastroenteritis due to rotavirus, *Scand. J. Infect. Dis.*, 8(4): 241-243 (1976).

17. E. P. Caul, W. K. Paver, and S. K. R. Clarke, Coronavirus particles in faeces from patients with gastroenteritis, *Lancet*, 1:1192 (1975).

18. S. Chiba, M. Akihara, R. Kogasaka, K. Horino, T. Nakao, T. Urasawa, S. Urasawa, and S. Fukui, An outbreak of gastroenteritis due to rotavirus in an infant home, *Tohoku J. Exp. Med.*, 127:265-271 (1979).

19. S. Chiba, R. Kogasaka, M. Akihara, K. Horino, and T. Nakao, Recurrent attack of rotavirus gastroenteritis after adenovirus-induced diarrhoea, *Arch. Dis. Child.*, 54:398-400 (1979).

20. I. L. Chrystie, B. M. Totterdell, and J. E. Banatvala, Asymptomatic endemic rotavirus infections in the newborn, *Lancet*, 1:1176-1178 (1978).

21. S. K. R. Clarke, G. T. Cook, S. I. Egglestone, T. S. Hall, D. L. Miller, S. E. Reed, D. Rubenstein, A. J. Smith, and D. A. J. Tyrrell, A virus from winter vomiting disease, *Br. Med. J.*, 2:86-89 (1972).

22. M. I. Cleton-Soeteman and B. C. van Pelt, Gastro-enteritis veroorzaakt door rotavirus en versprelding van deze infectie in het ziekenhuis, *Ned. Tijdschr. Geneeskd.*, 121:866-869 (1977).

23. C. F. Crouch and G. N. Woode, Serial studies of virus multiplication and intestinal damage in gnotobiotic piglets infected with rotavirus, *J. Med. Microbiol.*, 11:325-334 (1978).

24. W. D. Cubitt and H. Holzel, An outbreak of rotavirus infection in a long-stay ward of a geriatric hospital, *J. Clin. Pathol.*, 33:306-308 (1980).

25. W. D. Cubitt, D. A. McSwiggan, and W. Moore, Winter vomiting disease caused by calicivirus, *J. Clin. Pathol.*, 32:786-793 (1979).

26. G. P. Davidson, R. F. Bishop, R. R. W. Townley, I. H. Holmes, and B. J. Ruck, Importance of a new virus in acute sporadic enteritis in children, *Lancet*, 1:242-246 (1975).

27. G. Delage, B. McLaughlin, and L. Berthiaume, A clinical study of rotavirus gastroenteritis, *J. Pediatr., 93*:455–457 (1978).

28. P. Echevarria, N. R. Blacklow, C. Zipkin, J. J. Volkt, J. A. Olson, H. L. DuPont, and J. H. Cross, Etiology of gastroenteritis among Americans living in the Phillipines, *Am. J. Epidemiol., 109*:493–501 (1979).

29. M. M. Elias, Distribution and titres of rotavirus antibodies in different age groups, *J. Hyg. 79*(3):373–380 (1977).

30. Epidemiological report. Rotavirus gastroenteritis (notes complied by the Communicable Disease Surveillance Centre of the U.K. Public Health Laboratory Service), *Br. Med. J., 1*(6064):844 (1977).

31. D. G. Evans, J. Olarte, H. L. DuPont, D. J. Evans, E. Galindo, B. L. Portnoy, and R. H. Conklin, Enteropathogens associated with pediatric diarrhea in Mexico City, *J. Pediatr., 91*:65–68 (1977).

32. T. H. Flewett, Implications of recent virological researches. In *Acute Diarrhoea in Childhood*, Ciba Symposium 42. Amsterdam, Elsevier, 1976.

33. T. H. Flewett, A. S. Bryden, H. A. Davies, and C. A. Morris, Epidemic viral enteritis in a long-stay children's ward, *Lancet, 1*:4–6 (1975).

34. T. H. Flewett and H. Davies, Caliciviruses of man, *Lancet, 1*:311 (1976).

35. T. H. Flewett, H. A. Davies, A. S. Bryden, and M. J. Robertson, Diagnostic electron microscopy of faeces. II Acute gastroenteritis associated with reovirus-like particles, *J. Clin. Pathol., 27*:608–614 (1974).

36. J. L. Fonteyne, G. Zissis, J. P. Butzler, J. P. Lambert, D. de Kegel, A. Champenois, M. Dineur, H. R. van Goethem, and J. Jaumain, Diarrhoea with rotaviruses in a paediatric surgery in Brussels, *Acta Clin. Belg., 32*: 280–281 (1977).

37. J. Fonteyne, G. Zissis, and J. P. Lambert, Recurrent rotavirus gastroenteritis, *Lancet, 1*:983 (1978).

38. P. S. Gardner, E. G. Knox, S. D. M. Court, and C. A. Green, Virus infection and intussusception in childhood, *Br. Med. J., 2*:697–700 (1962).

39. P. N. Goldwater, Gastroenteritis in Auckland: An aetiological and clinical study, *J. Infect., 1*:339–351 (1979).

40. J. Halvorsrud and I. Ørstavik, An outbreak of rotavirus-associated gastroenteritis in a nursing home for the elderly, *Scand. J. Infect. Dis., 2*:161–164 (1980).

41. M. Hara, J. Mukoyama, T. Tsuruhara, Y. Saito, and I. Tagaya, Duovirus in school children with gastroenteritis, *Lancet, 1*:311 (1976).

42. B. M. Harrison, A. Kilby, J. A. Walker-Smith, N. E. France, C. B. S. Woode, Cows' milk protein intolerance: A possible association with gastroenteritis, lactose intolerance and IgA deficiency, *Br. Med. J., 1*:1501–1594 (1976).

43. J. P. Hieber, S. Shelton, J. D. Nelson, J. Leon, and E. Mohs, Comparison of human rotavirus disease in tropical and temperate settings, *Am. J. Dis. Child., 132*:853–858 (1978).

44. H. Holzel, D. W. Cubitt, D. A. McSwiggan, P. J. Sanderson, and J. Church, An outbreak of rotavirus infection among adults in a cardiology ward, *J. Infect., 2*:33–37 (1980).

45. R. I. Hutchinson, *Escherichia coli* (O-types III, 55 and 26) and their association with infantile diarrhoea. A five-year study, *J. Hyg., 55*:27–44 (1957).

46. A. Z. Kapikian, H. W. Kim, R. G. Wyatt, W. L. Cline, J. P. Arrobio, C. D. Brandt, W. J. Rodriguez, D. A. Sack, R. M. Chanock, and R. H. Parrott, Human reovirus-like agent as the major pathogen associated with "winter" gastroenteritis in hospitalized infants and young children, *N. Engl. J. Med., 294*(18):965–972 (1976).

47. H. W. Kim, C. D. Brandt, A. Z. Kapikian, R. G. Wyatt, J. P. Arrobio, W. J. Rodriguez, R. M. Chanock, and R. H. Parrott, Human reovirus-like agent infection. Occurrence in adult contacts of pediatric patients with gastroenteritis, *JAMA, 238/5*:404–407 (1977).

48. T. Konno, H. Suzuki, A. Imai, T. Kutsuzawa, N. Ishida, N. Katsushima, M. Sakamoto, S. Kitaoka, R. Tsuboi, and M. Adachi, A long-term study of rotavirus infection in Japanese children with acute gastroenteritis, *J. Infect. Dis., 138*:569–576 (1978).

49. T. Konno, H. Suzuki, T. Kutsuzawa, A. Imai, N. Katsushima, H. Sakamoto, S. Kitaoka, R. Tsuboi, and M. Adachi, Human rotavirus infection in infants and young children with intussusception, *J. Med. Virol., 2*: 265–269 (1978).

50. L. M. Kraft, Epizootic diarrhoea of infant mice and lethal intestinal infections of infant mice. In *Viruses of Laboratory Rodents,* National Cancer Institute Monograph No. 20, National Cancer Institute, Bethesda, 1966.

51. P. A. Krasilnikoff, P. C. Grauballe, J. Genner, A. Meyling, and A. Hornsleth, Den Kliniske betydning af rotavirus-infectioner hos born med akut diare. En preliminaer. *Ugeskr. Laeger, 139*(51):3049–3052 (1977).

52. J. B. Kurtz, T. W. Lee, J. W. Craig, and S. E. Reed, Astrovirus infection in volunteers, *J. Med. Virol., 3*:221–230 (1979).

53. Leading article: Viral cross-infection in children's wards, *Lancet, 1*:1391–1393 (1976).

54. T. W. Lee and J. G. Kurtz, Astroviruses detected by immunofluorescence, *Lancet, 2*:406 (1977).

55. H. M. Lewis, J. V. Parry, H. A. Davies, R. P. Parry, A. Mott, R. R. Dourmashkin, P. J. Sanderson, D. A. J. Tyrrell, and H. B. Valman, A year's experience of the rotavirus syndrome and its association with respiratory illness, *Arch. Dis. Child. 54*:339–346 (1979).

56. G. Maass, H. G. Baumeister, and N. Freitag, Viren Als Ursache der akuten Gastroenteritis bei Sauglingen und Kleinkindern, *Munch. Med. Wochenschr., 119*:1029–1034 (1977).

57. C. R. Madeley and B. P. Cosgrove, Viruses in infantile gastroenteritis, *Lancet, 2*(7295):124 (1975).

58. P. P. Maiya, S. M. Pereira, M. Mathan, P. Bhat, M. J. Albert, and S. J. Baker, Aetiology of acute gastroenteritis in infancy and early childhood in southern India, *Arch. Dis. Child., 52*(6):482–485 (1977).

59. P. D. Manuel and J. A. Walker-Smith, Decline of hypernatraemia as a problem in gastroenteritis, *Arch. Dis. Child., 55*:124-127 (1980).
60. M. Mathan, V. I. Mathan, S. D. Swaminathan, S. Yesudoss, and S. J. Baker, Pleomorphic virus-like particles in human faeces, *Lancet, 1*:1068-1069 (1975).
61. T. H. J. Matthews, M. K. Lawrence, C. D. G. Nair, and D. A. J. Tyrrell, Antiviral activity in milk of possible clinical importance, *Lancet, 2*:1387-1389 (1977).
62. O. H. Meurman and M. J. Laine, Rotavirus epidemic in adults, *N. Engl. J. Med., 296(22)*:1298-1299 (1977).
63. P. J. Middleton, M. T. Szymanski, G. D. Abbott, R. Bortolussi, and J. R. Hamilton, Orbivirus acute gastroenteritis of infancy, *Lancet, 1*:1241-1244 (1974).
64. D. H. Much and I. Zajak, Purification and characterization of epizootic diarrhea of infant mice virus, *Infect. Immun., 6*:1019-1024 (1972).
65. A. M. Murphy, M. B. Albrey, and E. G. Crewe, Rotavirus infections of neonates, *Lancet, 2*:1149-1150 (1977).
66. I. Ørstavik, K. W. Haug, and Søvde, Rotavirus-associated gastroenteritis in two adults probably caused by virus reinfection, *Scand. J. Infect. Dis., 8(4)*:277-278 (1976).
67. H. Peique, M. Beytout-Monghal, H. Laveran, and M. Bourges, Coronavirus et "Astrovirus" observés dans les selles d'enfants atteints de gastro-enterites, *Ann. Microbiol. (Inst. Pasteur), 129B*:101-106 (1978).
68. C. W. Potter, Adenovirus infection as an aetiological agent in intussusception of infants and young children, *J. Pathol. Bacteriol., 88*:263-274 (1964).
69. C. R. Pullan, H. Dellagrammatikas, and H. Steiner, Survey of gastroenteritis in children admitted to hospital in Newcastle-upon-Tyne in 1971-75, *Br. Med. J., 1*:619-621 (1977).
70. S. J. Richmond, S. M. Dunn, E. O. Caul, C. R. Ashley, and S. K. R. Clarke, An outbreak of gastroenteritis in young children caused by adenoviruses, *Lancet, 1*:1178-1180 (1979).
71. W. J. Rodriguez, H. W. Kim, J. O. Arrobio, C. D. Brandt, R. M. Chanock, A. Z. Kapikian, R. G. Wyatt, and R. H. Parrott, Clinical features of acute gastroenteritis associated with human reovirus-like agent in infants and young children, *J. Pediatr., 91*:188-193 (1977).
72. W. J. Rodriguez, H. W. Kim, C. D. Brandt, R. H. Yolken, J. O. Arrobio, A. Z. Kapikian, R. M. Chanock, and R. H. Parrott, Sequential enteric illnesses associated with different rotavirus serotypes, *Lancet, 2*:37 (1978).
73. K. B. Rogers, The spread of infantile gastroenteritis in a cubicled ward, *J. Hyg. (Cambridge), 49*:140-151 (1951).
74. D. Rubenstein, R. G. Milne, R. Buckland, and D. A. J. Tyrrell, The growth of the virus of epidemic diarrhoea of infant mice (EDIM) in organ cultures of intestinal epithelium, *Br. J. Exp. Pathol., 52*:442-445 (1971).

75. R. W. Ryder, J. E. McGowan, Jr., M. H. Hatch, and E. L. Palmer, Reovirus-like agent as a cause of nosocomial diarrhea in infants, *J. Pediatr., 90/5*: 698-702 (1977).

76. R. W. Ryder, D. A. Sack, A. Z. Kapikian, J. C. McLaughlin, J. Chakraborty, A. S. M. M. Rahman, M. H. Merson, and J. G. Wells, Enterotoxigenic *Escherichia coli* and reovirus-like agent in rural Bangladesh, *Lancet, 1*:659-662 (1976).

77. T. T. Salmi, P. Artsila, and A. Koivikko, Central nervous system involvement in patients with rotavirus gastroenteritis, *Scand. J. Infect. Dis., 19*: 29-31 (1978).

78. F. T. Saulsbury, J. A. Winkelstein, and R. H. Yolken, Chronic rotavirus infection in immunodeficiency, *J. Pediatr., 97*:61-65 (1980).

79. R. D. Schnagl, I. H. Holmes, and E. M. Mackay-Scollay, A survey of rotavirus associated with gastroenteritis in aboriginal children in Western Australia, *Med. J. Austr., 1*:304-307 (1978).

80. R. D. Schnagl, I. H. Holmes, and E. M. Mackay-Scollay, Coronavirus-like particles in aboriginals and nonaboriginals in Western Australia, *Med. J. Aust., 1*:307-309 (1978).

81. B. D. Schoub, H. J. Koornhof, G. Lecatsas, O. W. Prozesky, I. Freiman, E. Hartman, and H. Kassel, Viruses in acute summer gastroenteritis in black infants, *Lancet, 1*:1093 (1975).

82. D. S. Schreiber, N. R. Blacklow, and J. S. Trier, The mucosal lesion of the proximal small intestine in acute infectious non-bacterial gastroenteritis, *N. Engl. J. Med., 288*:1318-1323 (1973).

83. T. M. Scott, C. R. Madeley, B. P. Cosgrove, and J. P. Stanfield, Stool viruses in babies in Glasgow. 3. Community studies, *J. Hyg. (Cambridge), 83*:469-485 (1979).

84. T. Sebodo, Y. Soeharto, J. E. Rohde, N. J. Ryan, B. J. Taylor, R. J. K. Luke, R. F. Bishop, G. L. Barnes, I. H. Holmes, and B. J. Ruck, Aetiology of diarrhoea in children aged less than two years in central Java, *Lancet, 1*:490-491 (1977).

85. R. W. Shepherd, S. Truslow, J. A. Walker-Smith, R. Bird, W. Cutting, R. Darnell, and C. M. Barker, Infantile gastroenteritis: A clinical study of reovirus-like agent infection, *Lancet, 2*:1082-1084 (1975).

86. A. Simhon and L. Mata, Anti-rotavirus antibody in human colostrum, *Lancet, 1*:39-40 (1978).

87. A. K. Sinha and D. A. J. Tyrrell, Changes in the clinical pattern of gastrointestinal infection in North West London 1968-70, *Br. J. Clin. Pract., 27*: 45-48 (1973).

88. M. C. Steinhoff, Viruses and diarrhoea—a review, *Am. J. Dis. Child., 132*: 302-307 (1978).

89. M. C. Steinhoff and M. A. Gerber, Rotavirus infection of neonates, *Lancet, 1*:775 (1978).

90. S. Tallett, R. N. Mackenzie, P. Middleton, B. Kerzner, and R. Hamilton, Clinical, laboratory and epidemiological features of a viral gastroenteritis in infants and children, *Pediatrics, 60*:217-222 (1977).

91. P. R. Taylor, M. H. Merson, R. E. Black, A. S. M. Mizanur Rahman, M. D. Yunus, A. R. M. Alim, and R. H. Yolken, Oral rehydration therapy for treatment of rotavirus diarrhoea in a rural treatment centre in Bangladesh, *Arch. Dis. Child.*, *55*:376-379 (1980).

92. T. S. Thornhill, R. G. Wyatt, A. R. Kallen, R. Dolin, R. M. Chanock, and A. Z. Kapikian, Detection by immune electron microscopy of 26- to 27-nm viruslike particles associated with two family outbreaks of gastroenteritis, *J. Infect. Dis.*, *135(1)*:20-27 (1977).

93. M. E. Thouless, A. S. Bryden, and T. H. Flewett, Rotavirus neutralization by human milk, *Br. Med. J.*, *2*:1390 (1977).

94. B. M. Totterdell, I. L. Chrystie, and J. E. Banatvala, Rotavirus infections in a maternity unit, *Arch. Dis. Child.*, *51*:924-928 (1976).

95. J. H. Tripp, M. J. Wilmers, and B. A. Wharton, Gastroenteritis; a continuing problem of child health in Britain, *Lancet*, *2*:233-236 (1977).

96. B. Tufvesson, T. Johnsson, and B. Persson, Family infections by reo-like virus. Comparisons of antibody titres by complement fixation and immunoelectrophoosmophoresis, *Scand. J. Infect. Dis.*, *9(4)*:257-261 (1977).

97. J. J. Vollet, C. D. Ericsson, G. Gibson, L. K. Pickering, H. L. DuPont, S. Kohl, and R. H. Conklin, Human rotavirus in an adult population with travellers' diarrhea and its relationship to the location of food consumption, *J. Med. Virol.*, *4*:81-87 (1979).

98. J. A. Walker-Smith, Rotavirus gastro-enteritis, *Arch. Dis. Child.*, *53*:355-362 (1978).

99. J. A. Walker-Smith, *Diseases of the Small Intestine in Childhood*, Pitman Medical, London, 1979.

100. J. K. Welsh and J. T. May, Anti-infective properties of breast milk, *J. Pediatr.*, *94*:1-9 (1979).

101. A. Whitelaw, H. Davies, and J. Perry, Electron microscopy of fatal adenovirus gastroenteritis, *Lancet*, *1*:361 (1977).

102. R. H. Yolken, R. G. Wyatt, G. Zissis, C. D. Brandt, W. J. Rodriguez, H. W. Kim, R. H. Parrott, J. J. Urrutia, L. Mata, H. B. Greenberg, A. Z. Kapikian, and R.M. Chanock, Epidemiology of human rotavirus types 1 and 2 as studied by enzyme-linked immunosorbent assay, *N. Engl. J. Med.*, *299*: 1156-1161 (1978).

103. G. Zissis, Het Belang van Rotavirus in die Etiologie van Infantiele Diarree. M. D. Thesis, Vrije Universiteit, Brussel, 1979.

104. G. Zissis and J. P. Lambert, Different serotypes of human rotaviruses, *Lancet*, *1*:38-39 (1978).

105. G. Zissis, J. P. Lambert, J. Fonteyne, and D. de Kegel, Child-mother transmission of rotavirus? *Lancet*, *1*:96 (1976).

9

The Norwalk Group of Viruses—Agents Associated with Epidemic Viral Gastroenteritis

Albert Z. Kapikian, Harry B. Greenberg, Richard G. Wyatt, Anthony R. Kalica, and Robert M. Chanock National Institute of Allergy and Infectious Diseases, Bethesda, Maryland

Viral gastroenteritis can be divided into two distinct clinical entities with quite different epidemiologic characteristics. One, which may be designated *sporadic infantile gastroenteritis,* has been associated with severe diarrheal illness of infants and young children. This form of gastroenteritis, which may require hospitalization and parenteral or oral fluid replacement therapy, has been associated predominantly with the rotaviruses and was described in a previous chapter. The other form of viral gastroenteritis may be designated *epidemic viral gastroenteritis,* since it usually occurs in family or community-wide outbreaks, affecting adults, school-age children, family contacts, and some young children as well. This form of the disease, which is characteristically mild and self-limited, usually lasting 24-48 h, has been given various descriptive names, such as winter vomiting disease, epidemic diarrhea and vomiting, and acute infectious nonbacterial gastroenteritis [7,76]. The Norwalk group of viruses has been associated with this form of viral gastroenteritis and will be described in this chapter.

History

Although diarrheal diseases have been documented since pre-Hippocratic times, the etiologic agents of most such illnesses remained unknown until quite recently [13,14,38,52,75]. It was frequently assumed by exclusion, however, that viruses were responsible for many of the acute gastroenteric illnesses of unknown etiology. Indeed, in the 1940s and 1950s, this form of gastroenteritis was experimentally induced in volunteers following the administration of bacteria-free stool filtrates prepared from specimens from patients with the disease. Attempts to propagate an etiologic agent in vitro or to passage a filterable agent of epidemic gastroenteritis to animals were generally unsuccessful [21-25,37,46, 59,74] ; in one report a bacteria-free filtrate induced a diarrheal illness in cats [74]. A report in 1943 described the induction of diarrhea in calves with a filterable agent derived from stools of infants who developed diarrhea during outbreaks in premature or full-term nurseries [48]. (Over 30 years later, rotavirus was detected in a stool from one of these calves which had developed illness after such inoculation [35] .) Thus, in spite of extensive studies, by the early 1970s the etiologic agents of both epidemic gastroenteritis and infantile gastroenteritis were still unknown. However, since new methods for the detection of fastidious viruses, such as the use of organ cultures for detection of coronaviruses, had been developed in the 1960s, renewed attempts were made to elucidate the etiologic agents of viral gastroenteritis employing such newer techniques [69]. However, examination of specimens from different gastroenteritis outbreaks with the new techniques failed to reveal any etiologic agent [7]. Therefore, volunteer studies were undertaken once again in an attempt to generate study material known to contain an infectious agent as demonstrated by serial passage in volunteers [7,16,17].

One such study involved a specimen obtained from a gastroenteritis outbreak in Norwalk, Ohio, in which, within a period of 2 days, acute gastrointestinal illness developed in 50% of the students and teachers in an elementary school [1]. There was a secondary attack rate of 32% among family contacts of primary cases. The illness lasted about 24 h and had an incubation period of about 48 h; it was designated winter vomiting disease since vomiting and nausea were the predominant clinical findings, with diarrhea occurring in a lesser number of individuals. An etiologic agent could not be associated with this outbreak. A bacteria-free filtrate prepared from a rectal swab specimen from a secondary case was orally administered to three volunteers; two developed gastroenteritis [17]. Furthermore, known infectious material was generated, as the agent was serially passaged to other volunteers [16]. However, all attempts to propagate an agent in cell culture were unsuccessful, and such attempts in human embryonic intestinal organ culture were inconclusive [16,17]. Thus, it was clearly disappointing that in spite of the application of newer techniques, the search for an etiologic agent of viral gastroenteritis was still unsuccessful, and knowledge about such agents remained essentially as it was in the 1940s and 1950s.

However, in 1972, application of the technique of immune electron microscopy (IEM) led to the discovery of 27 nm particles in a known infectious stool filtrate derived from a volunteer who had developed illness following challenge with the Norwalk agent [44]. The particles were observed following incubation of this stool filtrate with a volunteer's convalescent-phase serum. Serologic evidence of infection with the 27 nm particle was shown by IEM not only in various experimentally infected individuals but also in certain affected individuals from the original outbreak. From these and other data it was suggested that the 27 nm particle was the etiologic agent of the Norwalk outbreak [44]. It was striking that the particles were discovered without the benefit of any in vitro or animal model system but in fact merely involved the examination of clinical material by electron microscopic techniques. This approach has been termed "direct virology"—a method which also enables the further characterization of a fastidious agent [4,39,40,43,45]. Soon afterward, morphologically similar particles were detected in diarrheal stool preparations by IEM and conventional electron microscopy, and it appeared that the etiology of the epidemic form of viral gastroenteritis was at least in part finally being elucidated. A description of the Norwalk and other viruses in this group, as well as several candidate viruses, is presented below [4,5,11,44,53,57,68].

Description of Norwalk-like Agents

Although the nucleic acid content of the Norwalk like agents has not yet been determined, these agents share certain characteristics which permit them to be grouped together: (1) they are associated with acute gastroenteritis; (2) they are morphologically similar, have a diameter of 25-27 nm, and bear a resemblance to the picornaviruses or parvoviruses and in certain preparations, to the caliciviruses as well (Fig. 1); (3) they have not been propagated in vitro; and (4) they have a density of 1.37-1.41 g/cm^3 in cesium chloride [4,5,30,36,41,44,68]. As shown in Table 1, in addition to the Norwalk virus, other members of this group include: (1) the Hawaii and (2) the Montgomery County (MC) agents which were both detected by IEM in stools from two separate family outbreaks of gastroenteritis [68]; the Norwalk and Hawaii agents appear to be distinct by IEM and cross-challenge studies, whereas the Norwalk and MC agents are related, and the relationship between the Hawaii and the Montgomery County is inconclusive [44,68,71]; (3) the Ditchling agent, which was visualized by EM in stools from a gastroenteritis outbreak in a primary school in Ditchling, England [4]; (4) the "W" agent, which was detected in the stool of a volunteer who developed a gastrointestinal illness following oral administration of a specimen derived from a gastroenteritis outbreak in a boy's boarding school in England [12]; the Ditchling and W agents are related to one another but distinct from the Hawaii and Norwalk agents by IEM [4,40]; and (5) the cockle agent which, as the name suggests, was detected by EM in stools from individuals who developed gastroenteritis following ingestion of cockles [5]; the cockle agent is

Table 1 Characteristics of Norwalk, Norwalk-like, and Possibly Related Agents Associated with Acute Epidemic Nonbacterial Gastroenteritis in Humans

Agent	Size (nm)	Buoyant density in cesium chloride (g/cm³)	Growth in cell culture	Administration of agent induces illness in: Humans	Animal(s)	Particle detected by	Serologic studies by	Antigenic relationships
Norwalk [16,17,32,41, 42,44,72]	27 X 32[a]	1.38–1.41	No	Yes	No	IEM[b]	IEM RIA IAHA	Distinct
Hawaii [18,44,68,71]	26 X 29[a]	1.37–1.39	No	Yes	No	IEM	IEM	Distinct
Montgomery County [44,68,71]	27 X 32[a]	1.37–1.41	No	Yes	No	IEM	IEM	Related to Norwalk agent by IEM and cross-challenge studies
Ditchling [4]	25–26	1.38–1.40	No	N.T.[c]	No	EM	IEM	Ditchling and W agents related to each other but appear to be distinct from Norwalk and Hawaii agents by IEM
W [4,12,40]	25–26	1.38–1.40	No	Yes	N.T.	EM	IEM	

Cockle [5]	25–26	1.40	No	N.T.	N.T.	EM	IEM	Appears to be distinct from Norwalk agent by IEM
Parramatta [11]	23–26	N.T.	No	N.T.	N.T.	EM	IEM	Distinct from Norwalk agent by IEM
Colorado[f] [53,57,77]	27–32	N.T.	No	Yes	N.T.	IEM	IEM	Distinct from Norwalk, Hawaii, and Marin County agents by IEM (and from Norwalk by RIA using Norwalk antigen[e])
Marin County [57]	27	N.T.	No	?[g]	No[g]	IEM	IEM	Distinct from Norwalk, Hawaii, and Colorado agents by IEM or RIA[e]

[a]Shortest X longest diameter.
[b]Immune electron microscopy.
[c]N.T. = not tested.
[d]By alimentary route.
[e]Greenberg et al., unpublished studies.
[f]Now designated Snow Mountain Agent [57,77].
[g]From H. B. Greenberg, N. Singh, L. Oshior, W. T. London, and D. L. Sly, unpublished studies.
Source: From Ref. 43 with additions.

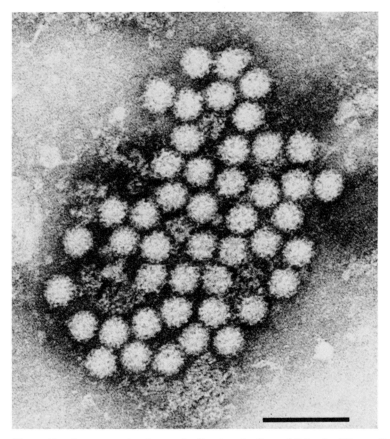

Figure 1 An aggregate observed after incubation of 0.8 ml of Norwalk (8FIIa) stool filtrate with 0.2 ml of a 1:5 dilution of prechallenge serum of a volunteer and further preparation for electron microscopy. The quantity of antibody on these particles was rated as 1+. The bar = 100 μm. (From Ref. 44.)

distinct from the Norwalk virus, but its relationship to the other agents is inconclusive [5].

Some further properties of two of these agents have been determined by studying the infectivity in volunteers of stool filtrates treated in various ways: the Norwalk agent was found to be acid stable and relatively heat stable, and both the Norwalk and the W agents were ether stable [12,16]. The term *parvo-virus-like* was suggested for the Norwalk group since they shared certain properties with the parvoviruses, such as morphology, ether, acid, and relative heat stability, and density in cesium chloride [16,41,44]. However, this classification was quite tentative since the nucleic acid content of the Norwalk agent was not

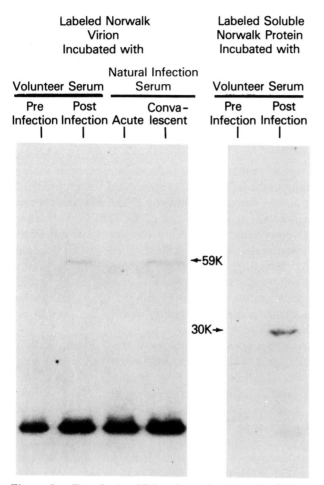

Figure 2 Tris-glycine-SDS polyacrylamide gel of Norwalk virion and soluble protein. Purified iodinated virion and soluble protein were incubated overnight with indicated serum, and the immune complex was precipitated with *Staphylococcus aureus A*. The resulting precipitate was dissociated and run on the gel as shown. Marker proteins (not shown) were run on the same gel for molecular weight estimates. (From Ref. 28.)

known. Recently the proteins of the Norwalk virion have been studied following purification of Norwalk antigens from fecal specimens obtained from volunteers who developed illness following Norwalk challenge [28,30]. Norwalk antigen activity was detected in the feces in both soluble and virion-associated forms. Purified virions and soluble proteins were iodinated and then specifically immunoprecipitated by Norwalk convalescent human sera; immunoprecipitation with preinfection and nonimmune serum was employed as the control. The dissociated immunoprecipitates were examined on polyacrylamide gels. As shown in Fig. 2, a single virion-associated protein with a molecular weight of 59,000 daltons and a single soluble protein with a molecular weight of 30,000 daltons were detected. It is noteworthy that among mammalian viruses in this size range only the caliciviruses possess a single structural protein of about 65,000 daltons [9,60,60a]. However, it should be noted that in some calicivirus preparations a small virion-associated protein with a molecular weight of about 15,000 has been described, and in addition, a 29,000 molecular weight, nonstructural virus-associated protein has been detected in calicivirus-infected cells [9,60,60a]. Moreover, as seen in Fig. 1, the Norwalk agent bears some resemblance morphologically to the caliciviruses, as observed in this preparation in which particles are only lightly coated with antibody [30,36,49]; there is a suggestion of small cuplike indentations on the surface of the Norwalk particle similar to but not nearly as pronounced as those observed on classic caliciviruses [28,30,49]. Perhaps in preparation without antibody these surface structures would be better defined. Thus, there is suggestive evidence that the Norwalk virus may indeed be a calicivirus. Moreover, recently several groups have described gastroenteritis outbreaks associated with calicivirus-like particles [10, 50,64]. Additional studies are needed to definitely classify the Norwalk and Norwalk-like viruses.

Table 1 also shows other potential members of the Norwalk family of agents: (1) the Parramatta agent, which was derived from a gastroenteritis outbreak in a primary school in Australia [11]; (2) the Marin County agent, which was derived from a gastroenteritis outbreak in elderly patients in a California convalescent home and which by IEM and/or radioimmunoassay (RIA) appears to be distinct from Norwalk, Hawaii, and Colorado agents [57]; and (3) the Colorado agent, which was associated with a waterborne outbreak of gastroenteritis in a resort camp and which appears to be distinct from Norwalk, Hawaii, and Marin County agents by IEM and/or RIA (Greenberg et al., unpublished studies) [53,57,77]. The Parramatta and Marin County agents were observed readily by EM and IEM, respectively [11,57]; the Colorado agent was observed by IEM and appeared to be present in low titer [53,77]. There is no information on the density of these three agents.

The Norwalk virus has also been administered to numerous animals, including mice, guinea pigs, rabbits, kittens, calves, baboons, chimpanzees, and various types of monkeys; none of these animals developed illness (Refs. 45, 73; Wyatt et al., unpublished studies). However, chimpanzees became infected, as they not only developed a seroresponse as demonstrated by IEM, immune adherence hemagglutination assay (IAHA), and RIA, but also shed Norwalk antigen as detected by RIA [32,40,42,72].

There is compelling evidence for the etiologic role of the Norwalk virus in viral gastroenteritis. For example, 30 of 52 volunteers (58%) challenged with

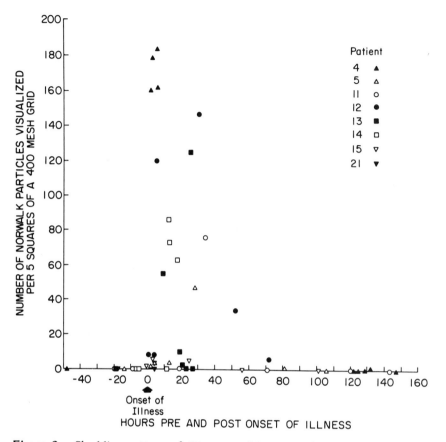

Figure 3 Shedding pattern of 27 nm particles in stool specimens from eight individuals experimentally infected with Norwalk agent. (From Ref. 67.)

this agent not only developed illness but also most of a sample of those who have been tested have developed serologic evidence of infection [27,32,42,44, 71]. In addition, certain individuals from the original Norwalk outbreak also developed seroresponses [44]. Additional evidence for an etiologic association was obtained when the shedding pattern of the Norwalk virus was studied in volunteers who developed illness following Norwalk virus challenge [67]. Figure 3 shows that the Norwalk virus was not observed prior to the onset of illness, whereas it was detected maximally around the onset of illness and only infrequently after 72 h following onset. Thus, the temporal pattern of virus shedding coincided closely with the presence of clinical manifestations. In later studies, Norwalk virus was also detected in vomitus from certain volunteers who developed illness following Norwalk challenge [31]. Illness has also been induced in volunteers inoculated with the Hawaii, MC, W, and Colorado agents [18,53,68,

71]. Serologic responses were documented in volunteers challenged with Hawaii and MC agents [18,68]. In addition, homologous IEM responses have been observed in most individuals who developed illness associated with the Parramatta and Marin County agents [11,57].

Epidemiology

The Norwalk virus has been the most thoroughly studied member of this group of agents since the development of both an IAHA and RIA has enabled large-scale seroepidemiologic studies. Thus, with one or both of these techniques, the prevalence of Norwalk antibody in the United States and abroad has been studied. The acquisition of Norwalk virus and rotavirus antibody was compared in pediatric, college, and adult age groups in the metropolitan Washington, D.C. area [42]. As shown in Fig. 4, the pattern of IAHA antibody acquisition was strikingly different for the two viruses. Norwalk antibody was acquired gradually beginning slowly in childhood and accelerating in adult years so that by the fifth decade of life, 50% of the individuals studied possessed Norwalk antibody. The acquisition of rotavirus antibody was in sharp contrast, as over 90% of the children had already acquired such antibody by the age of 36 months. This pattern of acquisition of Norwalk antibody was similar to that observed with hepatitis A and certain rhinovirus serotypes in similar populations [33,65,66]. The relative absence of Norwalk antibody in the pediatric age group is consistent with the view that the Norwalk virus is not an important cause of severe gastroenteritis in infants and young children, at least in the United States [8,42].

The prevalence of Norwalk antibody has also been studied in individuals from various parts of the world by an RIA blocking technique (Fig. 5) [29]. The prevalence of Norwalk antibody in adults in the United States and certain European and less developed countries was comparable, as at least a majority of those studied from each country had such antibody. It was of interest that one group of highly isolated Ecuadorian Indians in Gabaro lacked antibody to Norwalk virus, whereas most inhabitants of three less isolated Ecuadorian villages had such antibody. The prevalence of Norwalk virus antibody in adult male and female homosexuals was similar to that observed in other adults in the United States [29].

The prevalence of antibody to the Norwalk agent was also studied by the RIA blocking technique in children from various parts of the world [29]. As shown in Fig. 6, children in the United States and Yugoslavia acquired antibody more slowly than did children in the less developed countries of Ecuador and Bangladesh. It was of interest that children in the isolated village of Gabaro also lacked Norwalk virus antibody. The high prevalence of Norwalk antibody in children in Bangladesh and Ecuador was not anticipated and may indicate that the Norwalk or an antigenically related virus infects children early in life in these

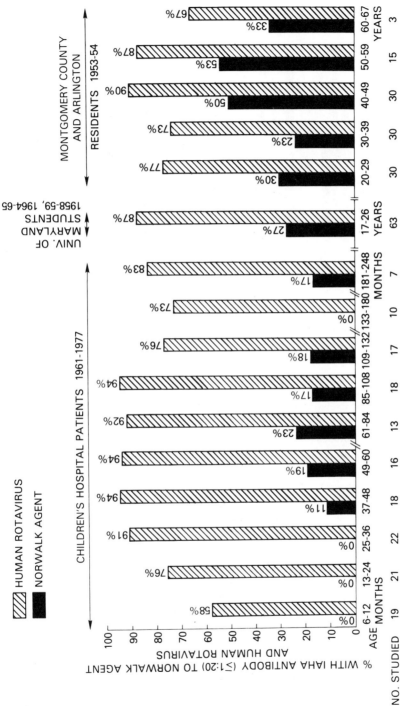

Figure 4 Prevalence of antibody to Norwalk agent and rotavirus by IAHA in three groups. (From Ref. 42.)

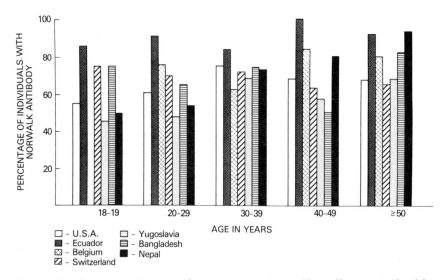

Figure 5 Prevalence by age of serum antibody to Norwalk virus in healthy adults from various parts of the world. Note that no specimens were tested in the 18 to 29 year age group of Belgians. (From Ref. 29.)

less developed countries. It should be stressed however, that the importance of the Norwalk or related virus in the etiology of infantile gastroenteritis in less developed countries has not yet been determined.

The prevalence of Norwalk antibody in Crohn's disease patients and in controls was studied by the RIA blocking technique. No significant differences in Norwalk antibody prevalence or in Norwalk antibody titers were observed between the test and control groups [26].

As noted before, the Norwalk group of viruses is associated with outbreaks of viral gastroenteritis occurring in families, schools, institutions, and communities, affecting adults, school-age children, family contacts, and some young children as well. Examination of the various outbreaks from which the Norwalk group and potential members of this group were detected serves to demonstrate clearly the setting which may yield these agents. The Norwalk agent was derived from an explosive outbreak of gastroenteritis in an elementary school in which 50% (116 of 232) of the students and teachers became ill, with the majority of the cases occurring within a 24 h period [1]. Although a common source exposure from well water was suspected, this could not be confirmed. Secondary cases were common as they occurred in 32% of the family contacts of primary cases. The W agent was derived from a gastroenteritis outbreak in a boys' boarding school which affected about 200 of the 830 pupils

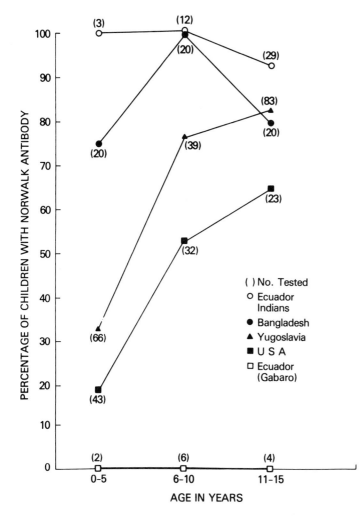

Figure 6 Age-related prevalence of serum antibody to Norwalk virus in children from various countreis. (From Ref. 29.)

(24%) in a period of less than 1 week [12]. Similarly, the Ditchling agent was derived from an outbreak of gastroenteritis in a primary school in Ditchling, England in which 33 of 138 individuals (24%) developed the illness in less than 1 week [4]. The Parramatta agent was also derived from a primary school outbreak which affected 207 of 381 children (54%), as well as 9 of 18 teachers in a period of about 1 month in Sydney, Australia [11].

Table 2 Epidemiologic Characteristics of 24 Norwalk Virus-Associated Gastroenteritis Outbreaks*

Location or source of outbreak	No. of outbreaks	Month of occurrence	Age range of affected individuals
Recreational camps	4	March, June August, November	Children (4–15 years) and adults
Cruise ships	4	January, April	Adults
Contaminated drinking or swimming water	4	May, July (2), October	Children (> 4 years) and young adults
Community or family	4	February, June, August, December	Children and adults
School (elementary or college)	3	May, October, November	Children and young adults
Nursing homes	2	November, April	Elderly adults
Shellfish	1	June (Australia)	All ages
Other	2	August?	Adults

*Clinical characteristics consisted of mild to moderate nausea, vomiting, diarrhea, or a combination.
Source: Adapted from Ref. [30].

The Hawaii and MC viruses were derived from family outbreaks of gastroenteritis [68,71]. The Hawaii outbreak involved both parents, a 2½-year-old child, and a student who lived with the family, all within a 4 day period. The MC agent involved both parents and two children, ages 4 and 5 years, all within a 7 day period.

As the name suggests, the cockle agent was derived from two outbreaks of gastroenteritis which affected groups of individuals within 24-30 h after ingestion of cockles [5]. It is noteworthy that recently a large outbreak of gastroenteritis involving more than 2000 persons has been associated with the ingestion of oysters in several Australian states [54-56]. Infection with the Norwalk virus has been demonstrated in certain individuals from the Australian outbreak.

Elderly patients also appear to be susceptible to these agents, as the Marin County virus was derived from a gastroenteritis outbreak in a convalescent home in Marin County, California affecting 51% of 187 residents and 12 of 180 employees [57]. Two of the elderly residents who had developed mild diarrhea died during the outbreak of causes apparently unrelated to the outbreak.

A contaminated water supply was suspected as the cause of the outbreak associated with the Colorado agent [53]. This outbreak occurred in a resort camp in Colorado affecting 418 of 760 individuals (55%). Secondary cases were recorded in 11% (82 of 772) of household contacts of ill individuals.

With the development of an RIA for the Norwalk agent, it has been possible to study the role of this virus in numerous outbreaks of viral gastroenteritis [30,32]. Paired sera from 70 such outbreaks have now been studied by this technique; 24 of the 70 (34%) have been found to be associated with the Norwalk agent. The diversity of outbreaks is shown in Table 2. Several of the outbreaks appear to be related to a common source. It is striking that 9 of 23 outbreaks occurred during the warmer months of the year. In addition, the high proportion of outbreaks associated with the Norwalk virus suggests that the number of serologically distinct epidemic gastroenteritis agents may be limited. When practical serologic assays are developed for the other members or potential members of the Norwalk group, it may well be that the majority of such outbreaks could then be associated with an infectious agent.

Pathogenesis

The pathogenesis of Norwalk and Hawaii-induced illness has been studied in volunteers [2,18,61,62]. Acute infection results in a histopathological lesion in the jejunum. By light microscopy, there is broadening and blunting of the villi of the proximal small intestine (Fig. 7). The mucosa itself is histologically intact. Mononuclear cell infiltration and cytoplasmic vacuolization have also been observed. By transmission EM, the epithelial cells are intact but the microvilli appear shortened. Convalescent-phase biopsies are normal. The extent of small intestinal involvement is not known, since studies have included only the proximal small intestine. Histologic lesions were not reported in the gastric fundus, antrum, or colonic mucosa of volunteers with Norwalk virus-induced illness [70]. The gastric emptying of liquids was recently studied in volunteers challenged with the Norwalk or Hawaii agents [51]. Volunteers who developed illness and/or the characteristic intestinal mucosal lesion observed with gastroenteritis associated with these agents demonstrated marked delays in gastric emptying. It was suggested that the nausea and vomiting associated with this form of viral gastroenteritis could be a result of the abnormal gastric motor function. Brush-border small intestinal enzyme studies (including alkaline phosphatase, sucrase, and trehalase) were decreased in comparison to baseline and convalescent-phase values [2]; jejunal adenylate cyclase activity was not elevated [47]. Interferon could not be detected in sera, jejunal aspirates, and jejunal biopsy specimens of volunteers challenged with either of these two viral agents [78].

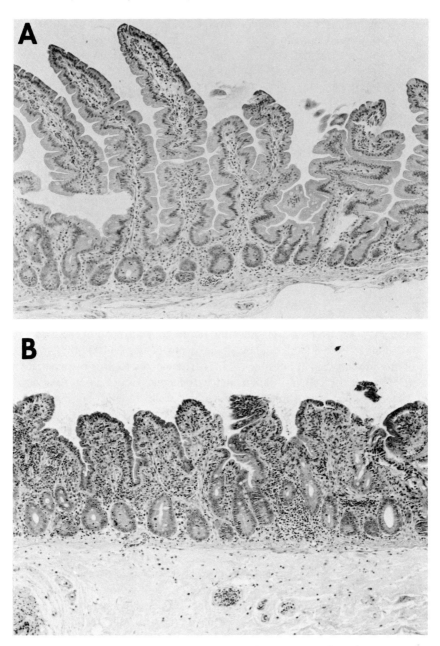

Figure 7 (A) Normal-appearing jejunal tissue from biopsy of a volunteer prior to challenge with Norwalk agent. (Hematoxylin and eosin, X 100). (B) Broadened and flattened villi in jejunal biopsy tissue from same volunteer during illness with Norwalk-induced gastroenteritis. (Hematoxylin and eosin, X 100). (From Ref. 2.)

Immunity

An understanding of the nature of immunity to this group of viruses remains one of the most perplexing aspects in the study of these agents. Volunteer studies have demonstrated that there are two forms of immunity to Norwalk virus-induced illness: one is short term and the other, long term [16,58,71]. Short-term homologous immunity was described in early studies when volunteers who had developed illness following an initial Norwalk virus challenge failed to become ill on rechallenge with the same inoculum 6--14 weeks later [16,71]. A series of volunteer studies later clearly demonstrated some of the complexities of immunity—especially long-term—to this agent [58]. Twelve volunteers were administered the Norwalk virus orally on two separate occasions 27-42 months apart, and 4 were challenged a third time with the same inoculum 4-8 weeks after the second study. As shown in Fig. 8, each of the 6 volunteers who became ill after initial challenge also developed illness following the second challenge. In contrast, however, 6 volunteers failed to develop illness following both initial and second challenges. In addition, 4 of the 6 volunteers who had developed illness following each of the two challenges were rechallenged a third time 4-8 weeks after the second inoculation and only one of them developed illness. The pre- and postchallenge serum antibody status of

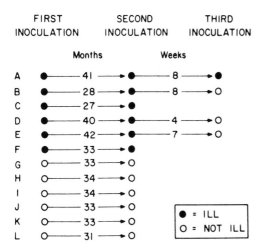

Figure 8 Sequence of Norwalk agent inoculation studies in 12 volunteers who are shown individually by an alphabetic letter. The numbers indicate the months or weeks between inoculations. The filled circles represent volunteers who experienced clinical illness, and the open circles those in whom clinical illness failed to develop. (From Ref. 58.)

Table 3 Level of Antibody to Norwalk Virus Prior to
Inoculation of Volunteers

Response of volunteers to oral administration of Norwalk virus	No. of volunteers	Geometric mean preinoculation antibody titer[a] (reciprocal)	
		Serum	Jejunal fluid
Diarrheal illness	11	291	53[b]
No illness	12	178	9[c]

[a]Measured by radioimmunoassay blocking technique.
[b]Only 7 of 11 volunteers tested successfully.
[c]Only 8 of 12 volunteers tested successfully.
Note: Jejunal Norwalk antibody titers standardized to 20 mg% IgA.
Source: From Ref. [30].

most of these volunteers were studied by IEM in an attempt to elucidate the role of serum antibody on susceptibility or resistance to Norwalk-induced illness. Such studies revealed that 4 of 5 volunteers who became ill after each of the first two challenges developed a seroresponse after the first challenge, lost most if not all such antibody in the interval prior to the second challenge, and had a marked antibody increase after the second challenge. However, the fifth volunteer in this group possessed a high level of antibody before and after each of the two challenges. Each of the 4 volunteers challenged a third time (only one developed illness following this inoculation) had high levels of antibody prior to and after this challenge. Paradoxically, antibody studies on sera from 3 of the volunteers who did not become ill following either of two challenges indicated that each had little, if any, Norwalk antibody prior to and after each of the inoculations. Thus, there was a clear lack of correlation between the level of prechallenge Norwalk antibody and susceptibility to illness following Norwalk challenge. One explanation for this might be that local intestinal antibody rather than circulating serum antibody is the prime determinant of resistance. However, this explanation seems rather unlikely since it requires the existence of at least two cohorts of individuals, one able and the other unable to produce sufficient local antibody for long-term protection. Another explanation would involve genetic mechanism(s) which govern susceptibility to Norwalk infection. For example, individuals refractory to Norwalk infection may lack a genetically specific receptor for this virus in epithelial cells in the small intestine [58].

The role of local intestinal Norwalk antibody and circulating serum Norwalk antibody on resistance to Norwalk virus infection was recently evaluated with the RIA blocking technique [30]. Prechallenge serum and local jejunal blocking antibody levels in another group of 23 volunteers challenged with Norwalk virus were studied (Table 3). It was striking that the 11 volunteers who developed illness had significantly greater geometric mean antibody titers in jejunal fluid than did the 12 who failed to develop illness. In addition, the geometric mean serum antibody titer of the volunteers who developed illness tended to be higher than that of the group who did not develop illness. A similar paradoxical relationship between prechallenge serum RIA antibody level and susceptibility to illness following Norwalk challenge has been described in additional volunteer studies [6]. Thus, both serum and local intestinal antibody failed to correlate with resistance to Norwalk challenge. The specific role of Norwalk IgA intestinal antibody has not been evaluated, but future studies in this regard should prove important.

Clinical Manifestations

The clinical manifestations in the original Norwalk outbreak were similar but not identical to those observed in the subsequent volunteer studies. The clinical characteristics observed in the 604 primary or secondary cases in the Norwalk, Ohio outbreak were tabulated as follows: 85% had nausea, 84% vomiting, 62% abdominal cramps, 57% lethargy, 44% diarrhea, 32% fever, and 5% chills. The illnesses were self-limited, as symptoms lasted 12-24 h and none of the patients had to be hospitalized. The mean incubation period was 48 h.

Clinical characteristics observed in 31 (of 52) volunteers who developed definite or probable illness following Norwalk virus challenge included fever $\geq$ 99.4°F in 45%, diarrhea in 81%, vomiting in 65%, abdominal discomfort in 68%, anorexia in 90%, headache in 81%, and myalgias in 58% [71]. The incubation period was 10-51 h. Illnesses were generally mild and self-limited and usually lasted 24-48 h; however, one volunteer vomited about 20 times within a 24 h period and required parenteral fluid therapy [17]. Characteristically, the diarrheal stools are not bloody, lack mucus, and do not contain leukocytes [15, 19,34]. A transient lymphopenia was observed in 14 of 16 ill volunteers challenged with Norwalk or Hawaii agents [19]. Figure 9 graphically demonstrates the clinical characteristics observed in two volunteers challenged with the same Norwalk inoculum [17]. A striking difference in clinical manifestations was observed, as one volunteer had an illness characterized by vomiting without diarrhea and the other had diarrhea without vomiting. As noted previously, studies by IEM revealed that virus shedding was maximal around the onset of illness and occurred only infrequently after 72 h following onset [67]. Illnesses induced in volunteers with the Hawaii, MC, and W agents appear clinically indistinguishable from those observed with the Norwalk virus [12,72]. Similarly, naturally occurring illnesses with each of the viruses in the Norwalk group are not distinguishable clinically.

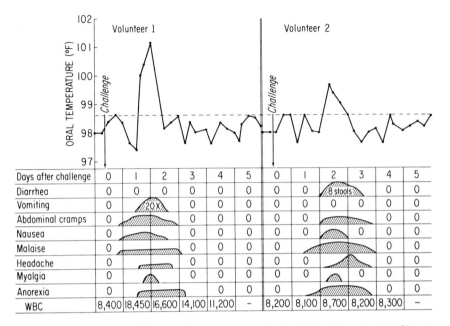

Days after challenge	0	1	2	3	4	5	0	1	2	3	4	5
Diarrhea	0	0	0	0	0	0	0	0	8 stools	0	0	
Vomiting	0	20X	0	0	0	0	0	0	0	0	0	0
Abdominal cramps	0		0	0	0	0	0	0		0	0	
Nausea	0		0	0	0	0	0	0		0	0	0
Malaise	0		0	0	0	0	0			0	0	
Headache	0		0	0	0	0	0	0		0	0	
Myalgia	0		0	0	0	0	0	0		0	0	
Anorexia	0			0	0	0	0			0	0	
WBC	8,400	18,450	16,600	14,100	11,200	–	8,200	8,100	8,700	8,200	8,300	–

Figure 9   Response of two volunteers to oral administration of stool filtrate derived from volunteer who received original Norwalk rectal swab specimen. The height of the curve is directly proportional to the severity of the sign or symptom. Volunteer 1 had severe vomiting without diarrhea, while volunteer 2 had diarrhea without vomiting, although both received the same inoculum. (From Ref. 17.)

Diagnosis

It is not possible to make a specific diagnosis of infection with the Norwalk group on the basis of patients' clinical manifestations. Unfortunately, establishing a specific diagnosis is still a research procedure, since none of these agents grows in cell culture or in a convenient laboratory animal model. Various methods which may be employed in the diagnosis of infection with this group of agents include: (1) EM and IEM for the entire group; (2) RIA for the Norwalk virus; and (3) IAHA for the Norwalk virus.

Electron Microscopy and Immune Electron Microscopy

None of the members of this group are distinctive enough morphologically to enable their identification by EM, although direct examination of negatively stained stool material with or without prior concentration may be useful in detecting the particles, in general. The Ditchling, W, and cockle agents were

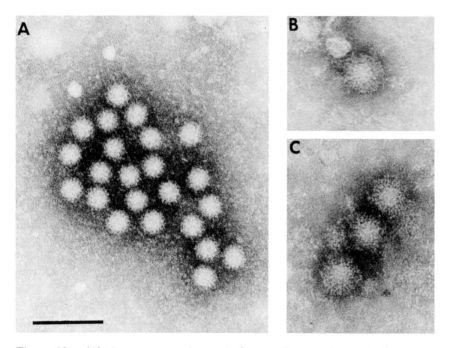

Figure 10   (A) An aggregate observed after incubation of 0.8 ml of Norwalk (8FIIa) stool filtrate with 0.2 ml of a 1:5 dilution of a volunteer's prechallenge serum and further preparation for electron microscopy. This volunteer developed gastroenteritis following challenge with a second-passage Norwalk filtrate which had been heated for 30 min at 60°C [16]. The quantity of antibody on the particles in this aggregate was rated 1-2-2+, and this prechallenge serum was given an overall rating of 1-2+. (B) A single particle, and (C) three single particles observed after incubating 0.8 ml of the Norwalk (8FIIa) stool filtrate with 0.2 ml of a 1:5 dilution of the volunteer's postchallenge convalescent serum and further preparation for EM. These particles are very heavily coated with antibody. The quantity of antibody on these particles was rated 4+, and the serum was also given an overall rating of 4+. The difference in the quantity of antibody coating the particles in the prechallenge and postchallenge sera of this volunteer is clearly evident. The bar = 100 nm and applies to A, B, and C. (From Ref. 40.)

observed initially after concentration by ultracentrifugation, density gradient centrifugation in cesium chloride, and further preparation for negative-stain electron microscopy [4,5]. However, IEM remains the most important procedure for specific identification of members of this group as a whole. This technique, which has been defined as the direct examination of antigen-antibody interaction by EM [3], is essential for the identification of this group of agents since stools contain numerous objects of about the same size as the members of this group. However, in IEM studies in which specific paired sera are employed, the significance of the particles observed may be determined. For example, Fig. 10 shows Norwalk particles following incubation with a pre- or postchallenge serum obtained from a volunteer who developed illness after Norwalk challenge [40]. The heavy antibody coating observed on the particles following incubation with the convalescent serum and further preparation for EM can be readily observed; comparison of the amount of antibody on the particles incubated with the prechallenge serum indicates that this volunteer developed a specific serum response to the particle. Studies of this type should be performed under code with appropriate paired sera to help establish the significance of particles observed in stools. It should be noted that simple aggregation of particles following incubation with serum and further preparation for EM should not be considered as indicative of a specific response, since certain particles such as the Norwalk agent aggregate spontaneously without the addition of serum. It is therefore essential to evaluate the amount of antibody coating the particles, even if they are aggregated. The significance of aggregation may be resolved by varying the dilutions of antigen or antibody to determine if aggregate size and amount of antibody coating the particles change as the reaction goes from antigen excess to antibody excess. Once the significance of an antigen has been established, IEM studies can be carried out to detect serologic evidence of infection in further tests with paired sera [39].

Radioimmunoassay

The RIA for detection of Norwalk virus appears to be more efficient than IEM [27,32]. The RIA is able to detect not only particulate but soluble antigens as well. This test is dependent on the availability of high-titered convalescent-phase Norwalk antiserum and antibody-negative preinfection Norwalk serum from the same source [32]. The second antibody is an IgG fraction of convalescent phase Norwalk serum which has been radioiodinated with ^{125}I. The RIA is based on the differential binding of Norwalk-positive stools to microtiter wells coated with either a convalescent-phase or a preinfection serum. Thus, nonspecific reactions between the infection serum and the stool material can be distinguished from the specific Norwalk antigen binding. The ratio of counts bound to wells coated with convalescent serum to that with preinfection serum is used to measure Norwalk antigen activity. A positive over negative (P/N) ratio equal to or greater than 2 is considered diagnostic for Norwalk antigen activity. A schematic presentation of the principle of the Norwalk RIA for antigenic detection is shown in Fig. 11 [32,45].

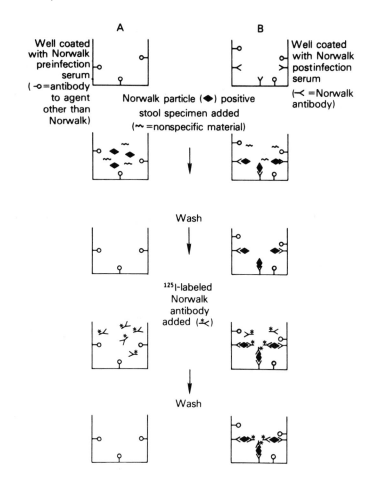

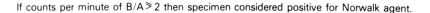
If counts per minute of B/A ≥ 2 then specimen considered positive for Norwalk agent.

Figure 11 Radioimmunoassay for Norwalk antigen detection. (From Ref. 45.)

The RIA test has been modified to detect Norwalk antibody [27,32]. This test is highly sensitive and specific and is at least as efficient as IEM for detecting serologic responses. However, it has the advantage of being more practical and thus enables the study of a larger number of specimens for epidemiologic studies. It is dependent on the availability of high-titered convalescent-phase Norwalk antiserum, the IgG fraction of convalescent-phase Norwalk serum iodinated

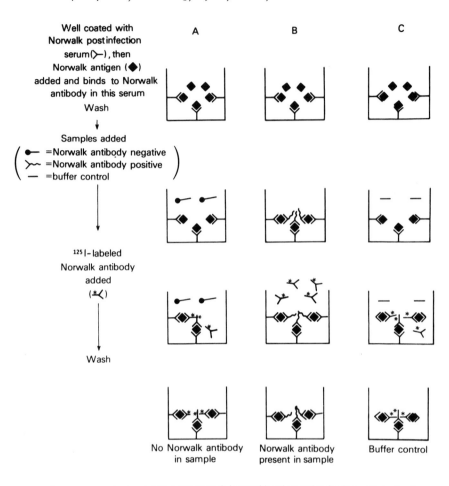

Well coated with
Norwalk postinfection
serum (>—), then
Norwalk antigen (◆)
added and binds to Norwalk
antibody in this serum
Wash

Samples added
(●— =Norwalk antibody negative
  >~ =Norwalk antibody positive
  — =buffer control)

125 I - labeled
Norwalk antibody
added
(*✓)

Wash

No Norwalk antibody
in sample

Norwalk antibody
present in sample

Buffer control

If counts per minute of A/C >0.5, then A is considered negative for Norwalk antibody.
If counts per minute of B/C ≤ 0.5, then B is considered positive for Norwalk antibody.

Figure 12 Blocking radioimmunoassay for Norwalk antibody measurement.
(From Ref. 45.)

with ^{125}I, and Norwalk antigen in the form of a partially purified preparation
or a crude stool suspension. This assay is based on the ability of a test serum to
block the binding of the ^{125}I-labeled IgG fraction of convalescent-phase Norwalk serum to the Norwalk antigen attached to the precoat on the solid phase.
A reduction of 50% in residual-bound radioactivity produced by a serum as compared to a buffer control is considered to be diagnostic for Norwalk antibody. A
schematic presentation of the RIA blocking test is shown in Fig. 12 [45].

Immune Adherence Hemagglutination Assay

The development of an IAHA for Norwalk virus has also enabled serologic studies of large numbers of specimens [42]. This assay was quite efficient for detecting serologic responses, but IEM and RIA were slightly more efficient. In addition, the IAHA was not able to be used successfully for detecting Norwalk antigen in stools, although relatively high-titered, purified virus could be detected. Although this test is very practical for large-scale epidemiologic studies, it has the disadvantage of requiring relatively purified and high-titered antigen. In addition, it requires considerably more antigen than the RIA. This is of practical importance, since the source of Norwalk antigen is not only limited but also, high-titered Norwalk virus-containing stools are found under natural conditions only rarely. It should also be noted that it may be necessary to screen various donors' red blood cells before finding one that reacts effectively in the IAHA, since not all human group O red blood cells react comparably in the IAHA. The procedure for this test has been described in detail elsewhere [42].

Treatment

Illnesses associated with the Norwalk group are generally self-limited and mild and characteristically resolve without sequelae [4,5,11,12,16,17,53,57,68,71]. Characteristically, oral fluid and replacement therapy with isotonic liquids is adequate to replace fluid loss. Parenteral fluid therapy may be necessary if severe vomiting or diarrhea occur. The role of this group of agents in debilitated hosts has not been studied extensively. However, it is obvious that clinical manifestations associated with these agents in such a host could lead to more severe sequelae.

Recently, the therapeutic effect of bismuth subsalicylate on experimentally induced Norwalk gastroenteritis was evaluated in a controlled double-blind study [63]. Volunteers who developed illness after challenge were administered either the test product or a placebo. Abdominal cramps were found to be significantly less severe and of significantly shorter duration in the group treated with bismuth subsalicylate; the median duration of gastrointestinal symptoms was also significantly shorter (14 h versus 20 h). However, the number, weight, and water content of stools, as well as the rate of viral excretion, did not differ between the test and control groups.

Control and Prevention

No methods are available for the prevention or control of infection and illness associated with the Norwalk group. In a family or group setting in which one member is ill with this form of gastroenteritis, effective hand washing and disposal or disinfection of contaminated material might limit the spread of this disease. In addition, increased awareness of the purity of drinking water or swimming pool water might also decrease the number of outbreaks. There are, as yet, many unanswered questions which hinder discussion of the development of methods of immunoprophylaxis for this group of agents. The number of serotypes of this group or the role of other agents in this form of epidemic gastroenteritis also needs to be determined. Of equal or even greater importance is the elucidation of the mechanism of immunity to this group of agents, especially in view of the suggestion that genetic factors may be of prime importance in susceptibility to Norwalk infection.

References

1. I. Adler and R. Zickl, Winter vomiting disease, *J. Infect. Dis., 119*:668–673 (1969).
2. S. G. Agus, R. Dolin, R. G. Wyatt, A. J. Tousimis, and R. S. Northrup, Acute infectious nonbacterial gastroenteritis: Intestinal histopathology. Histologic and enzymatic alterations during illness produced by the Norwalk agent in man, *Ann. Intern. Med., 79*:18–25 (1973).
3. J. D. Almeida and A. P. Waterson, The morphology of virus-antibody interaction, *Adv. Virus Res., 15*:307–338 (1969).
4. H. Appleton, M. Buckley, B. T. Thom, J. L. Cotton, and S. Henderson, Virus-like particles in winter vomiting disease, *Lancet 1*:409–411 (1977).
5. H. Appleton and M. S. Pereira, A possible virus etiology in outbreaks of food poisoning from cockles, *Lancet, 1*:780–781 (1977).
6. N. R. Blacklow, G. Cukor, M. K. Bedigian, P. Echeverria, H. B. Greenberg, D. S. Schreiber, and J. S. Trier, Immunoresponse and prevalence of antibody to Norwalk enteritis virus as determined by radioimmunoassay, *J. Clin. Microbiol., 10*:903–909 (1979).
7. N. R. Blacklow, R. Dolin, D. S. Fedson, H. DuPont, R. S. Northrup, R. B. Hornick, and R. M. Chanock, Acute infectious nonbacterial gastroenteritis: Etiology and pathogenesis. A combined clinical staff conference at the Clinical Center of the National Institutes of Health, *Ann. Intern. Med., 76*:993–1008 (1972).
8. C. D. Brandt, H. W. Kim, R. H. Yolken, A. Z. Kapikian, J. O. Arrobio, W. J. Rodriguez, R. G. Wyatt, R. M. Chanock, and R. H. Parrott, Comparative epidemiology of two rotavirus serotypes and other viral agents associated with pediatric gastroenteritis, *Am. J. Epidemiol., 110*:243–254 (1979).
9. J. N. Burroughs and F. Brown, Presence of a covalently linked protein in calicivirus RNA, *J. Gen. Virol., 41*:443–446 (1978).
10. S. Chiba, Y. Sakuma, R. Kogasaka, M. Akihara, K. Horino, T. Nakao, and S. Fukui. An outbreak of gastroenteritis associated with calicivirus in an infant home. *J. Med. Virol., 4*:249–254 (1979).
11. P. J. Christopher, G. S. Grohmann, R. H. Millsom, and A. M. Murphy,

Parvovirus gastroenteritis—a new entity for Australia. *Med. J. Aust., 1*: 121–124 (1978).

12. S. K. R. Clarke, G. T. Cook, S. I. Egglestone, T. S. Hall, D. L. Miller, S. E. Reed, D. Rubenstein, A. J. Smith, and D. A. J. Tyrrell, A virus from epidemic vomiting disease, *Br. Med. J., 3*:86–89 (1972).

13. J. D. Connor and E. Barrett-Connor, Infectious diarrheas, *Pediatr. Clin. North Am., 14*:197–221 (1967).

14. H. J. Cramblett and C. M. F. Siewers, The etiology of gastroenteritis in infants and young children with emphasis on the occurrence of simultaneous mixed viral-bacterial infection, *Pediatrics, 35*:885–889 (1965).

15. R. Dolin, Norwalk-like agents of gastroenteritis. In *Principles and Practice of Infectious Diseases* (G. L. Mandell, R. G. Douglas, Jr., and H. J. F. Bennett, eds.), J. Wiley and Sons, New York, 1979, pp. 1364–1370.

16. R. Dolin, N. R. Blacklow, H. DuPont, R. F. Buscho, R. G. Wyatt, J. A. Kasel, R. Hornick, and R. M. Chanock, Biological properties of Norwalk agent of acute infectious nonbacterial gastroenteritis, *Proc. Soc. Exp. Biol. Med., 140*:578–583 (1972).

17. R. Dolin, N. R. Blacklow, H. DuPont, S. Formal, R. F. Buscho, J. A. Kasel, R. P. Chames, R. Hornick, and R. M. Chanock, Transmission of acute infectious nonbacterial gastroenteritis to volunteers by oral administration of stool filtrates, *J. Infect. Dis., 123*:307–312 (1971).

18. R. Dolin, A. G. Levy, R. G. Wyatt, T. S. Thornhill, and J. D. Gordon, Viral gastroenteritis induced by the Hawaii agent. Jejunal histopathology and seroresponse, *Am. J. Med., 39*:761–769 (1975).

19. R. Dolin, R. C. Reichmann, and A. S. Fauci, Lymphocyte populations in acute viral gastroenteritis, *Infect. Immun., 14*:422–428 (1976).

20. H. L. DuPont and R. B. Hornick, Clinical approach to infectious diarrheas, *Medicine, 52*:265–270 (1973).

21. H. Fukumi, R. Nakaya, S. Hatta, H. Noriki, H. Yunoki, K. Akagi, T. Saito, K. Uchiyama, K. Kobari, and R. Nakanishi, An indication as to identity between the infectious diarrhea in Japan and the afebrile infectious nonbacterial gastroenteritis by human volunteer experiments, *Jpn. J. Med. Sci. Biol. 10*:1–17 (1957).

22. I. Gordon, H. S. Ingraham, and R. F. Korns, Transmission of epidemic gastroenteritis to human volunteers by oral administration of fecal filtrates, *J. Exp. Med., 86*:409–422 (1947).

23. I. Gordon, H. S. Ingraham, R. F. Korns, and R. E. Trussel, Gastroenteritis in man due to a filtrable agent, N.Y. State J. Med., *49:1918–1920 (1949)*.

24. I. Gordon, J. K. Meneely, Jr., G. D. Currie, and A. Chicone, Clinical laboratory studies in experimentally-induced epidemic nonbacterial gastroenteritis, *J. Lab. Clin. Med., 41*:133–141 (1953).

25. I. Gordon, P. R. Patterson, and E. Whitney, Immunity in volunteers recovered from nonbacterial gastroenteritis, *J. Clin. Invest., 35*:200–205 (1956).

26. H. B. Greenberg, R. L. Gebhard, C. J. McClain, R. D. Soltis, and A. Z.

Kapikian, Antibodies to viral gastroenteritis viruses in Crohn's disease, *Gastroenterology, 76*:349–350 (1979).

27. H. B. Greenberg and A. Z. Kapikian, Detection of Norwalk agent antibody and antigen by solid-phase radioimmunoassay and immune adherence hemagglutination assay, *J. Am. Vet. Med. Assoc., 173*:620–623 (1978).

28. H. B. Greenberg, J. Valdesuso, A. R. Kalica, R. G. Wyatt, V. J. McAuliffe, A. Z. Kapikian, and R. M. Chanock, Proteins of Norwalk virus, *J. Virol., 37*:994–999 (1981).

29. H. B. Greenberg, J. Valdesuso, A. Z. Kapikian, R. M. Chanock, R. G. Wyatt, W. Szmuness, J. Larrick, J. Kaplan, R. H. Gilman, and D. A. Sack, Prevalence of antibody to the Norwalk virus in various countries. *Infect. Immun., 26*:270–273 (1979).

30. H. B. Greenberg, R. G. Wyatt, A. R. Kalica, R. H. Yolken, R. Black, A. Z. Kapikian, and R. M. Chanock, New insights in viral gastroenteritis, *Perspect. in Virol., 11*:163–187 (1981).

31. H. B. Greenberg, R. G. Wyatt, and A. Z. Kapikian, Norwalk virus in vomitus, *Lancet, 1*:55 (1979).

32. H. B. Greenberg, R. G. Wyatt, J. Valdesuso, A. R. Kalica, W. T. London, R. M. Chanock, and A. Z. Kapikian, Solid-phase microtiter radioimmunoassay for detection of the Norwalk strain of acute nonbacterial epidemic gastroenteritis virus and its antibodies, *J. Med. Virol., 2*:97–108 (1978).

33. J. M. Gwaltney, Jr., Medical reviews. Rhinoviruses, *Yale J. Biol. Med., 48*: 17–45 (1975).

34. J. C. Harris, H. L. DuPont, and R. B. Hornick, Fecal leukocytes in diarrheal illness, *Ann. Intern. Med., 76*:697–703 (1972).

35. H. L. Hodes, American Pediatric Society presidential address, *Pediatr. Res., 10*:201–204 (1976).

36. I. H. Holmes, Viral gastroenteritis, *Prog. Med. Virol., 25*:1–36 (1979).

37. W. S. Jordan, I. Gordon, and W. R. Dorrance, A study of illness in a group of Cleveland families. VII. Transmission of acute nonbacterial gastroenteritis to volunteers: Evidence for two different etiologic agents, *J. Exp. Med., 98*:461–475 (1933).

38. A. Z. Kapikian, Enteroviral diseases. In *Cecil Textbook of Medicine*, 14th ed. (P. B. Beeson, W. McDermott, and J. B. Wyngarrden, eds.), W. B. Saunders, Philadelphia, 1975, pp. 216–222.

39. A. Z. Kapikian, J. L. Deinstag, and R. H. Purcell, Immune electron microscopy as a method for the detection, identification, and characterization of agents not cultivable in an in vitro system. In *Manual of Clinical Immunology* (N. R. Rose and H. Friedman, eds.), American Society for Microbiology, Washington, D.C., 2d ed., 1980, pp. 70–83.

40. A. Z. Kapikian, S. M. Feinstone, R. H. Purcell, R. G. Wyatt, T. S. Thornhill, A. R. Kalica, and R. M. Chanock, Detection and identification by immune electron microscopy of fastidious agents associated with respiratory illness, acute nonbacterial gastroenteritis and hepatitis A, *Perspect. Virol., 9*:9–47 (1975).

41. A. Z. Kapikian, J. L. Gerin, R. G. Wyatt, T. S. Thornhill, and R. M. Chanock, Density in ceisum chloride of the 27 nm "8FIIa" particle associated with acute infectious nonbacterial gastroenteritis: Determination by ultracentrifugation and immune electron microscopy, *Proc. Soc. Exp. Biol. Med., 142*:874–877 (1974).
42. A. Z. Kapikian, H. B. Greenberg, W. L. Cline, A. R. Kalica, R. G. Wyatt, H. D. James, Jr., N. L. Lloyd, R. M. Chanock, R. W. Ryder, and H. W. Kim, Prevalence of antibody to the Norwalk agent by a newly developed immune adherence hemagglutination assay, *J. Med. Virol., 2*:281–294 (1978).
43. A. Z. Kapikian, H. B. Greenberg, R. G. Wyatt, A. R. Kalica, H. W. Kim, C. D. Brandt, W. J. Rodriguez, R. H. Parrott, and R. M. Chanock. Viral gastroenteritis. In *Viral Infections of Humans,* 2d ed. (A. S. Evans, ed.), Plenum, New York (in press).
44. A. Z. Kapikian, R. G. Wyatt, R. Dolin, T. S. Thornhill, A. R. Kalica, and R. M. Chanock, Visualization by immune electron microscopy of a 27 nm particle associated with acute infectious nonbacterial gastroenteritis, *J. Virol., 10*:1075–1081 (1972).
45. A. Z. Kapikian, R. H. Yolken, H. B. Greenberg, R. G. Wyatt, A. R. Kalica, R. M. Chanock, and H. W. Kim, Gastroenteritis viruses. In *Diagnostic Procedures for Viral, Rickettsial, and Chlamydial Infections,* 5th ed. (E. H. Lennette and N. J. Schmidt, eds.), American Public Health Association, Washington, D.C., 1979, pp. 927–995.
46. S. Kojima, H. Fukumi, H. Kusama, S. Yamamoto, S. Suzuki, T. Uchida, T. Ishimaru, T. Oka, K. Kuretani, K. Ohmura, F. Nishikawa, J. Fujimoto, K. Fujita, A. Nakano, and S. Sunakawa, Studies on the causative agent of the infectious diarrhea. Records of the experiments on human volunteers, *Jpn. Med. J., 1*:467–476 (1948).
47. A. G. Levy, L. Widerlite, P. R. Schwartz, R. Dolin, N. R. Blacklow, J. Gardner, D. V. Kimberg, and J. S. Trier, Jejunal adenylate cyclase activity in human subjects during viral gastroenteritis, *Gastroenterology, 70*:321–325 (1976).
48. J. L. Light and H. L. Hodes, Studies on epidemic diarrhea of the newborn: Isolation of a filtrable agent causing diarrhea in calves, *Am. J. Public Health, 33*:1451–1454 (1943).
49. R. Madeley, Comparison of the features of astroviruses and caliciviruses seen in samples of feces by electron microscopy, *J. Infect. Dis., 139*:519–523 (1979).
50. D. A. McSwiggan, D. Cubitt, and W. Moore, Calicivirus associated with winter vomiting disease, *Lancet, 1*, 1215 (1978).
51. J. C. Meeroff, D. S. Schreiber, J. S. Trier, and N. R. Blacklow, Abnormal gastric motor function in viral gastroenteritis, *Ann. Intern. Med., 92*:370–373 (1980).
52. H. L. Moffet, H. K. Shulenberger, and E. R. Burkholder, Epidemiology and etiology of severe infantile diarrhea, *J. Pediatr., 72*:1–14 (1978).
53. D. M. Morens, R. M. Zweighaft, T. M. Vernon, G. W. Gary, J. J. Eslien,

B. T. Wood, R. C. Holman, and R. Dolin, A waterborne outbreak of gastroenteritis with secondary person-to-person spread. Association with a viral agent, *Lancet, 1*:964–966 (1979).

54. A. M. Murphy, G. S. Grohmann, P. J. Christopher, W. A. Lopez, G. R. Davey, and R. H. Millsom, An Australia-wide outbreak of gastroenteritis from oysters caused by Norwalk virus, *Med. J. Aust., 2*:329–332 (1979).

55. A. M. Murphy, G. S. Grohmann, P. J. Christopher, W. A. Lopez, and R. H. Millsom, Oyster food poisoning, *Med. J. Aust., 2*:439 (1978).

56. A. M. Murphy, G. S. Grohmann, R. H. Millson, and A. M. Murphy, Parvovirus gastroenteritis—a new entity for Australia, *Med. J. Aust., 1*:121–124 (1978).

57. L. S. Oshiro, C. E. Haley, R. R. Roberto, J. L. Riggs, M. Croughan, H. B. Greenberg, and A. Z. Kapikian, A 27 nm virus isolated during an outbreak of acute infectious nonbacterial gastroenteritis in a convalescent home: A possible new serotype, *J. Infect. Dis., 143*:791–795 (1981).

58. T. A. Parrino, D. S. Schreiber, J. S. Trier, A. Z. Kapikian, and N. R. Blacklow, Clinical immunity in acute gastroenteritis caused by the Norwalk agent, *N. Engl. J. Med., 297*:86–89 (1977).

59. H. A. Reimann, A. H. Prince, and J. H. Hodges, The cause of epidemic diarrhea, nausea and vomiting (viral dysentery?), *Proc. Soc. Exp. Biol. Med., 59*:8–9 (1945).

60. F. L. Schaffer and M. E. Soergel, Single major polypeptide of a calicivirus and characterization by polyacrylamide gel electrophoresis and stabilization of virions by cross-linking with dimethyl suberimidate, *J. Virol., 19*: 925–931 (1976).

60a. F. L. Schaffer, Calicivirus. In *Comprehensive Virology*, Vol. 14 (H. Fraenkel-Conrat and R. R. Wagner, eds.), Plenum, New York, pp. 249–281.

61. D. S. Schreiber, N. R. Blacklow, and J. S. Trier, The mucosal lesion of the proximal small intestine in acute infectious nonbacterial gastroenteritis, *N. Engl. J. Med., 288*:1318–1323 (1973).

62. D. S. Schreiber, N. R. Blacklow, and J. S. Trier, The small intestinal lesion induced by the Hawaii agent in infectious nonbacterial gastroenteritis, *J. Infect. Dis., 124*:705–708 (1974).

63. M. C. Steinhoff, R. G. Douglas, Jr., H. B. Greenberg, and D. R. Callahan, Bismuth subsalicylate therapy of viral gastroenteritis, *Gastroenterology* 78:1495–1499 (1980).

64. H. Suzuki, T. Konno, T. Katsuzawa, A. Imai, F. Tazawa, N. Ishida, N. Katsushima, and M. Sakamoto, The occurrence of calicivirus in infants with acute gastroenteritis, *J. Med. Virol., 4*:321–326 (1979).

65. W. Szmuness, J. L. Dienstag, R. H. Purcell, E. J. Harley, C. E. Stevens, and D. C. Wong, Distribution of antibody to hepatitis A antigen in certain adult populations, *N. Engl. J. Med., 295*:755–759 (1976).

66. W. Szmuness, J. L. Dienstag, R. H. Purcell, C. E. Stevens, D. C. Wong, H. Ikram, S. Bar-Shany, R. P. Beasley, J. Desmyter, and J. A. Gaon, The prevalence of antibody to hepatitis A antigen in various parts of the world: A pilot study, *Am. J. Epidemiol., 106*:392–398 (1977).

67. T. S. Thornhill, A. R. Kalica, R. G. Wyatt, A. Z. Kapikian, and R. M. Chanock, Pattern of shedding of the Norwalk particle in stools during experimentally induced gastroenteritis in volunteers as determined by immune electron microscopy, *J. Infect. Dis., 132*:28–34 (1975).

68. T. S. Thornhill, R. G. Wyatt, A. R. Kalica, R. Dolin, R. M. Chanock, and A. Z. Kapikian, Detection by immune electron microscopy of 26–27 nm virus-like particles associated with two family outbreaks of gastroenteritis, *J. Infect. Dis., 135*:20–27 (1977).

69. D. A. J. Tyrrell, M. L. Bynoe, and B. Hoorn, Cultivation of "difficult" viruses from patients with common colds, *Br. Med. J., 1*:606–610 (1968).

70. L. Widerlite, J. S. Trier, N. R. Blacklow, and D. S. Schreiber, Structure of the gastric mucosa in acute infectious nonbacterial gastroenteritis, *Gastroenterology, 68*:425–430 (1975).

71. R. G. Wyatt, R. Dolin, N. R. Blacklow, H. L. DuPont, R. F. Buscho, T. S. Thornhill, A. Z. Kapikian, and R. M. Chanock, Comparison of three agents of acute nonbacterial gastroenteritis by cross-challenge in volunteers, *J. Infect. Dis., 129*:704–714 (1974).

72. R. G. Wyatt, H. B. Greenberg, D. W. Dalgard, W. P. Allen, D. L. Sly, T. S. Thornhill, R. M. Chanock, and A. Z. Kapikian, Experimental infection of chimpanzees with the Norwalk agent of epidemic viral gastroenteritis, *J. Med. Virol., 2*:89–96 (1978).

73. R. G. Wyatt and A. Z. Kapikian, Viral agents associated with acute gastroenteritis in humans, *Am. J. Clin. Nutr., 30*:1857–1870 (1977).

74. A. Yamamoto, H. Zennyogi, K. Yanagita, and S. Kato, Research into the causative agent of epidemic gastroenteritis which prevailed in Japan in 1948, *Jpn. Med. J., 1*:379–384 (1948).

75. M. D. Yow, J. L. Melnick, R. J. Blattner, N. B. Stephenson, N. M. Robinson, and M. A. Burkhardt, The association of viruses and bacteria with infantile diarrhea, *Am. J. Epidemiol., 92*:33–39 (1970).

76. J. Zahorsky, Hyperemesis hiemis or the winter vomiting disease, *Arch. Pediatr., 46*:391–395 (1929).

77. R. Dolin, R. C. Reichman, K. Roessner, T. S. Tralka, R. T. Schooley, W. Gary, and D. Morens, Detection by immune electron microscopy of Snow Mountain agent of acute viral gastroenteritis. Abstract 232 in Program and Abstracts of the 21st Interscience Conference on Antimicrobial Agents and Chemotherapy, Nov. 4–6, 1981, Chicago, Illinois. Published by American Society for Microbiology, Washington, D.C.

78. R. Dolin and S. Baron, Absence of detectable interferon in jejunal biopsies, jejunal aspirates and sera in experimentally induced viral gastroenteritis in man, *Proc. Soc. Exp. Biol. Med., 150*:337–339 (1975).

10

Coronaviruses in Humans

E. O. Caul Public Health Laboratory,
Bristol, England

S. I. Egglestone* Public Health
Laboratory, Exeter, England

Coronaviruses belong to a distinct virus family, the Coronaviridae [34]. They are pleomorphic, enveloped RNA viruses possessing an approximately 20 nm fringe of widely spaced radiating surface projections. Virus replication occurs in the cytoplasm of infected cells, with mature particles budding from the endoplasmic reticulum. This group of viruses is well recognized as causal agents of both respiratory and intestinal disease in animals and respiratory disease in humans.

It was predicted in 1975 [18] that in view of the association of coronaviruses with the enteric tract of animals that it was likely that a human counterpart existed. This prediction was closely followed by two reports describing coronavirus-like particles in human feces following electron microscope examinations. The first report came from Vellore, Southern India where the particles were described as "myxovirus or coronavirus-like" but distinct from mycoplasmas [23]. The second report came from Bristol, England where they were described as coronaviruses on the basis that the particles possessed a fine structure which more closely resembled coronaviruses than any other known virus group [9]. Morphologically similar particles have been described in Australia

---

*Dr. Egglestone is now with the Public Health Laboratory, Bristol, England.

[25,32], Gambia [29], Germany [19], the Gilbert Islands [15], and South America [21].

All the above reports concern the identification of coronaviruses in fecal extracts, which by the very nature of the dynamic state of the intestinal environment will also contain various cell fragments possessing a variety of fringes. Thus at the electron microscope level the differentiation of fringed cellular particles from enteric coronaviruses, which also possess a fringe of projections, is of paramount importance, particularly since a suitable sensitive culture system is not available at present. These culture problems have hindered the work with the human enteric coronavirus (HECV) described by the Bristol laboratory. Nevertheless, progress has been made with its characterization, and the following sections outline the approaches undertaken to establish these particles as coronaviruses and the attempts to determine their role, if any, in gastroenteritis.

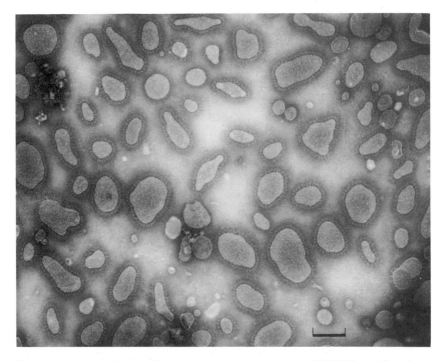

Figure 1 Morphology of human enteric coronaviruses (HECV) purified from feces in a 20%/60% w/w sucrose gradient. Preparation stained with 1.5% phosphotungstic acid, pH 6.5. Bar represents 100 nm.

Morphologic Studies

The presence of fringed particles in fecal extracts is well known to anyone familiar with the electron microscope appearance of fecal preparations. Many of these particles are likely to be fragments of bursh-border membranes or possibly submitochondrial particles released from lysed cells shed from the villous lining during the normal turnover of the mucosal surface. Other fringed fragments may be derived from the membranes of disintegrated gut bacteria. Increased proliferation and migration of epithelial cells, induced by infectious agents, can undoubtedly result in a concomitant increase in cellular fragments. In addition one should be aware that mycoplasmas can appear as fringed particles in similar preparations [13]. With these possibilities in mind, the initial studies were directed toward characterizing the particles morphologically and finding criteria that differentiated them from normal cellular fragments. Prior to these initial investigations no known coronavirus strains were held in the laboratory, and as a matter of policy none were introduced at this stage of the studies.

A striking feature of many of the fecal preparations examined was that they contained large numbers of quite distinct coronavirus-like particles (Fig. 1) which in our experience were not normally present in fecal extracts. It was estimated that these fecal specimens often contained as many as 10^8 coronavirus particles per gram of feces, and many of the particles were very pleomorphic. Other fringed bodies likely to be found in fecal extracts and purified mitochondrial fractions were examined in detail, and these fringes showed marked differences from the "solar corona" of the surface projections of HECV (5,10].

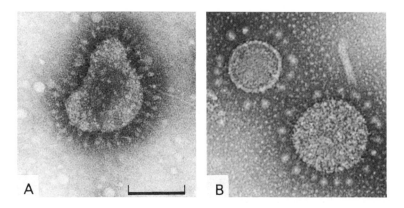

Figure 2 Morphology of HECV following staining with: (A) 1.5% phosphotungstic acid, pH 6.5, or (B) 1.0% ammonium molybdate, pH 5.0. Note the differences in the *shape* of the surface projections. Bar represents 100 nm.

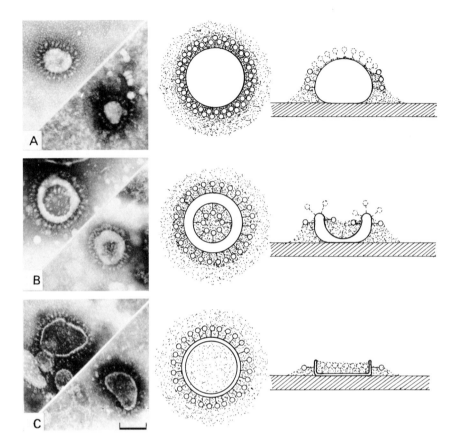

Figure 3 Variation in the appearance of HECV particles at different stages of collapse of the envelope. A diagrammatic interpretation of each stage of this collapse is shown. (A) Solid (uncollapsed) HECV particle. (B) Partially collapsed HECV particle. Note the central pool of negative stain and delineation of the surface projections against this central area. (C) Totally collapsed, stain-penetrated, HECV particle. In each case the upper micrograph represents HECV particles which should be compared with the lower micrograph in each case showing the morphology of a well-characterized coronavirus (A, transmissible gastroenteritis virus; B, avian infectious bronchitis virus; C, human respiratory coronavirus 229E). Preparations stained with 1.5% phosphotungstic acid, pH 6.5. Bar represents 100 nm. Line drawings are not to scale.

The most salient characteristic for the morphologic identification of HECV particles is the widely spaced, approximately 20 nm radiating projections which give rise to the solar corona appearance. Studies have shown that the staining regime is important for the morphologic identification of coronaviruses. Staining with uranyl acetate and prior fixation have been shown to be highly unsatisfactory, whereas ammonium molybdate or phosphotungstic acid (PTA) staining gave excellent resolution of the surface projections [5]. Following PTA staining the surface projections appear as thin stalks with a teardrop-like dilatation at the distal end (Fig. 2A). Following staining with ammonium molybdate the distal dilatations appeared spherical, and often the thin stalk is invisible (Fig. 2B).

It is common to find the majority of HECV particles collapsed either totally or partially, and only rarely were they not collapsed. This interpretation is based on the increasing accumulation of negative stain on the surface of a spherical solid particle as it collapses (Fig. 3). Partial collapse of the viral envelope gives rise to a central pool of negative stain and results in the delineation of the surface projections against this central area (Fig. 3B). When particles which are not collapsed are visualized the resultant image of the fringe is likely to be a composite of many layers of projections (Fig. 3A), and this multilayer gives rise to the appearance of closely packed projections. This appearance resembles more closely the appearance of known coronaviruses. The first description of the morphology of a coronavirus (avian infectious bronchitis virus, AIBV) by negative staining highlighted the petal-shaped radiating surface projections possessed by this virus [2]. The authors further noted variation in the shape of the projections within the population of virus particles examined. Since this original description, comparative studies with known coronaviruses have confirmed that variation in the shape of coronavirus projections does occur [11].

In a recent study of simian feces we have found coronavirus-like particles with surface projections indistinguishable from those possessed by HECV [8], the coronavirus-like particles reported by Mathan et al. [23] and Maas et al. [19] and the recent coronavirus-like particles found in Australian aborigines and dogs [31,32]. Coronavirus-like particles with similar projection morphology have also been visualized in the feces of calves [24] and cows [16]. The HECV may therefore be a member of a subgroup of coronaviruses whose projection morphology differs from that of the classic animal enteric coronaviruses, but further work is required to support this hypothesis.

The observation that many HECV particles were collapsed raised interesting questions regarding the internal structure of the virus. One explanation was that these collapsed particles lacked an internal component. Thin sections of purified HECV particles have shown that only a few particles contained substantial amounts of internal material, indicating that the majority were "empty." This result could explain the collapsed appearance of many of the particles following negative staining, since particles lacking an internal component would be more prone to physical stress following ultracentrifugation and electron microscope preparative techniques.

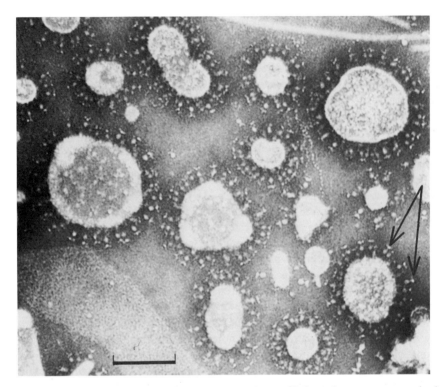

Figure 4 HECV particles showing *additional* T- or Y-shaped structures attached to the distal end of the projections (arrows). Preparation stained with 1.5% phosphotungstic acid, pH 6.5. Bar represents 100 nm. (Courtesy of Mr. C. I. Ashton.)

Of relevance to these findings are the recent observations of M. R. Macnaughton (personal communication) who separated AIBV into two populations of differing densities. The lighter particles on examination were collapsed and lacked any RNA, in contrast to the more dense particles which were not collapsed and did contain RNA. A limited amount of information is available on the internal component of HECV. We have shown that purified HECV particles contain RNA but not DNA, and studies using the nonionic detergent NP-40 demonstrated a clearly resolved tubular, internal component, 9-10 nm in diameter (unpublished observations). The diameter of this tubular component is the same as that of the internal component of the human respiratory coronavirus 229E [6,17] and that of avian infectious bronchitis virus described by Apostolov et al. [1]. From these studies it would appear that only a small proportion of virus particles contain an internal component and that a large proportion of

HECV particles in feces are defective possibly because intracytoplasmic maturation was faulty. This may be linked to the low-grade persistent type of excretion which is often found [10,23,25,32].

A few fecal specimens, which were obtained from patients of Far Eastern extraction, contained coronavirus particles with projections identical to those described above but with an *additional*, delicate, T- or Y-shaped structure attached to the distal end of the projection (Fig. 4). The rarity of these coronavirus particles with modified projections in the U.K. population is in sharp contrast to the situation in the Indian population where this additional structure appears to be very common (Prof. Mathan, personal communication). Similar T- or Y-shaped structures, which were attached to rotavirus particles present in fecal preparations, have been visualized (Dr. A. Curry, personal communication). We believe they are not an integral part of the virus structure but rather that they may represent attached IgA molecules since they closely resemble the electron microscope appearance of the IgA molecules described by Munn et al. [26]. If this turns out to be the case it is intriguing to know what implication this virus-host interaction has, if any, in terms of intestinal abnormalities. Present theories for the release of IgA molecules into the gut allow for a stage when IgA components enter and assemble within columnar epithelial cells [3], with movement from the lamina propria to the lumen of the gut probably occurring at the same time within the cisternae of the endoplasmic reticulum. It is conceivable that coronaviruses, which mature and bud into cisternae of the endoplasmic reticulum, could become attached to IgA molecules, producing transportable antigen-antibody complexes. The consequence of immune complexes in relationship to cellular pathology is well recognized and warrants consideration, particularly in the severe intestinal abnormalities seen in Southern Indian communities with tropical sprue. In these communities reinfection of the mucosal surface with infectious agents is probably common, and thus there is an increased possibility that antigen-antibody complexes may occur.

In Vitro Replication

Clearly the morphologic appearance of HECV particles supported their classification within the Coronaviridae, but it was necessary to show replication in vitro. Attempts were therefore made to demonstrate the infectivity of these particles by propagation in a suitable system. Earlier, organ cultures had been used to propagate transmissible gastroenteritis virus of pigs [30] and some human respiratory coronaviruses [35]. Our initial studies used human fetal intestinal organ cultures to propagate HECV. Virus replication was demonstrated by an increase in the number of extracellular virus particles in the organ culture fluids, positive immunofluorescence in the cells, and the appearance in the columnar epithelial cells of ultrastructural changes characteristic of coronavirus replication [7].

Table 1 Comparison of Ultrastructural Changes in Studies In Vitro and In Vivo of the Small Intestine from Different Animals Infected with Different Coronaviruses

Ultrastructural changes in columnar epithelial Cells	In vitro		In Vivo			
	HECV [7]	NCDV [4]	CET [28][a]	TGEV [27][b]	NCDCV [12]	CCV [33][c]
Cell desquamation	+	+	+	+	+	+
Loss of microvilli	+	+	+	+	+	+
Vacuolation	+	+	+	+	+	+
Nuclear changes	–	–	–	–	–	–
Budding from cell surface	–	–	–	–	–	–
Virus in vesicles	+	+	+	+	+	+
Virus in dilated smooth endoplasmic reticulum	+	+	+	+	+	+
Virus in large vacuoles	+	+	+	–	+	–
Free nucleocapsids	+	–	–	–	–	–
Tubular inclusions	+	–	–	–	+	–

[a]Coronavirus enteritis of turkeys.
[b]Transmissible gastroenteritis virus.
[c]Canine coronavirus.

As this was the first ultrastructural study of the intracellular development of an enteric coronavirus in intestinal organ cultures, the changes were compared with those resulting from infection of a similar system with a known enteric coronavirus, that is, bovine intestinal organ cultures infected with the bovine enteric coronavirus (neonatal calf diarrhea virus (NCDCV)) [4,10]. These comparative ultrastructural studies showed changes indistinguishable from those which occurred in HECV-infected human intestinal organ cultures and from those which have been reported by other workers in their in vivo studies of the small intestine of animals infected with different coronaviruses (Table 1). The end product of virus replication is the release of large numbers of virus particles from lysing desquamated cells (Fig. 5). The large virus-containing vacuoles in these cells presumably arise as a result of the coalescence of endoplasmic vesicles containing coronavirus particles [7].

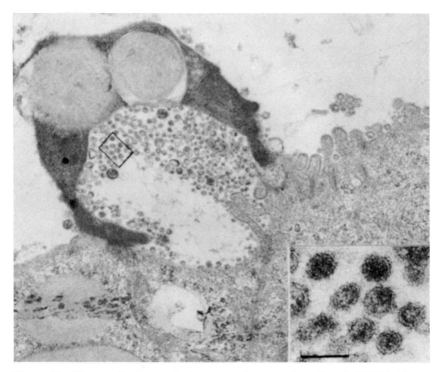

Figure 5   Human fetal intestinal organ cultures infected with HECV. Micrograph shows a desquamating mucosal cell containing large numbers of HECV particles. Inset is an enlargement of these intracytoplasmic HECV particles. Bar represents 100 nm.

Epidemiology

A further part of the investigation was directed toward resolving the etiologic role of HECV in human gastroenteritis. Accordingly, four groups of people were studied: patients with sporadic gastroenteritis, normal subjects, people involved in outbreaks of gastroenteritis in closed or semiclosed communities, and patients with known bacterial gastroenteritis [10]. The frequency with which coronavirus particles were seen in the feces of patients with sporadic gastroenteritis is shown in Table 2. In this study they were not found in feces from infants less than 1 year of age, although more recently they have been detected but never in early neonatal life. The absence of an association of HECV with gastroenteritis in neonates is in sharp contrast to the situation in animals, where the highest incidence of morbidity and mortality due to coronaviruses occurs in early neonatal life. The incidence of rotaviruses and adenoviruses

Table 2 Sporadic Cases of Gastroenteritis

Age (years)	No. tested	HECV (no.)	Positive (%)	Rotavirus (no.)	Positive (%)	Adenovirus (no.)	Positive (%)
1	230	0	0	32	14	12	5.2
1–4	164	2	1.2	32	19	12	7.3
5–14	63	3	4.8	6	9.5	0	0
15–24	62	4	6.5	1	1.6	0	0
25–44	144	6	4.2	5	3.5	0	0
45–64	78	1	1.3	2	2.5	0	0
>64	71	4	5.7	3	4.2	0	0

in acute gastroenteritis in comparison with HECV is also shown in Table 2, where the importance of the former viruses in young children is apparent. The incidence of HECV in adults with sporadic gastroenteritis and normal adults was similar (4.2 and 5.6%, respectively). In outbreaks of gastroenteritis in closed and semiclosed communities (Table 3), HECV was found in association with 8 of the 34 outbreaks. Detailed studies on these 8 outbreaks suggested that HECV did not have a causal role, as overall HECV was found in 20% of cases and 15% of contacts (Table 4).

Fecal samples were also examined from patients with diarrhea known to be caused by *Salmonella agona* to determine whether infection with a known bacterial pathogen affected the excretion of HECV particles in the feces. The incidence in this group (5.1%) was similar to that in asymptomatic adults (5.6%) and to that in sporadic cases (4.2%). Similar studies in India have shown that the incidence of HECV is reduced following enteric infection with other known pathogens [22].

In the course of these epidemiologic studies it became apparent that HECV could be excreted in the feces over a long period of time. In a specific study to determine the duration of excretion, 22 patients representing both sporadic cases of gastroenteritis and cases from outbreaks were followed. It was found that 77% of patients were still excreting HECV 2–85 weeks later. Of these persistent excretors, 40% had chronic gastroenteritis on follow-up. However these results are biased, as many of the follow-up specimens were examined because of continuing diarrhea. Since HECV is excreted for so long it is not surprising that they are detected in the apparently asymptomatic population. Furthermore, it makes the comparison of the incidence of HECV excretion in cases of gastroenteritis with that in asymptomatic controls difficult to interpret.

During the course of the above studies an opportunity arose to investigate endemic nonbacterial gastroenteritis problems in a psychogeriatric assessment

Table 3 Outbreaks of Gastroenteritis in Closed or Semiclosed Communities

Type of community	Number of outbreaks		Total no. of subjects tested
	Tested	Coronavirus positive[a]	
General hospital	7	1	58
Geriatric unit	6	2	79
Institution for for ESN†[b]	4	2	47
Hotel/holiday camp	2	2	48
Services camp	3	1	21
School	9	0	108
Family	3	0	8
Total	34	8	369

[a]Coronavirus excreted by one or more patients or contact.
[b]Educationally subnormal.
Source: From Ref. 10.

ward. It was known that patients admitted to this ward developed diarrhea soon after admission. At the onset of this study 80% of patients with gastroenteritis were excreting HECV particles as compared to 17% of patients without gastroenteritis; the overall incidence among patients was 56% and among the nursing staff, 6%. The high incidence of HECV excretion in this ward suggested that the low standard of personal hygiene among the inmates was an important factor in the acquisition of infections. Patients examined prior to admission were not excreting HECV particles. Although the patients both acquired the virus and developed gastroenteritis soon after admission, this does not prove that the virus caused the disease.

We suggest that infection can become endemic under low standards of personal hygiene, and this agrees with the high incidence found in the rural population of Southern India [23] and among Australian aborigines [32]. The Southern Indian workers reported HECV in 90% of stool specimens of children and adults, both in apparently healthy subjects and in those with tropical sprue. In Australia the incidence of HECV in the aboriginal population with gastroenteritis rose from 17% in those under 6 months to 63% in those 2-6 years old. A similar incidence was found by these authors in aboriginal children without gastroenteritis. The incidence of HECV in nonaboriginals was lower, and there was a less marked increase with age. In addition, Mata et al. [21] reported HECV particles in association with endemic gastroenteritis in populations of

Table 4 Outbreaks of Gastroenteritis in Which Coronaviruses Were Excreted by Patients or Contacts

Type of Community	Gastroenteritis		No illness	
	No. patients tested	No. HECV positive	No. contacts tested	No. HECV positive
General hospital nurses	2	1	0	
Institution for ESN	3	0	2	2
Institution for ESN	6	3	27	3
Geriatric unit	1	1	5	0
Geriatric unit	7	0	8	3
Hotel	5	1	9	0
Holiday camp, nursery nurses	18	2	16	2
RAF apprentices	9	2	0	
Total	51	10	67	10

Source: From Ref. 10.

South America but no mention was made of the incidence in normal or asymptomatic individuals, since the incidence is so high in "normal" populations throughout the world they are apparently well tolerated and it becomes impossible to assess their importance in acute gastroenteritis. In contrast, Maas et al. [19] concluded that HECV was a cause of neonatal gastroenteritis, but this has not yet been confirmed. Mathan et al. [23] suggested that HECV could be causally related to the widespread intestinal morphologic abnormalities and malabsorption found in Southern India. More recent studies by these workers on jejunal biopsies from patients with tropical sprue, who were excreting HECV particles in the feces, have shown ultrastructural changes in damaged mucosal cells similar to those produced by known coronaviruses [22]. They concluded that HECV was a cause of some cases of tropical sprue. In this respect it is interesting to note that a spruelike condition has been described in the small intestine of pigs infected with transmissible gastroenteritis virus [14,20,36]. In view of the persistent excretion of HECV in the above studies, a chronic low-grade infection may result in chronic abnormality of the small intestine. Whether repeated insults to the mucosal surface with other enteric pathogens, in addition to the preexisting chronic HECV infection, is necessary to precipitate the pathological lesion seen in tropical sprue is at present unclear.

Future Work

It is apparent from the above that many questions remain unanswered, in particular the role of HECV, if any, in both acute and chronic intestinal disease. It is appreciated that one unexplored approach to this problem is the use of volunteers to provide the definitive proof of transmission. However, human volunteer studies have not been done because of the persistent excretion of these viruses and their association with long-lasting intestinal abnormalities. The possibility of using monkeys as an animal model is currently under examination [8]. Dogs may provide an alternative animal model in view of the observation in dog feces of particles morphologically similar to HECV [31].

Intriguing questions concerning the pathogenesis of these viruses remain to be answered. What is the mode of entry into the gastrointestinal tract? Evidence from most of the studies suggests fecal-oral spread as the method of transmission, but the subsequent route to the intestine is unknown. It may be directly down the alimentary tract, or by the viremic route, or indeed by both. Having reached the mucosal surface, are the enterocytes the only cells involved in virus replication? Whatever cells are involved, the large number of "empty" particles produced suggests that replication is occurring in nonpermissive cells. Since virus replication involves internal membranes of the host cell and the subsequent production of large numbers of coronavirus particles, it is difficult to envisage that it is entirely nonpathological.

Finally, as with other human enteric viruses, we do not know how to propagate them in a susceptible system in vitro. One approach may be to extract the viral RNA, which in other coronaviruses has been shown to be infectious, in an attempt to infect cells in vitro. However, in view of the low efficiency of the procedure at present and the apparently small number of infectious HECV particles, this may prove to be difficult. In addition, autointerference may be a limiting factor in their direct cultivation, although defective particles could be separated to overcome this problem. Once adaptation has been achieved it opens new avenues for comparative biologic, biochemical, and serologic studies which will in turn enhance our knowledge of relationships within the family Coronaviridae and clarify the role of HECV in human intestinal disease.

References

1. K. Apostolov, T. H. Flewett, and A. P. Kendal. In *The Biology of Large RNA Viruses* (R. D. Barry and B. W. Mahy, eds.), Academic, New York, 1970, pp. 3–26.
2. D. M. Berry, J. G. Cruickshank, H. P. Chu, and R. J. H. Wells, The structure of infectious bronchitis virus, *Virology, 23*:403–407 (1964).
3. P. Brandtzaeg and K. Bakien. In *Immunology of the Gut.* CIBA Foundation Symposium No. 46, Elsevier/Excerpta Medica/North Holland, Amsterdam, 1977, pp. 77–113.

4. J. C. Bridger, E. O. Caul, and S. I. Egglestone, Replication of an enteric bovine coronavirus in intestinal organ cultures, *Arch. Virol., 57*:43–51 (1978).

5. E. O. Caul, C. R. Ashley, and S. I. Egglestone, Recognition of human enteric coronaviruses by electron microscopy, *Med. Lab. Sci., 34*:259–263 (1977).

6. E. O. Caul, C. R. Ashley, M. Ferguson, and S. I. Egglestone, Preliminary studies on the isolation of coronavirus 229E nucleocapsids, *FEMS Microbiol. Lett., 5*:101–105 (1979).

7. E. O. Caul and S. I. Egglestone, Further studies on human enteric coronaviruses, *Arch. Virol., 54*:107–117 (1977).

8. E. O. Caul and S. I. Egglestone, Coronavirus-like particles present in simian faeces, *Vet. Rec., 104*:168–169 (1979).

9. E. O. Caul, W. K. Paver, and S. K. R. Clarke, Coronavirus particles in faeces in patients with gastroenteritis, *Lancet, 1*:1192 (1975).

10. S. K. R. Clarke, E. O. Caul, and S. I. Egglestone, The human enteric coronaviruses, *Postgrad. Med. J., 55*:135–142 (1979).

11. H. A. Davies and M. R. MacNaughton, Comparison of the morphology of three coronaviruses, *Arch. Virol., 59*:25–33 (1979).

12. A. M. Doughri, J. Storz, I. Hajer, and H. S. Fernando, Morphology and morphogenesis of a coronavirus infecting intestinal epithelial cells of newborn calves, *Exp. Mol. Pathol., 25*:355–370 (1976).

13. R. N. Gourlay and S. G. Wyld, Isolation of mycoplasmas from bovine faeces, *Lancet 2*:231 (1975).

14. E. O. Haelterman and B. E. Hooper, Transmissible gastroenteritis of swine as a model for the study of enteric disease, *Gastroenterology, 53*:109–113 (1970).

15. I. H. Holmes, Viral gastroenteritis, *Prog. Med. Virol., 25*:1–36 (1979).

16. G. W. Horner, R. Hunter, and C. A. Kirkbride, A coronavirus-like agent present in faeces of cows with diarrhoea, *N. Zealand Vet. J., 23*, 98 (1975).

17. D. A. Kennedy and C. M. Johnson-Lussenburg, Isolation and morphology of the internal component of human coronavirus, strain 229E, *Intervirology, 6*:197–206 (1976).

18. Leading article, Rotaviruses of man and animals, *Lancet, 1*:257–259 (1975).

19. G. Maas, H. H. Baumeister, and N. Freitag, Viren als Ursache der akuten Gastroenteritis bei Säuglingen und Kleinkindern, *Munch. Med. Wochenschr., 119*(32/33):1029–1033 (1977).

20. R. R. Maronpot and C. K. Whitehair, Experimental sprue-like small intestinal lesions in pigs, *Can. J. Comp. Med. Vet. Sci., 31*:309–316 (1967).

21. L. Mata, J. J. Urrutia, G. Serrato, E. Mohs, and T. D. Y. Chin, Viral infections during pregnancy and in early life, *Am. J. Clin. Nutr., 30*:1834–1842 (1977).

22. M. Mathan and V. I. Mathan, Fourth International Congress in Virology (Hague), Abstract, 1978, p. 469.

23. M. Mathan, V. I. Mathan, S. P. Swaminathan, S. Yesudoss, and S. J. Baker, Pleomorphic virus-like particles in human faeces, *Lancet,* *1*:1068-1069 (1975).

24. M. S. McNulty, W. L. Curran, and J. B. McFerran, Virus-like particles in calves faeces, *Lancet,* *2*:78 (1975).

25. B. Moore, P. Lee, M. Hewish, B. Dixon, and T. Mukherjee, Coronaviruses in Training Centre for intellectually retarded, *Lancet,* *1*:261 (1977).

26. E. A. Munn, A. Feinstein, and A. J. Munro, Electron microscope examination of free IgA molecules and of their complexes with antigen, *Nature,* *231*:527-529 (1971).

27. M. B. Pensaert, E. O. Haelterman, and E. J. Hinsman, Transmissible gastroenteritis virus of swine. Virus-intestinal cell interactions, II. Electron microscopy of the epithelium in isolated jejunal loops, *Arch. Ges. Virusforsch.,* *31*:335-351 (1970).

28. K. A. Pomeroy, B. L. Patel, C. T. Larsen, and B. S. Pomeroy, Combined immunofluorescence and transmission electron microscopic studies of sequential intestinal samples from turkey embryos and poults infected with turkey enteritis coronavirus, *Am. J. Vet. Res.,* *39*(8):1348-1354 (1978).

29. M. G. M. Rowland, H. Davies, S. Patterson, R. R. Dourmashkin, D. A. J. Tyrrell, T. H. J. Mathews, J. Parry, J. Hall, and H. E. Larson, Viruses and diarrhoea in West Africa and London: A collaborative study, *Trans. R. Soc. Trop. Med. Hyg.,* *72*(1):95-98 (1978).

30. D. Rubenstein, D. A. J. Tyrrell, J. B. Derbyshire, and A. P. Collins, Growth of porcine transmissible gastroenteritis (TGE) virus in organ cultures of pig tissue, *Nature,* *227*:1348-1349 (1970).

31. R. D. Schnagl and I. H. Holmes, Coronavirus-like particles in stools from dogs, from some country areas of Australia, *Vet. Rec.,* *102*:528-529 (1978).

32. R. D. Schnagl, I. H. Holmes, and E. M. Mackay-Scollay, Coronavirus-like particles in aboriginals and non-aboriginals in Western Australia, *Med. J. Aust.,* *1*:307-309 (1978).

33. A. Takeuchi, L. N. Binn, H. R. Jervis, K. P. Keenan, P. K. Hildebrandt, R. B. Valas, and F. F. Bland III, Electron microscope study of experimental enteric infection in neonatal dogs with a canine coronavirus, *Lab. Invest.,* *34*:539-549 (1976).

34. D. A. J. Tyrrell, D. J. Alexander, J. D. Almeida, C. H. Cunningham, B. C. Easterday, D. J. Garwes, J. C. Hierholzer, A. Kapikian, M. R. Macnaughton, and K. McIntosh, Coronaviridae: Second report, *Intervirology,* *10*: 321-328 (1978).

35. D. A. J. Tyrrell and M. L. Bynoe, Cultivation of a novel type of common-cold virus in organ cultures, *Br. Med. J.,* *1*:1467-1470 (1965).

36. G. L. Waxler, Lesions of transmissible gastroenteritis in the pig as determined by scanning electron microscopy, *Am. J. Vet. Res.,* *33*:1323-1328 (1972).

11

Other Small Virus-like Particles in Humans

Ruth F. Bishop   Royal Children's Hospital,
Melbourne, Victoria, Australia

Virus-like particles abound in negative stains of fecal extracts examined with an electron microscope. This is not surprising, since the gut lumen serves as a repository for solid and liquid food residues, desquamated cells, bacteria, fungi, yeasts, and their phages, as well as for viruses that have multiplied in gut cells, or have been shed into the gut lumen from other sites.

The "stool-gazing" electron microscopist must first learn to distinguish between debris and virus particles, and then to identify viruses (including bacteriophages) by morphology. This presents few problems for large viruses >50 nm in diameter, with characteristic structural features (e.g., rotaviruses, adenoviruses). Identification of small viruses can be extremely difficult.

The increasing use of electron microscopy to locate viral infection of the intestinal tract has resulted in numerous reports of small virus-like particles in tissues and feces from neonates, children, and adults with and without acute gastroenteritis. These small particles form a very heterogeneous group. Some may be phages or viruses that cause "silent" infections of the intestinal tract. Others may prove to be new animal viruses capable of producing symptomatic enteric infection in humans and animals.

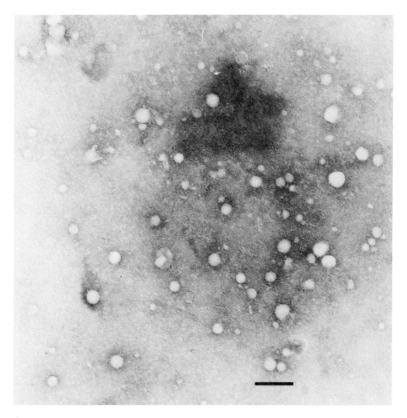

Figure 1 Negative stain of fecal extract showing collection of small hetero-geneous nonviral particles (bar = 100 nm).

Nonviral Particles in Feces

Small round particles of varying shapes and sizes occur in ultrathin sections of tissues, and in negative stains of fecal extracts (Fig. 1). These particles often bear a close resemblance to viruses. There is a dual risk in identification of these particles. Nonviral objects may be wrongly identified as viruses [11,26], or virus particles present in small numbers ($< 10^6$ per milliliter) may be indistinguishable from background debris [19].

Round bodies (20–50 nm) in tissue sections from small and large intestine may be remnants of degenerating microvilli, or other cellular structures [8,11, 36]. Small round particles seen in fecal extracts are unmistakably viruses if they exhibit cubic symmetry, possess some distinctive surface feature, such as spikes, knobs, or capsomeres, or are present as clumps of particles that are homogeneous in outline (Fig. 2). Small round particles scattered singly throughout an

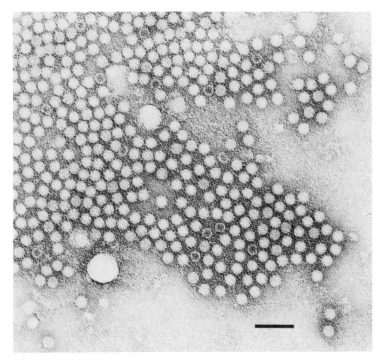

Figure 2 Negative stain of fecal extract showing collection of virus particles with homogeneous outline (bar = 100 nm).

extract are more difficult to identify. Viruses < 50 nm in diameter often lack characteristic structural detail, even when stains are prepared from cell culture [11,26], so it is likely that these small viruses are frequently unrecognized in negative stains of fecal extracts.

Viral Particles Seen by Electron Microscopy of Feces

Identification of small viruses seen in feces is assisted by growth in cell culture, e.g., enteroviruses, or by serologic assay, e.g., radioimmunoassay for Norwalk agent and related agents [17]. The majority of small viruses seen by electron microscopy have resisted cultivation in routine cell culture, fetal cell culture, and in suckling mice. The identification of these viruses rests solely on recognition of morphology. This is a very imprecise art, since the size and shape of viruses can vary according to techniques used for storage, extraction, and staining of specimens.

The identification of viruses seen in feces allows their potential role in the etiology of gastroenteritis to be assessed. For example, rotaviruses seen in diarrheal feces can usually be assumed to be etiologically related to symptoms. However, the same assumption of "blame" or "innocence" cannot yet be made with many of the small noncultivable viruses. Few of the criteria required to implicate these viruses in causation of disease [18] have been satisfied. In addition, there have been few surveys of noncultivable viruses seen by electron microscopy of feces from healthy neonates, children, or adults [14,27,32].

Bacteriophages

These are an unlikely cause of acute enteritis, although theoretically, lysis of microorganisms colonizing the gut lumen could release toxins capable of damaging gut mucosa [12]. Most of the morphologic varieties of phages have been detected in feces in health and disease [14]. Tailed phages are readily recognized. It is not possible at present to be sure that many of the small round viruses seen in feces are not tailless phages [13].

Cultivable Viruses

Cultivable viruses are excreted in feces of neonates, children, and adults with or without gastroenteritis [22,33,35,43,51]. Most are carried silently by their hosts, although some have been associated with epidemics of gastroenteritis [35]. Some of the small round viruses seen in fecal extracts by electron microscopy may be silent enteroviruses. These are difficult to recognize since they show little or no surface detail. They are identified by routine cell culture followed by serologic tests.

Noncultivable Viruses

Some of the small particles seen in feces remain obstinately noncultivable in routine cell culture, in fetal cell culture, and in suckling mice. It is possible that some of these particles are enteroviruses that are nonviable after passage along the gut, or after long storage of specimens before examination. However, some may represent new animal viruses that infect the gut. These particles are at present "classified" by morphology, and much remains to be determined about their physicochemical nature, growth requirements, and pathogenicity. Norwalk agent and antigenically related agents will be excluded from this chapter as they are described in Chap. 9.

Astroviruses

Astroviruses were first described in 1975 in the feces of newborn babies in Glasgow, Scotland with and without acute gastroenteritis [29]. The 28 nm particles were shed in feces in very large numbers, often in quasicrystalline array. Careful observation of some of the particles showed a faint surface

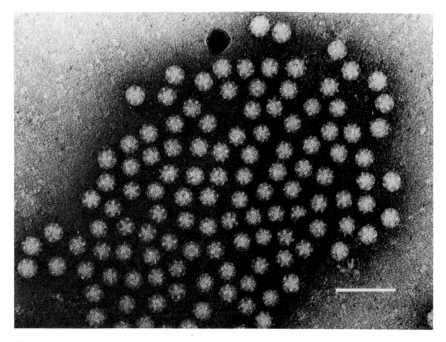

Figure 3   Astroviruses in intestinal contents of gnotobiotic lambs (bar = 100 nm). (From Ref. 45.)

structure resembling a star. This morphologic feature was suggested as the basis for naming the particles *astrovirus* [30]. Astrovirus particles have since been observed in feces from children and adults with diarrhea [5,21,33]. Morphologically indistinguishable particles have been reported in diarrheal feces from lambs [44] and calves [49].

The identification of astrovirus particles rests on recognition of the star shape and on precise differentiation from calicivirus structure [28]. The method of preparation of stool extracts may be critical. Most particles show a smooth circular entire edge, but 10-15% of particles in any one specimen exhibits the typical astrovirus morphology (Fig. 3). These show a faint structure, assumed to be due to the presence of stain-filled hollows arranged to give the impression of a five- or six-pointed star. These hollows appear triangular when assessed from photographs. The particle never exhibits a central hollow, but may show a white center that appears raised.

Astroviruses fail to grow in cells from monkey kidney or human amnion [21,30]. Human astrovirus infects monolayers of primary human embryo kidney cells without producing cytopathic changes [23]. Similarly, bovine astrovirus can be demonstrated by indirect immunofluorescence in primary calf kidney and calf testicular cells [49]. The lamb astrovirus failed to grow in monolayers of primary fetal lamb kidney. Human, bovine, and lamb astroviruses remain unclassified. They are serologically unrelated to each other [44,49] and to W agent, or to Ditchling agent [23]. Lamb astrovirus contains single-stranded RNA (D. R. Snodgrass and A. J. Herring, personal communication, 1979) and may prove to be a picornavirus.

Evidence that astroviruses are human enteric pathogens is equivocal. Infection in neonates 4–7 days after birth is usually asymptomatic but may be associated with loose stools [29,32]. Sporadic infection was observed in 15% of older children admitted to the hospital in Glasgow with diarrhea [33]. No other surveys of etiology of sporadic diarrhea record similar findings, but difficulties with identification of astrovirus particles may partly explain the discrepancy.

Astroviruses have been seen in two outbreaks of nosocomial diarrhea in children [5,21], accompanied by spread to adult ward staff in one outbreak [21]. Coincident infection with rotavirus, or *Salmonella bredeny* complicates the etiology of this outbreak. Seroconversion to astrovirus occurred in a number of infected children and adults [5,21], and IgM antibodies to astrovirus were demonstrated in one child [5].

Attempts to transmit astrovirus infection to adult volunteers have had partial success [20]. Fecal filtrate from a nosocomial outbreak in children was fed to 17 adult volunteers. Only 1 developed acute diarrhea and simultaneously shed astrovirus particles. Rises in serum antibody to astrovirus were detected in 12 of the 17 volunteers. The presence of serum antibody before ingestion of the filtrate appeared to give some protection against symptomatic illness [20].

Evidence that astroviruses are human enteric pathogens is strengthened by comparative studies proving astrovirus to be an enteric pathogen of lambs. Astrovirus particles from 4 to 6-week-old lambs with diarrhea were fed to gnotobiotic lambs and produced mild diarrhea coincident with astroviruses in feces or intestinal contents [45]. Astroviruses infected epithelial cells of the villi of the small intestine and subepithelial macrophages, producing villous atrophy and depression of lactase levels in mid-small intestine [44]. By contrast, astroviruses from calves did not cause diarrhea when fed to two gnotobiotic calves [49].

In summary, small noncultivable viruses identified by the starlike shape of some of the particles (astroviruses) infect humans, sheep, and cattle. Infection of lambs causes mild diarrhea. Astroviruses may prove to be human enteric pathogens, causing mild diarrhea and/or vomiting in children and adults.

Calicivirus-like Particles

Caliciviruses comprise a genus within the family Picornaviridae. Members of the genus are small spherical viruses (30–40 nm), often showing an ill-defined edge with a "feathery" appearance. The surface is indented by round or oval

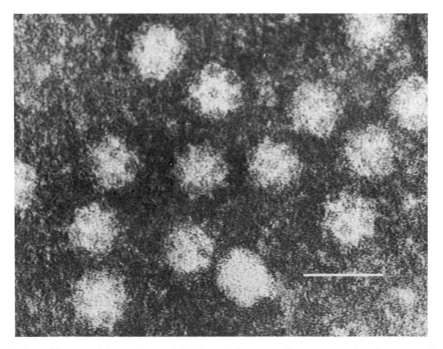

Figure 4   Calicivirus-like particles in stool extract (bar = 50 nm). (Courtesy of Dr. D. A. McSwiggan, Public Health Laboratory, Central Middlesex Hospital, England.)

cup-shaped hollows (calyx = cup or chalice). These often form a "star of David" configuration, with six hollows surrounding a seventh central hollow (Fig. 4). Caliciviruses have a density of 1.36-1.38 g/cm^3 in cesium chloride, contain single-stranded RNA, and are composed of a single major polypeptide [3,47, 48].

Caliciviruses infect mucous membranes, particularly of the nose and throat, and occasionally the intestinal tract of cats, pigs, and sea mammals [47]. Infection is rarely accompanied by enteritis. Particles indistinguishable from caliciviruses have been seen in feces from children [15,24,31-34,46] and calves [49] with diarrhea. Identification is mainly based on morphology alone, and the term *calicivirus-like* should be retained until physicochemical evaluations of the particles are made.

Characteristic calicivirus morphology is often seen on only a minority of particles after thorough searching, and can be confused with astrovirus morphology [28]. Although caliciviruses from cats, pigs, and sea mammals grow readily in cell culture, calicivirus-like particles associated with enteritis in humans and cattle have not yet been cultured in vitro [31-46,49].

The calicivirus-like particles seen in human feces have been described in children with acute gastroenteritis in the United Kingdom [15,25,31] and in Canada [24,34,46]. It is not known what, if any, antigenic relationships exist between these particles. Their relationship to Norwalk agent has not been defined.

Their involvement in the etiology of acute gastroenteritis is difficult to evaluate. Calicivirus-like particles are only an occasional finding in children admitted to the hospital with sporadic acute diarrhea [24,31,34]. Their presence does not always parallel the presence of enteric symptoms [31–46], and they are often associated with rotaviruses or adenoviruses [31]. The most convincing evidence that calicivirus-like particles cause human enteritis comes from the temporal association of calicivirus excretion with an outbreak of winter vomiting disease in an infants' school in London [25]. This "London-agent" (Fig. 4) has a morphology and buoyant density consistent with caliciviruses, but bears no antigenic relationship to feline or porcine caliciviruses (D. A. McSwiggan, personal communication, 1979). Rising antibody titers were demonstrated in several children during the outbreak [25].

Calicivirus-like particles have also been seen in feces from calves with diarrhea [49]. Ingestion of this "Newbury agent" produced diarrhea in 12 gnotobiotic calves, after an incubation period of 1-3 days. Infection was associated with a reduction in absorption of D-xylcse and with hemorrhagic lesions and villous atrophy in mid-small intestine. No virus particles were seen in gut cells from infected calves.

In summary, noncultivable particles closely resembling known caliciviruses have been seen in feces from calves and children with diarrhea or vomiting. Classification of these particles cannot be attempted until physicochemical studies are carried out. The particles differ antigenically, and in symptoms of disease, from known caliciviruses. Proof of their involvement in the etiology of human enteritis requires further study.

Small Round Viruses (Picorna-Parvovirus-like)

A heterogeneous collection of small round viruses has been described by different laboratories in feces from neonates [4,6,7], children [9,14,24,33,34, 37,46,50], and adults [1,2,38] with or without gastroenteritis. The particles have an entire edge with no detectable surface structure, and a diameter of 20-30 nm. They are most easily distinguished as clumps against a background of fecal debris, and visualization has been aided by the reaction of fecal extracts with human sera [1,2,38]. The particles have not grown in vitro in routine cell culture and, when tested, have failed to grow in suckling mice or in human fetal cell cultures.

Evaluation of the relationship of these particles to each other, to known viral genera, and to the etiology of gastroenteritis, is frustrated by an almost

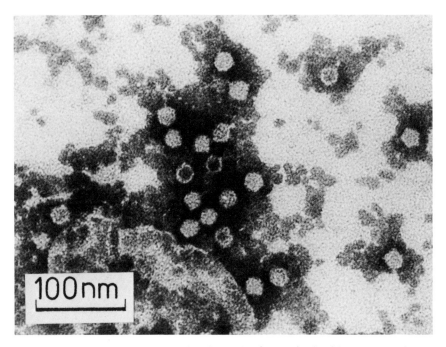

100 nm

Figure 5 Parvovirus-like particles from the feces of a healthy neonate (bar = 100 nm). (Courtesy of Virus Laboratory, Bristol Public Health Laboratory, England.)

total lack of information of their physicochemical nature. Some may be tailless phages. Some may be enteroviruses that are coated with antibody and unable to grow in tissue culture. Others may be adeno-associated viruses [13], although adenovirus particles have seldom been seen in the same specimens. Some may be new animal viruses that cause silent or symptomatic infections of the gastrointestinal tract.

The best characterized of these small round viruses is the 22 nm particle seen in Bristol, England (Fig. 5) in stools from adults with or without acute gastroenteritis [38]. Further studies on this particle showed it to have a buoyant density of 1.34-1.42 g/cm^3 in CsCl, to be distinguishable morphologically from representatives of each of two groups of small spherical phages, but indistinguishable from parvoviruses of pigs and mink [39]. It is considered that this particle is a human parvovirus [41,42] unrelated serologically to parvovirus-like particles found in normal human sera [10,40,42]. The frequency of antibody to this human parvovirus in an adolescent population is on the order of 30-40% [40,41]. Parvoviruses cause enteritis in calves, rodents, pigs, cats, and dogs [16] but none have yet been shown to cause human enteritis.

Small round viruses have frequently been observed in feces from neonates [6,7], children [14,33,37], and adults [1,2] with no symptoms of gastrointestinal disease. It is likely that small round viruses are ubiquitous in the human intestine. However, it does not follow that all small round viruses seen in feces are innocent of causation of disease. Particles seen in surveys of sporadic cases of acute enteritis should be regarded as dubious pathogens, unless further evidence of pathogenicity is available. For example, the small picorna–parvovirus-like particles shed by a small percentage of children with acute gastroenteritis in Canada [24,34,46] and Glasgow [33] could represent the normal fecal occurrence of these particles in those communities. Particles seen in common-source outbreaks are more likely to be enteric pathogens, particularly if excretion can be temporally related to enteric symptoms [4], or if seroconversion to the particles can be demonstrated during infection [9]. Although such evidence is suggestive, it is disturbing that many of these common-source outbreaks have not excluded infection with pathogenic or toxigenic *Escherichia coli*. Diarrhea due to bacterial infection could perhaps "flush out" viruses ubiquitous in the gut, so that the appearance of these viruses in feces became a secondary phenomenon.

The small round viruses seen in feces of neonates might form a special group (Fig. 2). Morphologically similar particles have been seen in newborn babies with diarrhea in the United Kingdom [4] and Australia [6,7]. They may be associated with mild diarrhea and vomiting that is not due to infection with pathogenic or toxigenic *E. coli* [6]. The particles are shed in clumps, are temporally related to the onset of diarrhea [4], and are absent from feces after cessation of diarrhea [7]. The Australian particles were often excreted asymptomatically, and were more common during the winter months. Perhaps these particles are the same ubiquitous parvoviruses that are often shed silently by older children and adults.

In summary, small round viruses have been frequently seen in feces from neonates, children, and adults. Some of these particles may be ubiquitous in the human intestinal tract and cause only silent infections. Surveys of etiology of sporadic gastroenteritis should be wary of assigning an etiologic role to any of these particles until techniques exist to identify them more precisely. Information of this kind will probably accumulate from studies of common-source outbreaks of enteritis.

Minireovirus

This 30 nm particle has been described in Canada in feces from children with acute gastroenteritis [34,46]. Although it is similar in size to other small round viruses it is distinguished from them by its morphology. The intact particles appear to possess a double capsid (Fig. 6). Some stain-penetrated particles have a complete anterior capsid, while others appear as rims with sparsely spaced external projections 2-3 nm long [34].

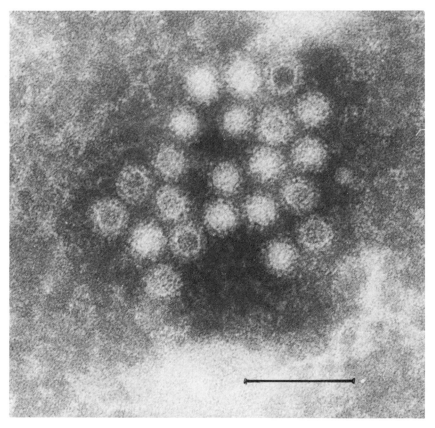

Figure 6 Minireovirus (MRV) particles in feces from child with acute diarrhea (bar = 100 nm). (Courtesy of the Virology Department, The Hospital for Sick Children, Toronto, Ontario, Canada.)

Minireovirus (MRV) or minirotavirus particles [46] were seen in stools from 7% of children admitted to the hospital from August 1975 to July 1976 with acute gastroenteritis [34], and in infants with nosocomial diarrhea [46]. Evidence that MRV is an enteric pathogen is incomplete. These particles are temporally associated with diarrhea, and "breedtrue" in ward outbreaks; i.e., subsequent cases of gastroenteritis in the same room yield the same virus as the index patient. Immune electron microscopy [34] has shown a seroresponse to infection in a few patients.

Conclusion

There have been numerous reports of small noncultivable viruses of less than 50 nm in fecal extracts examined by electron microscopy.

Systematic, and occasional, examinations of healthy neonates, children, and adults make it clear that small noncultivable viruses are ubiquitous in fecal extracts. Nevertheless, there is reason to believe that some small noncultivable viruses are etiologic agents of acute gastroenteritis. These "candidate" viruses are classified by morphology into astroviruses, calicivirus-like particles, minireovirus particles, and small round viruses (picorna-parvovirus-like). It is not clear what relation these viruses bear to each other, or to accepted genera of viruses. All require further physicochemical evaluation. This may show that some of the particles are identical, and that differences in morphology are more apparent than real.

Astroviruses are enteric pathogens in lambs, and there is considerable evidence that they are also human enteric pathogens. Of the remaining groups, the evidence linking calicivirus-like particles with enteric infection is more convincing than for the remaining particles. None should be described as enteric pathogens until further studies prove a causal relationship between infection and symptomatic illness.

References

1. J. D. Almeida, F. Deinhardt, and A. J. Zuckerman, Virus-like particles in hepatitis-A-positive faecal extracts, *Lancet, 2*:1083–1084 (1974).
2. J. D. Almeida, F. W. Gay, and T. G. Wreghitt, Pitfalls in the study of hepatitis A, *Lancet, 2*:748–751 (1974).
3. J. D. Almeida, A. P. Waterson, J. Prydie, and E. W. L. Fletcher, The structure of a feline picornavirus and its relevance to cubic viruses in general, *Arch. Virusforsch., 25*:105–114 (1968).
4. H. Appleton and P. G. Higgins, Viruses and gastroenteritis in infants, *Lancet, 1*:1297 (1975).
5. C. R. Ashley, E. O. Caul, and W. K. Paver, Astrovirus associated gastroenteritis in children, *J. Clin. Pathol., 31*:939–943 (1978).
6. D. J. S. Cameron, R. F. Bishop, A. A. Veenstra, and G. L. Barnes, Noncultivable viruses and neonatal diarrhoea. A fifteen month survey in a newborn special care nursery, *J. Clin. Microbiol., 8*:93–98 (1978).
7. D. J. S. Cameron, R. F. Bishop, A. A. Veenstra, G. L. Barnes, I. H. Holmes, and B. J. Ruck, Pattern of shedding of two non-cultivable viruses in stools of newborn babies, *J. Med. Virol., 2*:7–13 (1978).
8. R. L. Chandler, R. G. Bird, and A. P. Bland, Particles associated with microvillous border of intestinal mucosa, *Lancet, 2*:931–932 (1975).
9. P. J. Christopher, G. S. Grohmann, R. H. Millsom, and A. M. Murphy, Parvovirus gastroenteritis—a new entity for Australia, *Med. J. Aust., 1*: 121–124 (1978).
10. Y. E. Cossart, A. M. Field, B. Cant, and D. Widdows, Parvovirus-like particles in human sera, *Lancet, 1*:72–73 (1975).

11. A. J. Dalton and F. Haguenau, *Ultrastructure of Animal Viruses and Bacteriophages: An Atlas.* Academic, New York, 1973.
12. A. G. Dean, R. B. Couch, T. C. Jones, and R. G. Douglas, Jr., Seasonal gastroenteritis and malabsorption at an American military base in the Philippines. III. Microbiologic investigations and volunteer experiments, *Am. J. Epidemiol., 95*:451–463 (1972).
13. T. H. Flewett, Diagnosis of enteritis virus, *Proc. R. Soc. Med., 69*:693–696 (1976).
14. T. H. Flewett, A. S. Bryden, and H. Davies, Diagnostic electron microscopy of faeces. I. The viral flora of the faeces as seen by electron microscopy. *J. Clin. Pathol., 27*:603–614 (1974).
15. T. H. Flewett and H. Davies, Caliciviruses in man, *Lancet, 1*:311 (1976).
16. J. H. Gillespie, Feline panleucopenia and other parvoviruses. In *Hagan's Infectious Diseases of Domestic Animals,* 6th ed. (D. W. Brunner and J. H. Gillespie, eds.), Cornell University Press, Ithaca, New York, 1973, pp. 1086–1098.
17. H. B. Greenberg and A. Z. Kapikian, Detection of Norwalk agent antibody and antigen by solid-phase radioimmunoassay and immune adherence hemagglutination assay, *J. Am. Vet. Med. Assoc., 173*:620–623 (1978).
18. R. J. Huebner, The virologist's dilemma, *N.Y. Acad. Sci. Ann., 67*:430–439 (1967).
19. A. Z. Kapikian, S. M. Feinstone, R. H. Purcell, R. G. Wyatt, T. S. Thornhill, A. R. Kalica, and R. M. Chanock, Detection and identification by immune electron microscopy of fastidious agents associated with respiratory illness, acute non-bacterial gastroenteritis and hepatitis A. The Gustav Stern Symposium; Antiviral Mechanisms, *Perspect. Virol., 9*:9–20 (1975).
20. J. B. Kurtz, T. W. Lee, J. W. Craig, and S. E. Reed, Astrovirus infection in volunteers, *J. Med. Virol., 3*:221–230 (1979).
21. J. B. Kurtz, T. W. Lee, and D. Pickering, Astrovirus associated gastroenteritis in a children's ward, *J. Clin. Pathol., 30*:948–952 (1977).
22. Leading article, Viruses and reclaimed water, *Br. Med. J., 4*:1662 (1978).
23. T. W. Lee and J. B. Kurtz, Astroviruses detected by immunofluorescence, *Lancet, 2*:406 (1977).
24. D. M. McLean, K. S. K. Wong, and S. K. A. Bergman, Virions associated with acute gastroenteritis in Vancouver, 1976, *CMA J., 5*:1035–1036 (1977).
25. D. A. McSwiggan, D. Cubitt, and W. Moore, Calicivirus associated with winter vomiting disease, *Lancet, 1*:1215 (1978).
26. C. R. Madeley, *Virus Morphology,* Churchill Livingstone, London, 1972.
27. C. R. Madeley, Viruses in the stools, *J. Clin. Pathol., 32*:1–10 (1979).
28. C. R. Madeley, A comparison of the features of astroviruses and caliciviruses seen in samples of faeces by electron-microscopy, *J. Infect. Dis. 139*:519–523 (1979).

29. C. R. Madeley and B. P. Cosgrove, Viruses in infantile gastroenteritis, *Lancet, 2*:124 (1975).

30. C. R. Madeley and B. P. Cosgrove, 28 nm particles in faeces in infantile gastroenteritis, *Lancet, 2*:451–452 (1975).

31. C. R. Madeley and B. P. Cosgrove, Caliciviruses in man, *Lancet, 1*:199–200 (1976).

32. C. R. Madeley, B. P. Cosgrove, and E. J. Bell, Stool viruses in babies in Glasgow. 2. Investigation of normal newborns in hospital, *J. Hyg. Camb., 82*:285–294 (1978).

33. C. R. Madeley, B. P. Cosgrove, E. J. Bell, and R. J. Fallon, Stool viruses in babies in Glasgow. 1. Hospital admissions with diarrhoea, *J. Hyg. Camb., 78*:261–273 (1977).

34. P. J. Middleton, M. T. Szymanski, and M. Petric, Viruses associated with acute gastroenteritis in young children, *Am. J. Dis. Child., 131*:733–737 (1977).

35. H. L. Moffett, H. K. Shulenberger, and E. R. Burkholder, Epidemiology and etiology of severe infantile diarrhoea, *J. Pediatr., 72*:1–14 (1968).

36. R. L. Owen, Pseudomembranous colitis: Viral etiology discussed, *Gastroenterology, 70*:1185–1186 (1976).

37. S. Patterson, J. Parry, T. H. J. Matthews, R. R. Dourmashkin, D. A. J. Tyrrell, R. G. Whitehead, and M. G. M. Rowland, Viruses and gastroenteritis, *Lancet, 2*:451 (1975).

38. W. K. Paver, E. O. Caul, C. R. Ashley, and S. K. R. Clarke, A small virus in human faeces, *Lancet, 1*:237–240 (1973).

39. W. K. Paver, E. O. Caul, and S. K. R. Clarke, Comparison of a 22 nm virus from human faeces with animal parvoviruses, *J. Gen. Virol., 22*:447–450 (1974).

40. W. K. Paver, E. O. Caul, and S. K. R. Clarke, Parvovirus-like particles in human sera, *Lancet, 1*:232 (1975).

41. W. K. Paver, E. O. Caul, and S. K. R. Clarke, Parvovirus-like particles in human faeces, *Lancet, 1*:691 (1975).

42. W. K. Paver and S. K. R. Clarke, Comparison of human fecal and serum parvo-like viruses, *J. Clin. Microbiol., 4*:67–70 (1976).

43. A. B. Sabin, The significance of viruses recovered from the intestinal tracts of healthy infants and children, *N. Y. Acad. Sci. Ann., 66*:226–230 (1956).

44. D. R. Snodgrass, K. W. Angus, E. W. Gray, J. D. Menzies, and G. Paul, Pathogenesis of diarrhoea caused by astrovirus infections in lambs, *Arch. Virol. 60*:217–226 (1979).

45. D. R. Snodgrass and E. W. Gray, Detection and transmission of 30 nm virus particles (astroviruses) in faeces of lambs with diarrhoea. *Arch. Virol. 55*:287–291 (1977).

46. H. C. Spratt, M. I. Marks, M. Gomersall, P. Gill, and C. H. Pai, Nosocomial infantile gastroenteritis associated with minirotavirus and calicivirus, *J. Pediatr., 93*:922–926 (1978).

47. M. J. Studdert, Caliciviruses—brief review, *Arch. Virol.*, *58*:157–191 (1978).

48. J. Wawrzkiewicz, C. J. Smale, and F. Brown, Biochemical and biophysical characteristics of vesicular exanthema virus and the viral ribonucleic acid, *Arch. Virusforsch.*, *25*:337–351 (1968).

49. G. N. Woode and J. C. Bridger, Isolation of small viruses resembling astroviruses and caliciviruses from acute enteritis of calves, *J. Med. Microbiol.*, *11*:441–452 (1978).

50. A. P. Wyn-Jones, Virus associated gastroenteritis in children, *Lancet, 2*: 559 (1975).

51. M. D. Yow, J. L. Melnick, R. J. Blattner, W. B. Stephenson, N. M. Robinson, and M. A. Burkhardt, The association of viruses and bacteria with infantile diarrhoea, *Am. J. Epidemiol.*, *92*:33–39 (1970).

_12

Role of Viruses in Pediatric Gastrointestinal Disease and Epidemiologic Factors

Peter J. Middleton   The Hospital for Sick Children, Toronto, Ontario, Canada

Scope of the Problem

Infectious gastroenteritis in developed countries is second only to respiratory infections as a cause of morbidity in childhood [1,2]. Besides causing a great deal of morbitity [3-6], rotavirus and adenovirus infection may also cause fatal disease [4,7-11]. During the interval from May 1972 through February 1979 we have documented 26 fatal rotavirus infections and 2 fatal adenovirus enteritis infections in Metropolitan Toronto. Viral gastroenteritis accounts for a substantial number of pediatric hospital admissions [3-6] and adds enormously to the load of nosocomially acquired infections [3,12]. In developing countries the impact of enteritis is even more devastating; it has been estimated that 5-18 million childhood deaths occur each year in Asia, Africa, and South America [13]. Although rotavirus has been documented as causing enteritis on each of these continents, the contribution of viral enteritis to this staggering mortality figure has yet to be established.

In addition to rotavirus, several other candidate etiologic viral agents are known. These include the Norwalk-like group of agents [14,15], adenoviruses [3,7,12], astroviruses [16,17], calicivirus [17,18], minireovirus [3,71], and coronavirus [20]. Each year at The Hospital for Sick Children in Toronto, approximately 700 patients are diagnosed by the laboratory as having a virus infection associated with their gastroenteritis. Making up this total are 360 rotaviruses, 100 minireoviruses, 90 adenoviruses, 100 picorna-parvoviruses, 25 astroviruses, and 25 caliciviruses. These figures underestimate the prevalence of virus gastroenteritis in our institution since only one stool specimen is examined per patient; few outpatients are investigated, and many inpatients cannot be diagnosed because our single electron microscope already operates at full capacity.

Proof of Causation

Several lines of evidence suggest that at least certain of the viruses listed above are in fact the etiologic agents causing enteritis. Workers throughout the world have observed morphologically identical virions in association with acute gastro-enteritis but not during convalescence; other causative organisms and toxins have been excluded; serologic responses have been demonstrated; human volunteer studies and animal inoculation experiments have indicated virus shedding, production of disease, and serologic responses; natural epidemics have been witnessed and nosocomial spread of these various viruses documented [3,12,18, 21,22,23,24,25,28].

Clinically it is sometimes possible to distinguish viral diarrhea from certain bacterial diarrheas. Thus in the case of *Campylobacter* enteritis prominent early vomiting and dehydration generally never occur, but blood in the stools is common [26].

Finally, counterpart animal viruses often cause enteritis in their natural hosts, and that disease may be prevented by either vaccination or the administration of colostrum which contains appropriate antibodies [27,29-32].

Incubation Period

The incubation periods for the several viral enteritis agents are of brief duration, i.e., 1-7 days. Thus, Davidson et al. [4] considered that the incubation period for rotavirus in children was less than 48 h. Woode et al. [31] found that porcine rotavirus given to gnotobiotic piglets caused diarrhea within 20-48 h. When human rotavirus was given to gnotobiotic piglets, diarrhea and virus shedding was observed after 1-5 days by one group of workers [33] and from 2 to 7 days by another group [34]. In a human volunteer study using human rotavirus, symptoms first occurred on day 2 following the ingestion of virus [35]. Dolin [36] found that volunteers who received the Norwalk agent by the oral route developed symptoms 18-54 h later. Experimental coronavirus diarrhea in gnotobiotic calves occurred about 20 h after oral administration of virus [32]. From our observations of hospital room and ward outbreaks of enteritis associated with astrovirus, calicivirus, adenovirus, and minireovirus, the incubation periods appear to be of 1-5 days' duration.

Age and Sex

Viral enteritis is generally a disease of infants and young children. Animal diarrhea viruses also chiefly affect very young animals. Reinfection in later childhood and adult life is probable, since a durable immunity is unlikely to follow a superficial mucosal infection. Repeated small bowel infections (often subclinical) might be anticipated from studies that indicate reinfections throughout life with respiratory syncytial viruses and parainfluenza viruses in the respiratory mucosa [37]. Tables 1 and 2 show the sex ratios and age ranges of hospitalized Toronto children with acute gastroenteritis. Rotavirus disease is most common in the interval between 6 months and 1 year. The average age of our rotavirus patients is 1 year. With the exception of calicivirus, disease caused by the other agents listed in Table 2 occurs most frequently in the first 12 or 24 months of life. These figures probably do not reflect what happens in a nonhospital setting, since a high percentage of recorded cases represent nosocomially acquired infections [3]. It would seem that by admitting a child to the hospital we guarantee uncontrolled but "supervised" active immunization with one or more of the diarrhea-producing agents. Other workers have also shown that rotavirus infection and disease occur chiefly in children less than 3 years old [4,38-41]. Newborn nursery studies have shown that rotavirus infection may be acquired in the first few days of life. Infection at this age is either subclinical or expressed

Table 1 Sex and Age Range of 326 Consecutive Rotavirus Patients

Patients (no.)	Sex (%)		Age groups (%)					
	M	F	0-6 mo.	6-12 mo.	12-18 mo.	18-24 mo.	2-3 y.	>3 y.
Patients admitted with enteritis (257)	55	45	21.4	40.1	18	5	8.2	7.3
Nosocomial enteritis patients (69)	61	39	56	34	6	1	3	—
Total patients (326)	57	43	29	39	15	4	7	6

Table 2 Sex and Age Range of 322 Nonrotavirus Enteritis Patients

Virus	Sex (%) M	Sex (%) F	Age groups (%) 0-6 mo.	6-12 mo.	12-18 mo.	18-24 mo.	2-3 y.	>3 y.
Adenovirus	56	44	46	34.7	8.3	9.7	–	1.3
Picorna-parvovirus	55	45	34.3	34.3	19.2	8.5	2.6	2.6
Minireovirus	60	40	49	26	5	4	8	8
Astrovirus	50	50	41	31.5	6	12.5	6	3
Calicivirus	53	47	6.3	33	6.3	20	27	6.3

as a very mild disease [42,43]. By way of contrast, infection by the Norwalk group of agents occurs in older children and adults [44]. In fact, by the fifth decade of life only 50% of the population in developed and developing countries possesses antibody [44].

Adenovirus-associated gastroenteritis probably occurs in the first few years of life [12,38]. Caul and others [45] described an outbreak of coronavirus gastroenteritis in servicemen aged 16-20 years. Coronavirus enteritis of swine (transmissible gastroenteritis, TGE) tends to involve very young animals. A good deal more about the role of a human coronavirus in acute enteritis needs to be learned. Astrovirus infection has been demonstrated in both children and adults [23]. The bulk of our so-called minireovirus infections was seen in infants and young children (Table 2). However, these figures reflect a hospital rather than a community population.

Tables 1 and 2 indicate the "superiority" of the male child in acquiring viral gastroenteritis. Taking all gastroenteritis patients admitted to our hospital into account each year, we find 58% are male and 42% are female [25]. Rotavirus patients have a similar ratio of males to females.

Season

In temperate climates it has been abundantly demonstrated that rotavirus disease occurs with much greater prevalence in the cold season [3-6]. Figure 1 demonstrates the seasonal pattern of rotavirus over a 2 year span in our hospital. This picture is duplicated in many other developed countries with temperate climates. Murphy and others [42] in Sydney, Australia found no seasonal variation when rotavirus infection was studied in newborn nurseries. De Torres and co-workers

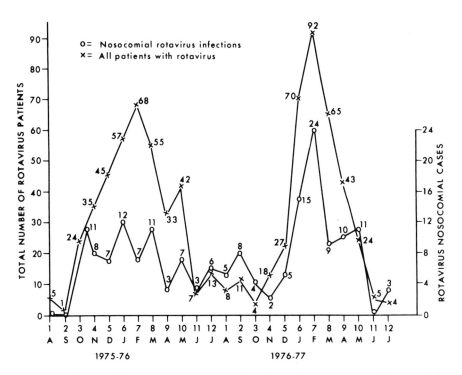

Figure 1 Seasonal frequency of hospital-based rotavirus gastroenteritis patients over a 2 year period. The numbers forming the plot represent patients diagnosed each month.

[40] during a 14 month study period found that rotavirus was detected throughout the year in tropical Caracas, Venezuela. The mean temperature in Caracas was 20.1°C, with a range of 17.9-21.6°C. They also showed that there was no relationship between rainfall and rotavirus infection. Enterovirus infections in Caracas were also evenly distributed throughout the year, unlike the summer and early autumn distribution seen in temperate climates. Mata [46] in Costa Rica during a 2 year period could find no correlation between rotavirus activity and temperature. However, outbreaks were concomitant with the dry season. Similarly, Wyatt and others [47] found no seasonal incidence in semitropical Guatemala.

Table 3 records the number of enteritis patients diagnosed as adenovirus, picorna-parvovirus, minireovirus, astrovirus and calicivirus during a 12 month period. No seasonal trends are evident with the exception of minireovirus. In previous years [3] we have noted that this same virus shows a cold season prev-

Table 3 Number of Nonrotavirus Enteritis Patients per Month

Month	Virus*				
Sept. 77–Aug. 78	Adeno	P/P	MRV	A	C
S	13	13	1	5	–
O	4	18	15	4	–
N	6	10	9	–	–
D	9	17	18	–	2
J	7	7	21	1	1
F	4	8	10	1	4
M	4	5	18	6	1
A	6	5	7	6	–
M	1	9	–	6	2
J	10	6	–	2	2
J	3	2	–	1	2
A	5	4	–	–	1
Totals	72	104	99	32	15

*P/P = Picorna/parvo; MRV = minireovirus, A = astrovirus, C = calicivirus.

alence pattern. The original Norwalk, Hawaii, and Montgomery County outbreaks occurred in October, March, and June, respectively [48]. Other Norwalk-like agents are referred to as the W agent and the Ditchling agent. These
agents have caused epidemics in the winter and autumn. Christopher and others
[50] described an outbreak of parvovirus enteritis in Australia during the winter
months. An outbreak of astrovirus on a children's ward in England also occurred
during the cold season [51].

Socioeconomic Status

Very little has been written on this aspect of viral enteritis disease. Therefore,
instead of solid data I offer some impressions and speculations. When the home
addresses of patients admitted to the hospital with rotavirus diseases were
plotted on a map of Metropolitan Toronto it became evident that patients
mainly originated from the poorer and ethnic areas of the City. If an infection
spreads by the fecal-oral route then it seems reasonable to assume higher rates
of infection would occur at an earlier age under conditions of overcrowding
and poor hygiene.

Our in-hospital studies have indicated that the average age of nosocomially
acquired rotavirus infection is considerably less than the average age of patients

admitted with the disease. Variations in the severity of disease and the age at which infection is first acquired might also be determined in part by the degree that breast feeding is practiced in a given geographic area by a particular socioeconomic group. Actual rotavirus disease versus rotavirus infection in relation to age, geographical area, and socioeconomic status has yet to be studied in a rigorous fashion.

Serosurveys in Different Age Groups

In a study from Washington, D.C. by Wyatt and others [38], rotavirus antibody was detected by complement fixation and immunofluorescence in over 90% of institutionalized children after the second year of life.

Gust and others [52] in Melbourne, Australia using a complement fixation (CF) test for rotavirus antibody detection found that 40% of infants 2 months of age or less possessed rotavirus antibody. By 3-5 months of age the percentage with antibody had fallen to 15%. Thereafter the percentage with antibody increased and approached 70% by 3 years of life. Approximately 70% of adults were shown to have antibody. Middleton and others [53] in Toronto, Canada also using CF generated a similar set of figures. In both these latter studies sera for testing were collected from hospitalized patients with nondiarrheal diseases. When sera from infants and children without diarrhea in Vellore, India were tested for rotavirus antibody by counterimmunoelectrophoresis, 85% of newborns were shown to have antibody. By the fifth month 30% had antibody, and by the third year of life nearly 90% possessed evidence of previous infection [54]. Ghose and co-workers [55], using the enzyme-linked immunosorbent assay (ELISA), determined the rotavirus antibody prevalence in European and aboriginal populations living in the same outback area in Australia. The results of this ELISA survey showed that 100% of both populations possessed antibody throughout the age range—2-60 years. The geometric means of rotavirus ELISA titers in the different age groups were greater in the aboriginal as opposed to the European population. Yolken et al. [56] in Washington, D.C., also using ELISA, found that by 18 months of age 85% of children possessed rotavirus antibody to serotype 1 and serotype 2 viruses.

By way of contrast, Norwalk antibody is acquired gradually so that by the fifth decade 50% had such antibody [57]. Kurtz and Lee [58], using immunofluorescence, found that 75% of children aged 5-10 years possessed astrovirus antibody.

Family Studies

Rotavirus infection along with many other virus infections involve other members of the family unit. Studies by Kim et al. [59], Tallett et al. [60], Tufvesson et al. [61], and Haug et al. [62] suggest that up to one-third of older siblings, parents, and grandparents show evidence of infection or reinfection on a basis of serologic and/or virus demonstration studies. The question has not yet been answered as to whether it is the infected younger child or the (usually) asymptomatic adult members who are responsible for the introduction of rotavirus into the family unit.

The Norwalk group of agents also spreads among children and adults in family units or students and teachers in a school setting [48]. In the original Norwalk outbreaks gastroenteritis developed in 50% of the students and teachers and in 32% of family contacts.

McSwiggan and others [18] described a small outbreak of calicivirus infection involving young children, a teacher, and a home contact. The serologic responses of infected subjects were demonstrated by immune electron microscopy.

Reinfection and Multiple Serologic Types

Both long-stay pediatric patients (see Table 5) and adults in a home environment experience reinfection with rotavirus. Evidence for the existence of more than one human rotavirus comes from several groups of workers. Flewett et al. [64], using a fluorescent-neutralization test system, defined four rotavirus serotypes from Great Britain and elsewhere in the world. Zissis and Lambert [65] in Belgium employed complement fixation and immune electron microscopy and described two rotavirus serotypes. Yolken and others [56] developed an enzyme-linked immunosorbent assay to differentiate serotype-specific rotavirus antigen and antibody. They defined two distinct serotypes both in Washington, D.C. and in other parts of the world. Sera of most children aged 2 years in the Washington, D.C. area contained rotavirus antibodies to both serotypes. An analysis of children who experience sequential infections revealed that an illness caused by one serotype did not provide resistance to illness caused by the other serotype. Espejo et al. [66] in Mexico City and Kalica et al. [67] in Washington, D.C. defined two different rotaviruses on a basis of gel electrophoresis of viral RNA. Similarly, bovine rotaviruses may be divided into at least two different strains on a basis of viral hemagglutinin production [68]. The genetic diversity of rotaviruses may be much greater than the serotyping studies related above would suggest. Thus Rodger and Holmes [69], using gel electrophoresis to separate the double-stranded RNA segments of bovine rotavirus isolates, found four electropherotypes on one farm during a single outbreak of disease.

The Norwalk group of agents comprises several distinct serotypes: (1) the original Norwalk agent (an identical agent has recently been found in an outbreak of gastroenteritis from the ingestion of oysters in Australia) and the related Montgomery County agent; (2) the Hawaii agent; and (3) the Ditchling agent and the antigenically similar W agent [14,15,21,36,48,49,63].

Parrino and others [70] working with volunteers challenged with the Norwalk agent demonstrated that some subjects displayed short-term immunity while others showed long-term immunity. Of the 12 volunteers initially challenged with the Norwalk agent, 6 became ill. These same 6 volunteers were re-challenged 27-42 months later and all 6 again developed clinical illness. Four of these volunteers received a third dose of the Norwalk agent 4-8 weeks later and 1 of the 4 developed enteritis.

It has not yet been established if the so-called enteric adenoviruses found in stools by EM but which do not replicate in cell cultures represent a single or multiple serotypes.

Mode of Spread

Previously it has been stated that rotavirus infection spreads by way of the fecal-oral pathway. Volunteer and animal experiments back up this statement. There is no evidence to suggest that rotavirus multiplies with the production of infectious particles in other than small bowel enterocytes. Observations by both physicians and veterinarians lead us to the conclusion that rotavirus-diseased subjects "generously" contaminate their environment. This in turn acts as a source of oral contamination for those who are not immune. In the elegant studies by Lecce and co-workers [71] involving piglets in a nursery it was shown that contamination of the facility with porcine rotavirus increased with continuous use, causing a progressive increase in the incidence of enteritis and death. Piglets after 1 day's nursing on the sow were placed in a nursery for 2 weeks. Every 10 days new litters entered the nursery. Thus there was an overlap of younger and older piglets with no opportunity to clean and fumigate the facility. A repeatable pattern of events emerged: the first few litters introduced into the nursery were asymptomatic and showed a satisfactory weight gain; however, by the time the eighth lot of piglets were introduced (after 5 weeks of continuous operation) a mild diarrhea was noticed in older piglets. As additional piglets moved in the diarrhea became more pronounced and of longer duration. Between 7 and 9 weeks of continuous operation piglets started vomiting at 3-5 days of age, then became dehydrated; 50% died. At this time all piglets were removed from the nursery to allow for cleaning and fumigation. The first batch of new piglets entered the nursery 1 week later. The pattern of events described above recurred by the time the eighth lot of piglets was placed in the facility.

Nosocomial Infection

Outbreaks of diarrhea are a common occurrence in any pediatric institution. Rotavirus infection may be endemic in newborn nurseries [42,43]. In our own hospital one-third of laboratory-diagnosed gastroenteritis cases are nosocomially acquired. This amounts to 250 cases per year [3]. Moreover, we believe this

Table 4 Successive Bouts of Viral Enteritis
in a Long-Stay Hospital Patient

Date	Virus
December 21, 1977	Calicivirus
December 29, 1977	Rotavirus
January 19, 1978	Adenovirus

figure to be a considerable underestimation of the problem since our diagnostic facility cannot provide an EM examination of all patients who develop in-house diarrhea. Figure 1 reveals the extent of nosocomial rotavirus infections in our hospital. Long-stay pediatric patients develop successive bouts of enteritis. Tables 4 and 5 illustrate two such patients.

In a study of nosocomial infantile gastroenteritis by Spratt and others [19] it was shown that 11 index minirotavirus patients infected 10 room contact subjects and that 8 index calicivirus patients infected 7 room contacts. Flewett et al. [12] described two outbreaks of gastroenteritis in a long-stay children's ward. One outbreak was caused by rotavirus and the other by adenovirus. Astroviruses were also shown to cause nosocomial infections [23,72].

It is speculated that nosocomial infection is acquired by the patient coming into contact with virus-contaminated furniture or articles, which is then followed by the transfer of contaminated articles or fingers to the mouth. Alternatively, virus also seems to spread from a "dirty" area in the hospital to a noninfected area via staff with contaminated hands or garments.

Table 5 Successive Bouts of Viral Enteritis
in a Long-Stay Hospital Patient

Date	Virus
January 11	Rotavirus
January 19	Minireovirus
January 26	Picorna-Parvovirus
February 3	Rotavirus

References

1. J. H. Dingle, L. P. McCorkle, G. F. Badger, et al. A study of illness in a group of Cleveland families. XIII. Clinical description of acute nonbacterial gastroenteritis, *Am. J. Hyg., 64*:368–375 (1956).
2. J. H. Dingle, G. F. Badger, W. S. Jordan, Jr., *Illness in the Home: A Study of 25,000 Illnesses in a Group of Cleveland Families,* Case Western Reserve University Press, Cleveland, Ohio, 1964.
3. P. J. Middleton, M. T. Szymanski, and M. Petric, Viruses associated with acute gastroenteritis in young children, *Am. J. Dis. Child., 131*:733–737 (1977).
4. G. P. Davidson, R. F. Bishop, R. R. W. Townley, I. H. Holmes, and B. J. Ruck, Importance of a new virus in acute sporadic enteritis in children, *Lancet, 1*:242–246 (1975).
5. A. S. Bryden, H. A. Davies, R. E. Hadley, T. H. Flewett, C. A. Morris, and P. Oliver, Rotavirus enteritis in the West Midlands during 1974, *Lancet, 2*:241–243 (1975).
6. A. Z. Kapikian, H. W. Kim, R. G. Wyatt, W. L. Cline, J. O. Arrobio, C. D. Brandt, W. J. Rodriguez, D. A. Sack, R. M. Chanock, and R. H. Parrott, Human reo-like agent as a major pathogen associated with "winter" gastroenteritis in hospitalized infants and young children, *N. Engl. J. Med., 294*: 965–972 (1976).
7. H. L. Moffett, H. K. Shulenberger, and E. R. Burkholder, Epidemiology and etiology of severe infantile diarrhea, *J. Pediatr., 72*:1–14 (1968).
8. J. A. K. Carlson, P. J. Middleton, M. T. Szymanski, J. Huber, and M. Petric, Fatal rotavirus gastroenteritis: An analysis of 21 cases, *Am. J. Dis. Child., 132*:477–479 (1978).
9. E. Palmer, M. Martin, and S. Foster, Reo-like virus epidemic enteritis in 1964, *Abstracts, Am. Soc. Microbiol.,* p. 53, C110 (1977).
10. A. Whitlow, H. Davies, and J. Parry, Electron microscopy of fatal adenovirus gastroenteritis, *Lancet, 1*:361 (1977).
11. Public Health Laboratory Report, United Kingdom and Republic of Ireland, *Br. Med. J., 1*:1346 (1976).
12. T. H. Flewett, A. S. Bryden, A. Davies, and C. A. Morris, Epidemic viral enteritis in a long-stay children's ward, *Lancet, 1*:4–5 (1975).
13. K.M. Elliot, *Acute Diarrhoea in Childhood,* Ciba Foundation Symposium No. 42. Elsevier/North Holland/Excerpta Medica, Amsterdam, 1976, p. 1.
14. T. S. Thornhill, G. Wyatt, A. R. Kalica, R. Dolin, M. Chanock, and A. Z. Kapikian, Detection by immune electron microscopy of 26 to 27 nm virus particles associated with two family outbreaks of gastroenteritis, *J. Infect. Dis., 135*:20–27 (1977).
15. H. Appleton, M. Buckley, B. T. Thom, J. L. Cotton, and S. Henderson, Virus-like particles in winter vomiting disease, *Lancet, 1*:409–414 (1977).
16. C. R. Madeley and B. P. Cosgrove, 28 nm particles in faeces in infantile gastroenteritis, *Lancet, 2*:451–452 (1975).

17. E. Kjeldsberg, Small spherical viruses in faeces from gastroenteritis patients, *Acta Pathol. Microbiol. Scand* [B] *,85*:351–354 (1977).

18. D. A. McSwiggan, D. Cubitt, and W. Moore, Calicivirus associated with winter vomiting disease, *Lancet, 1*:1215 (1900).

19. H. C. Spratt, M. I. Marks, M. Gomersall, P. Gill, and H. P. Chik, Nosocomial infantile gastroenteritis associated with minirotavirus and calicivirus, *J. Pediatr., 93*:922–926 (1978).

20. E. O. Caul and S. I. Egglestone, Further studies on human enteric coronaviruses, *Arch. Virol., 54*:107–117 (1977).

21. A. Z. Kapikian, H. W. Kim, R. G. Wyatt, W. L. Cline, R. H. Parrott, R. M. Chanock, J. O. Arrobio, C. D. Brandt, W. J. Rodriguez, A. R. Kalica, and D. H. Vankirk, *Acute Diarrhea in Childhood,* Ciba Foundation Symposium No. 43, Elsevier/North Holland/Excerpta Medica, Amsterdam, 1976, pp. 273–309.

22. T. H. Flewett, Diagnosis of enteritis virus, *Proc. R. Soc. Med., 69*:693–696 (1976).

23. J. B. Kurtz, T. W. Lee, and D. Pickering, Astrovirus associated gastroenteritis in a children's ward, *J. Clin. Pathol., 30*:948–952 (1977).

24. C. R. Madeley, B. P. Cosgrove, E. J. Bell, and R. J. Fallon, Stool viruses in babies in Glasgow. 1. Hospital admissions with diarrhoea, *J. Hyg. Camb., 78*:261–273 (1977).

25. P. J. Middleton, Rotavirus: Clinical observations and diagnosis of gastroenteritis. In *Comparative Diagnosis of Viral Diseases I. Human and Related Disease, Part A* (E. Kurstak and C. Kurstak, eds.), Academic, New York, 1977, pp. 423–445.

26. M. A. Karmali and P. C. Fleming, Campylobacter enteritis in childhood, *J. Pediatr., 94*:527–534 (1979).

27. R. G. Wyatt, H. B. Greenberg, D. W. Dalgard, W. P. Allen, D. L. Sly, T. S. Thornhill, R. M. Chanock, and A. Z. Kapikian, Experimental infection of chimpanzees with the Norwalk agent of epidemic viral gastroenteritis, *J. Med. Virol., 2*:89–96 (1978).

28. S. E. Reed, J. B. Kurtz, and T. W. Lee, Inoculations of human volunteers with a human astrovirus, *Abstracts IV International Congress for Virology,* The Hague, *W35/7* p. 461 (1978).

29. D. R. Snodgrass and P. W. Wells, Passive immunity in rotaviral infections, *J. Am. Vet. Med. Assoc., 173* (Part 2):565–568 (1978).

30. E. P. Bass and R. L. Sharpee, Coronavirus and gastroenteritis in foals, *Lancet, 2*:822 (1975).

31. G. N. Woode, J. Bridger, G. A. Hall, J. M. Jones, and G. Jackson, The isolation of reovirus-like agents (rotaviruses) from acute gastroenteritis of piglets, *J. Med. Microbiol., 9*:203–209 (1976).

32. C. A. Mebus, Pathogenesis of coronavirus infection in calves, *J. Am. Vet. Med. Assoc., 173* (2):631–632 (1978).

33. P. J. Middleton, M. Petric, and M. T. Szymanski, Propagation of infantile gastroenteritis virus (orbi-group) in conventional germfree piglets, *Infect. Immun., 12*:1276–1280 (1975).

34. A. Torres-Medina, R. G. Wyatt, C. A. Mebus, N. R. Underdahl, and A. Z. Kapikian, Diarrhea caused in gnotobiotic piglets by the reovirus-like agent of human infantile gastroenteritis, *J. Infect. Dis., 133*:22–27 (1976).

35. P. J. Middleton, M. T. Szymanski, G. D. Abbott, R. Bortolussi, and J. R. Hamilton, Orbivirus acute gastroenteritis of infancy, *Lancet, 1*:1241–1244 (1974).

36. R. Dolin, Norwalk agent-like particles associated with gastroenteritis in human beings, *J. Am. Vet. Med. Assoc., 173*(2):615–619 (1978).

37. F. J. Tyeryar, Jr., L. S. Richardson, and R. B. Belshe, Report of a workshop on respiratory syncytial virus and parainfluenza viruses, *J. Infect. Dis., 137*:835–846 (1978).

38. R. G. Wyatt, A. R. Kalica, C. A. Mebus, H. W. Kim, W. T. London, R. M. Chanock, and A. Z. Kapikian, Reovirus-like agents (rotaviruses) associated with diarrheal illness in animal and man, *Perspect. Virol., 10*:121–145 (1978).

39. C. J. Birch, F. A. Lewis, M. L. Kennett, H. Pritchard, and I. D. Gust, A study of the prevalence of rotavirus infection in children with gastroenteritis admitted to an infectious diseases hospital, *J. Med. Virol., 1*:69–77 (1977).

40. B. V. De Torres, R. M. De Ilja, and J. Esparza, Epidemiological aspects of rotavirus infection in hospitalized Venezuelan children with gastroenteritis, *Am. J. Trop. Med. Hyg., 27*:567–572 (1978).

41. T. Konno, H. Suzuki, A. Imai, T. Kutsuzawa, N. Ishida, N. Katsushima, M. Sakamoto, S. Kitaoka, R. Tsuboi, and M. Adachi, A long-term survey of rotavirus in Japanese children with acute gastroenteritis, *J. Infect. Dis., 138*:569–576 (1978).

42. A. M. Murphy, M. B. Albrey, and E. B. Crewe, Rotavirus infections of neonates, *Lancet, 2*:1149–1150 (1977).

43. J. E. Banatvala, I. L. Chrystie, and B. M. Totterdell, Rotaviral infections in human neonates, *J. Am. Vet. Med. Assoc., 173*(1):527–530 (1978).

44. H. B. Greenberg and A. Z. Kapikian, Detection of Norwalk agent antibody and antigen by solid-phase radioimmunoassay and immune adherence hemagglutination assay, *J. Am. Vet. Med. Assoc., 173*:620–623 (1978).

45. E. O. Caul, W. K. Paver, and S. K. R. Clarke, Coronavirus particles in faeces from patients with gastroenteritis, *Lancet, 1*:1192 (1975).

46. L. Mata, Rotavirus disease in Costa Rica, *Abstracts IV International Congress for Virology*, The Hague. *P.35*:469 (1978).

47. R. G. Wyatt, R. H. Yolken, J. J. Urrutia, L. Mata, H. B. Greenberg, R. M. Chanock, and A. Z. Kapikian, Diarrhea associated with rotavirus in rural Guatemala: A longitudinal study of 24 infants and young children, *Am. J. Trop. Med. Hyg., 28*:325–328 (1979).

48. R. G. Wyatt, R. Dolin, N. R. Blacklow, H. L. DuPont, R. F. Buscho, T. S. Thornhill, A. Z. Kapikian, and R. M. Chanock, Comparison of three agents in acute infectious non-bacterial gastroenteritis by cross-challenge in volunteers, *J. Infect. Dis., 129*:709–714 (1974).

49. A. Z. Kapikian, S. M. Feinstone, R. H. Purcell, R. G. Wyatt, T. S. Thornhill, A. R. Kalica, and R. M. Chanock, Detection and identification by immune electron microscopy of fastidious agents associated with respiratory illness, acute nonbacterial gastroenteritis and hepatitis A, *Perspect. Virol.,* 9:9-47 (1975).

50. P. J. Christopher, G. S. Grohmann, R. M. Millsom, and A. M. Murphy, Parvovirus gastroenteritis—a new entity for Australia, *Med. J. Aust., 1:* 121-124 (1978).

51. J. B. Kurtz, T. W. Lee, and D. Pickering, Astrovirus associated gastroenteritis in a children's ward, *J. Clin. Pathol., 30:*948-952 (1977).

52. I. D. Gust, R. C. Pringle, G. L. Barnes, G. P. Davidson, and R. F. Bishop, Complement-fixing antibody response to rotavirus infection, *J. Clin. Microbiol., 5:*125-130 (1977).

53. P. J. Middleton, M. Petric, C. M. Hewitt, M. T. Szymanski, and J. S. Tam, Counter-immunoelectro-osmophoresis for the detection of infantile gastroenteritis virus (orbi-group) antigen and antibody, *J. Clin. Pathol., 29:*191-197 (1976).

54. E. S. Jesudoss, T. J. John, M. Mathan, and L. Spence, Prevalence of rotavirus antibody in infants and children, *Indian J. Med. Res., 68:*383-386 (1978).

55. L. H. Ghose, R. D. Schnagl, and I. H. Holmes, Comparison of an enzyme-linked immunosorbent assay for quantitation of rotavirus antibodies with complement fixation in an epidemiological survey, *J. Clin. Microbiol., 8:* 268-276 (1978).

56. R. H. Yolken, R. G. Wyatt, G. Zissis, C. D. Brandt, W. J. Rodriguez, H. W. Kim, R. H. Parrott, J. J. Urrutia, L. Mata, H. B. Greenberg, A. Z. Kapikian, and R. M. Chanock, Epidemiology of human rotavirus types 1 and 2 as studied by enzyme-linked immunosorbent assay, *N. Engl. J. Med., 299:* 1156-1161 (1978).

57. A. Z. Kapikian, H. B. Greenberg, W. L. Cline, A. R. Kalica, R. G. Wyatt, H. D. James, Jr., N. L. Lloyd, R. M. Chanock, R. W. Ryder, and H. W. Kim, Prevalence of antibody to the Norwalk agent by a newly developed immune adherence hemagglutination assay, *J. Med. Virol., 2:*281-294 (1978).

58. J. Kurtz and T. Lee, Astrovirus gastroenteritis age distribution of antibody, *Med. Microbiol. Immunol., 166:*227-230 (1978).

59. H. W. Kim, C. D. Brandt, A. Z. Kapikian, A. G. Wyatt, J. O. Arrobio, W. J. Rodriguez, R. M. Chanock, and R. H. Parrott, Human reovirus-like agent infection: Occurrence in adult contacts of pediatric patients with gastroenteritis, *JAMA, 238:*404-407 (1977).

60. S. Tallett, C. Mackenzie, P. Middleton, B. Kerzner, and R. Hamilton, Clinical, laboratory, and epidemiological features of a viral gastroenteritis in infants and children, *Pediatrics, 60:*217-222 (1977).

61. B. Tufvesson, T. Johnsson, and B. Persson, Family infections by reo-like virus: Comparison of antibody titres by complement fixation and immune-electrophoresis, *Scand. J. Infect. Dis., 9:*257-261 (1977).

62. K. W. Haug, I. Orstavik, and G. Kvelstad, Rotavirus infections in families: A clinical and virological study, *Scand. J. Infect. Dis., 10*:265–269 (1978).

63. A. M. Murphy, G. S. Grohmann, P. J. Christopher, W. A. Lopez, G. R. Davey, and R. H. Millsom, An Australia-wide outbreak of gastroenteritis from oysters caused by Norwalk virus, *Med. J. Austr., 2*:329–332 (1979).

64. T. H. Flewett, M. E. Thouless, J. N. Pilford, A. S. Bryden, and J. A. N. Candeias, More serotypes of human rotavirus, *Lancet, 2*:632 (1978).

65. G. Zissis and J. P. Lambert, Different serotypes of human rotavirus, *Lancet, 1*:38–39 (1978).

66. R. T. Espejo, E. Calderon, and N. Gonzalez, Distinct reo-like agents associated with acute infantile gastroenteritis, *J. Clin. Microbiol., 6*:502–506 (1977).

67. A. R. Kalica, M. M. Sereno, R. G. Wyatt, C. A. Mebus, R. M. Chanock, and A. Z. Kapikian, Comparison of human and animal rotavirus strains by gel electrophoresis of viral RNA, *Virology, 87*:247–255 (1978).

68. L. Spence, M. Fauvel, and R. Petro, Comparison of rotavirus strains by hemagglutination inhibition, *Can. J. Microbiol., 24*:353–356 (1978).

69. S. M. Rodger and I. H. Holmes, Comparison of the genomes of simian, bovine and human rotaviruses by gel electrophoresis and detection of genomic variation among bovine isolates, *J. Virol., 30*:839–846 (1979).

70. T. A. Parrino, D. S. Schreiber, J. S. Trier, A. Z. Kapikian, and N. E. Blacklow, Clinical immunity in acute gastroenteritis caused by the Norwalk agent, *N. Engl. J. Med., 297*:86–89 (1977).

71. J. G. Lecce, M. W. King, and W. B. Dorsey, Rearing regimen producing piglet diarrhea (rotavirus) and its relevance to acute infantile diarrhea, *Science, 199*:776–778 (1978).

72. P. J. Middleton, Analysis of the pattern of infections. In *Etiology, Pathophysiology and Treatment of Acute Gastroenteritis*, Seventy-fourth Ross Conference, (H. J. McClung, ed.), Ross Laboratories, Columbus, Ohio, 1978, pp. 18–23.

_13

Pathophysiological and Clinical Features of Viral Enteritis

J. Richard Hamilton and D. Grant Gall* Research Institute, The Hospital for Sick Children, and University of Toronto, Toronto, Ontario, Canada

To adequately understand and treat the vomiting and diarrhea that characterize viral enteritis, some insight into small intestinal transport processes and their response to these invasive infections is needed. The small intestine accounts for most of the intestinal capacity for water and solute transport, and it is the extent and severity of the disturbances of ion and sugar transport there that determine the severity and course of these diseases. This chapter discusses clinical features in the light of current pathophysiological concepts of commonly recognized viral enteritis.

Normal Small Intestine

Relatively mature in its structure at birth, the human small intestinal mucosa is characterized by a lush villus structure. The villus epithelium is composed largely of columnar absorptive cells possessing a microvillus brush border at the luminal surface. An important point to remember in the context of the discussion that follows is that renewal of the epithelium is a constant process. Cells divide in the crypts, and absorptive cells migrate up the villi to be shed from the tips [1]. This process, which in adults has been estimated to take 4–5 days, may be slower in infants. In fact, it is not yet clear at what stage in pre- or postnatal development that mitoses cease on villi and become confined to crypts. Villus enterocytes

*Present affiliation: University of Calgary, Calgary, Alberta, Canada

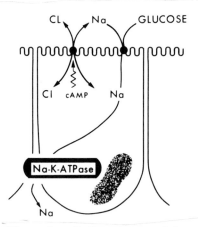

Figure 1   Sodium transport in enterocyte. Glucose-stimulated Na transport and neutral NaCl transport located in brush border, (NA$^+$-K$^+$)-ATPase confined to basolateral membrane. cAMP impairs NaCl uptake but has no effect on glucose-stimulated Na transport.

differ from crypt enterocytes not only in their structure but also in their function. In the crypt the epithelium is composed of poorly differentiated cells, rich in thymidine kinase activity. As these cells migrate to the villus tip many proteins are synthesized, among them the glucose-Na$^+$ carrier and several enzymes, the disaccharidases, alkaline phosphatase, and (Na$^+$-K$^+$)-ATPase, for example [2].

It is estimated that all but 10-15% of the water transported by the gut is absorbed in the small intestine [3]. Water flux across the intestinal epithelium is passive in the small bowel and determined by solute transport, particularly the active transport of Na$^+$ and glucose. Sodium transport is facilitated by a protein carrier at the brush border where glucose and amino acids exert stimulatory effects; a separate mechanism for the coupled influx of sodium and chloride at the brush border is inhibited by cyclic AMP (Fig. 1) [4]. The active Na pump, (Na$^+$-K$^+$)-ATPase, is located in the basolateral membrane of the enterocyte (Fig. 1) [4].

Sugars are hydrolyzed either in the bowel lumen or, in the case of dietary disaccharides, on the surface of the microvillus membrane. Transport of the constituent monosaccharides, largely glucose, into the enterocyte is facilitated by carriers; the most important appears to be the one shared with sodium.

Viral Enteritis

Timing and Site of Infection

Most of the known viral enteric pathogens invade the small intestinal epithelium. Human rotavirus (HRV) has been shown by immunofluorescence to be capable of massive invasion of the epithelium of the jejunum, particularly villus cells [5]. This infection may involve the entire small bowel, but gastric infection has not been noted and colonic involvement is unlikely. Infection can probably be patchy, but in severe cases it has been diffuse. A similar pattern of infection has been noted in parvo-like virus infection in humans [6], transmissible gastroenteritis (TGE) in swine [7], and epizootic diarrhea of infant mice (EDIM) [8]. The extent to which submucosa and regional lymph nodes can be infected is not known and probably varies in different infections, but the epithelium is the major site. Experience with TGE, produced experimentally in 2 to 3-week-old pigs, shows early invasion of the intestinal epithelium after placing the virus in the stomach; shedding of most virus-infected cells occurs within the first 24 h, before diarrhea becomes severe. In piglets infected experimentally with either TGE virus or HRV, virus was shed from the mucosa by the time diarrhea was severe [7,9]. In TGE-infected pigs ileal infection can occur almost simultaneously with invasion of the jejunal epithelium, and virus shed from the upper intestine does not reinfect the ileum [7]. Neither in infants with HRV nor in piglets experimentally infected with TGE have significant abnormalities of enteric bacterial flora been noted [10,11].

The Mucosal Lesion

Lesions of the upper intestinal mucosa have been described in HRV enteritis in infants [12] and in pigs [9], in adult volunteers infected with picorna-parvovirus [6], and in young pigs with TGE [7]. The light microscope features in all are similar: shortening of villi, elongation of crypts, and increased numbers of round cells in the lamina propria. Even under controlled experimental conditions the severity of the lesion is variable, and severe diarrhea may occur in the absence of a lesion visible with light microscopy [10]. Shortening and irregulariity of the brush border in TGE is inconsistent. In TGE or HRV piglet enteritis virus can be seen in villus enterocytes by electron microscopy early in the disease.

Functional Disturbances

Gastrointestinal

Invasion of the proximal small intestinal mucosa presumably is the stimulus for vomiting. Neither direct infection nor inflammatory involvement of the gastric mucosa can be implicated [13]. In infants with HRV enteritis [14] and in piglets with TGE [15], diarrhea is characterized by profuse watery stools containing increased concentrations of sodium, potassium, and chloride. Some patients with HRV enteritis may have excessive fecal sugar, but this has not been a consistent finding and steatorrhea has not been noted. Clearly, dietary sugar and fat consumption will affect fecal excretion of these nutrients.

Table 1 Mucosal Enzymes, Ion and Water Flux in 3-Week-Old Piglets with Acute Transmissible Gastroenteritis (Mean ± 5.0)

	Control	TGE	P
Enzyme activity in jejunal mucosal homogenate			
Sucrase (U/g protein)	7.9 ± 3.2	1.3 ± 0.5	<0.001
Alkaline phosphatase (U/g protein)	9.6 ± 1.6	4.2 ± 0.9	<0.01
$(Na^+\text{-}K^+)$-ATPase (U/g protein)	1.4 ± 0.4	0.9 ± 0.3	<0.001
Net flux, jejunum (in vivo)*			
Na (mM/cm per h)	0.009 ± 0.049	-0.119 ± 0.092	<0.005
K (mM/cm per h)	0.029 ± 0.015	0.003 ± 0.013	<0.01
Cl (mM/cm per h)	0.020 ± 0.058	-0.104 ± 0.073	<0.005
H_2O (ml/cm per h)	0.153 ± 0.430	-0.920 ± 0.752	<0.005

*(-) = Net secretion.
Source: From Ref. 15, with permission of the authors and publisher.

In a series of experiments we have attempted to define the defect in intestinal Na^+ transport in viral enteritis, using as a model transmissible gastroenteritis produced by experimental administration of TGE virus to young pigs [15]. A constant clinical pattern occurs with fever, vomiting, and diarrhea beginning 16-24 h after infection; fever and vomiting subside quickly, while the diarrhea reaches a zenith at 40 h. Table 1 summarizes data on activities of some enzymes in mucosal homogenates and on marker perfusion experiments measuring net absorption of water and electrolytes in the proximal small intestine at the 40 h stage of TGE [10,15]. The activities of the disaccharidases and $(Na^+\text{-}K^+)$-ATPase were significantly diminished and net absorption of sodium, potassium, chloride, and water were significantly decreased in the jejuna of infected animals, but tissue levels of adenylate cyclase and cyclic AMP were normal. We also measured active Na^+ transport in the jejunal epithelium in vitro in Ussing short-circuit chambers [16]. As shown in Fig. 2, tissue obtained 40 h after experimental TGE infection did not differ from control tissue under basal conditions but in the presence of 30 mM glucose the normal stimulation of sodium absorption was significantly blunted. Additional evidence to support the existence of defective glucose-stimulated Na transport has come from studies of epithelial cells isolated in suspension from villi and loaded with ^{22}Na. At the same 40 h stage of TGE infection, efflux rate constants for Na^+ from enterocytes responded less well than controls to glucose (Table 2), confirming the impression of a specific epithelial defect gained from the short-circuit chamber

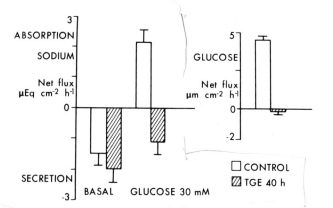

Figure 2 Na⁺ and glucose flux in control and TGE jejunal epithelium measured in Ussing short-circuit chambers. Response of net Na⁺ flux to 30 mM glucose, blunted in TGE (left panel). Net glucose flux impaired in TGE, compared with control (right panel).

experiments. Our observations in this invasive viral enteritis contrast with those found in cholera, where choleragen stimulated adenyl cyclase activity and increases epithelial cell cAMP levels leading to secretion of sodium chloride, but glucose-stimulated Na transport remains intact [4].

Studies from our laboratory in which young conventional piglets were successfully infected with human rotavirus have shown a pattern of pathophysiological abnormalities, identical to those described above for TGE [9]. While diarrhea occurs later, reaching a peak at 72 h, the enzyme and Na⁺ transport abnormalities observed are identical to those outlined for the TGE experiments.

Fecal sugar losses in viral enteritis have not been impressive, but a pathogenic role for glucose malabsorption in viral diarrhea was suggested by the defect observed in glucose-stimulated Na⁺ transport. In a recently completed series of experiments, marker perfusion in vivo and epithelial membranes in vitro

Table 2 Sodium Efflux Rate Constants in Piglet Enterocytes Isolated from Jejunal Villi, 40 h after TGE Infection (Mean ± 5.0)

	Na+ efflux rate constant per hour		
	Control	TGE	P
Basal	11.1 ± 0.4	9.6 ± 0.5	<0.01
Glucose	12.8 ± 0.4	9.5 ± 0.5	<0.001

Source: From Ref. 15 © 1976 The Williams & Wilkins Company, Baltimore, Maryland

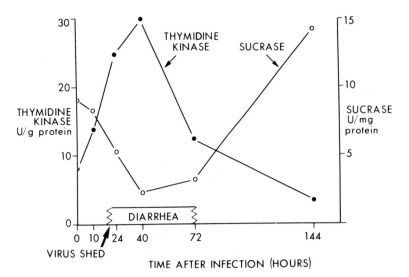

Figure 3 In experimental TGE infection, virus is shed from mucosa by 20 h when diarrhea begins. When diarrhea is worst (40 h) cells isolated from jejunal villi are rich in thymidine kinase, deficient in sucrase activity.

were used to assess glucose transport in acute TGE [17]. As anticipated, the data demonstrated defective glucose absorption which can be attributed to defective enterocyte transport of glucose (Fig. 2). In perfusion studies Na and water absorption were not stimulated by infusing increased concentrations of glucose in TGE, a result predicted from the Ussing chamber data described above.

When intestinal transport was assessed during the course of TGE it became apparent that the defect in glucose-stimulated Na^+ transport was maximal 40 h after infection, the stage in the disease when diarrhea was most severe [18]. However, immunofluorescence studies by Pensaert et al. [19], and in our own laboratory [7] have shown shedding of virus-infected cells within the first 24 h. A clue to this apparent paradox comes from studies of populations of enterocytes isolated from villi at different stages of the disease [18]. As shown in Figure 3, villus cells from pigs 40 h after infection are rich in thymidine kinase activity but deficient in sucrase activity. The pattern for activities of the other disaccharidases, alkaline phosphatase and $(Na^+\text{-}K^+)$-ATPase, resembles that of sucrase. Villus cells at the stage of acute diarrhea have an enzyme profile similar to that of normal crypt cells, suggesting that they have failed to fully differentiate as they migrated along the villi. Further support for this concept comes from Na^+ and glucose transport in small bowel epithelium after invasive virus infection. These functional abnormalities appear to be a result not of direct viral damage but rather of altered epithelial renewal leading to accelerated migration of enterocytes from the crypts and defective differentiation during the migration process. This sequence of events is triggered by an initial viral invasion of the villus epithelium which may occur almost simultaneously along the length of the small intestine. Undoubtedly the extent of the bowel infected affects the severity of the clinical problem, but in addition our data suggest that factors controlling migration and differentiation of the epithelium are also important determinants of the severity and course of viral diarrhea.

Systemic

Because of reduced nutritional reserves and decreased capacity to withstand a fast [19], decreased nutrient intake that accompanies viral enteritis is a particularly significant problem for the infant. In addition to vomiting, anorexia may be severe. Diarrhea is also a particular concern in the young; in this age group water losses can be massive in relation to body size, and although fluid reserves and the proportion of total water found in the extracellular compartment are relatively large, dehydration can progress quickly to shock and death. Dehydration is usually isotonic, but either hypernatremia or hyponatremia can occur. Bicarbonate is lost as organic acids are produced in the intestinal lumen during the acute illness, leading to a systemic metabolic acidosis [20]; Whatever the nature of the deficiency induced by these acute infections, the young infant's capacity to compensate is less than that of the older child or adult. Since renal function is relatively immature at birth and continues to mature during the first year, the renal capacity to conserve water and bicarbonate, when stressed, is likely to be compromised early in life.

Clinical Features

Human Rotavirus Enteritis

Rotavirus is a major cause of acute enteritis in infants and children throughout the world. As more is learned about this infection distinct clinical patterns are being recognized.

Asymptomatic Newborn Infants

In the newborn infant, HRV can be associated with an acute diarrheal illness, but several studies have demonstrated fecal rotavirus excretion in asymptomatic infants in newborn nurseries. Earlier studies in England of healthy full-term babies found that only 8-28% of HRV excretors had symptoms [22,23]. In a more recent report from Melbourne, 77% of infants with HRV, many of whom were immature, had diarrhea [24]. These discrepancies may be attributed in part to differences in the definition of diarrhea and the fact that the Melbourne patients were in a special care facility. The role of immunity acquired transplacentally or by breast milk in determining the clinical response to infection is not known, but one study showed that 75-80% of neonates have serum antibodies to HRV [25], and anti-HRV antibodies have been detected in breast milk [26].

Acute Enteritis in Infants and Children

The major clinical features of a group of 27 infants requiring admission to the hospital because of HRV enteritis, all had vomiting and diarrhea, 23 were febrile, and 13 dehydrated [14]. The disease was most common in the 6-36 month age group, and the clinical syndrome was remarkably consistent. Low-grade fever and vomiting preceded or accompanied diarrhea and lasted 24–48 h, while diarrhea persisted 3-6 days. Although the virus has not been isolated from the respiratory tract, mild respiratory symptoms were noted early in several cases. The emesis rarely if ever contained obvious bile or blood. Stools were watery and at times massive in volume without solid content; mucus, pus, or blood, features of lower intestinal inflammation, were rarely seen in HRV enteritis. At times liquid stool pooled in the baby's gut causing distention and audible borborygmus, and in some patients, watery stool was mistaken for urine. In fulminant cases dehydration and electrolyte imbalance occurred before parents realized their child had diarrhea. Useful early clues to dehydration were decreased general activity and diminished urine volume.

Physical examination of these children should focus on the assessment of their fluid, electrolyte, and acid-base balance. Rectal examination will immediately determine whether fecal water is pooling in the distal bowel and provide a specimen for microbiologic and microscopic study. Signs of dehydration—sunken eyes and fontanelle and diminished skin turgor—may be noted, but the most important quantitative sign of fluid loss is a sudden drop in body weight, anything over 5% signifying serious dehydration. Of course, a rapid thready pulse and a fall in systemic blood pressure indicate shock. Tachypnea may be seen if acidosis has developed. The hypernatremic infant is said to have a skin of "doughy" texture.

To date, clinical descriptions of HRV enteritis in children have focused on severely affected cases but there may be a wide spectrum of clinical severity. In most cases the disease is mild and medical attention is not sought, but at the other end of the clinical spectrum we now realize that in a few patients this infection can pursue a malignant course, progressing rapidly to death almost before diarrhea is recognized [27]. Between these two extremes lies a clinical state representing one of the more common health problems in infants and young children.

In an otherwise healthy child the course of even a severe episode of HRV enteritis is relatively short and self-limited. Although stool consistency may remain altered for weeks, severe diarrhea usually ceases and appetite improves when the virus disappears from stools within a week of onset.

Laboratory data from severely affected patients show a raised fecal Na^+ in the acute stage of the disease, with isotonic dehydration and a low plasma bicarbonate in most cases. Hyponatremia or hypernatremia occurred. Usually peripheral white blood cell counts and erythrocyte sedimentation rates were normal.

Recurrent Enteritis

Young children, particularly when confined to an institution, may be subject to recurrent attacks of acute enteritis. In some cases, HRV may be identified in stools from consecutive illnesses in the same child. It is now recognized that at least two immunologically distinct serotypes of HRV exist, and infection with one fails to protect against subsequent infection with the others [28].

Chronic Enteritis

Two patients in our hospital with severe combined immunodeficiency and severe persisting diarrhea have continued to excrete HRV in stools for several months. We have noted this phenomenon only in the face of profound immunoincompetence. In one patient virus disappeared from the stools when successful immunologic reconstitution was achieved by organ transplant.

HRV Enteritis in Adults

Our limited experience leads us to believe that the disease in adults is rather different than that occurring in the young. Human rotavirus can cause severe symptoms in an adult, but usually the disease is milder than that occurring in the young and the infection may even be asymptomatic. In a single adult volunteer given HRV by nasogastric tube, nausea and crampy abdominal pain developed after 48 h associated with the finding of the virus in stools and viral antigen fluorescence in the jejunal epithelium [11]; there was no diarrhea, and symptoms lasted less than 2 days.

In a study of 57 household contacts of patients with acute HRV, 8 adults with an apparently related diarrheal illness were noted [14]. One of these, an elderly grandparent, was very ill. Virus had also been detected in asymptomatic adult contacts but rarely in a child contact.

Human Parvo-like Viruses

Circumscribed epidemics of acute enteritis involving children and adults have been caused by these agents, of which at least three immunologically distinct strains are recognized [29]; one of these, the Norwalk agent, has been used to induce infection in healthy adult volunteers [30]. The clinical response to experimental infection was varied in that approximately half the subjects developed symptoms; some vomited, some had watery diarrhea, and others had both. Low-grade fever, anorexia, abdominal cramps, and myalgia were common accompanying symptoms. The incubation period for this invasive infection of the upper intestine varied between 28 and 48 h. Symptoms lasted for 48 h at the most, and virus particles had disappeared from the stools by 72 h. Laboratory studies were normal apart from a mild transient leukocytosis. Prolonged illness and long-term sequelae were not seen in the subjects studied.

Others

In the course of virologic investigations of young children with acute diarrhea, negative-stain electron microscopy has identified several other candidate viral etiologic agents; adenovirus, picorna-parvovirus, minireovirus, and calicivirus are among the terms used to describe these structurally distinct viruses [31]. Proof that any of these is a true human pathogen is not yet available, but clinical observations are suggestive, particularly where the pattern of nosocomial spread has been observed. The clinical features of the diseases assumed to be caused by these viruses have been indistinguishable from those seen in infants with HRV enteritis—an acute-onset and self-limited vomiting and watery diarrhea.

Course and Treatment

In an otherwise healthy patient, acute viral enteritis follows a brief, 3-6 day course and leaves no sequelae. The major hazards of these disorders are the dehydration and the electrolyte and acid-base imbalances that may result. In the young, deterioration may be rapid because of the relatively large volumes of fecal loss and immature capacity for compensation.

Obviously for such a prevalent, global health problem, preventive treatment must receive a high priority. No effective preventive measure is yet available, but possible approaches are considered elsewhere in this volume. The main goal of active therapy has been to maintain or restore fluid, electrolyte, and acid-base balance. Extra water must be given, if possible, by the enteric route. Since some solute is needed for water absorption, a sugar solution (2-3% glucose or 4-6% sucrose) is used to which some sodium chloride may be added (approximately 40 mEq/L). At present the ideal mixture has not been designed, but in the light of the pathophysiological findings described above it is sensible not to administer a hyperosmolar solution since transport of both sugars and ions is impaired.

The course of the diarrhea appears to depend to some extent on the normal migration and differentiation of the epithelium during convalescence, functions which are affected by malnutrition in experimental animals.

There is much to be learned about interactions between various nutritional factors and enteric infection, but it is rational to provide adequate nutrients during convalescence. It is usually necessary to limit nutrient intake early in the acute disease, but within 48-72 h of onset, particularly in the infant, there should be a concerted effort to encourage nutrient intake.

Since the major functional disturbances in acute viral enteritis are those of ion transport, antidiarrheal drugs, most of which affect motility, would not be expected to be beneficial. In fact these drugs can be hazardous in young infants. It goes without saying that antimicrobial agents are ineffective in these viral infections and no place has been found for their use even when symptoms persist.

References

1. G. L. Eastwood, Gastrointestinal epithelial renewal, *Gastroenterology, 72*: 962 (1977).
2. D. G. Gall, D. Chapman, M. Kelly, et al: Sodium transport in jejunal crypt cells, *Gastroenterology, 72*:452 (1977).
3. J. S. Fordtran and F. J. Ingelfinger, Absorption of water, electrolytes and sugar from the human gut. In *Handbook of Physiology, Sect. 6, Alimentary Canal,* Vol. 3, (C. F. Code and W. Hudel, eds), American Physiological Society, Washington D.C., 1968, pp. 1457–1490.
4. S. G. Schultz, R. A. Frizzell, and H. N. Nellans, Ion transport by mammalian small intestine, *Ann. Rev. Physiol., 36*:51–91 (1974).
5. G. P. Davidson, I. Galler, and R. F. Bishop, Immunofluorescence in duodenal mucosa of children with acute enteritis due to a new virus, *J. Clin. Pathol., 28*:263 (1975).
6. D. S. Schreiber, N. R. Blacklow, and J. S. Trier, The mucosal lesion in acute infectious nonbacterial gastroenteritis, *N. Engl. J. Med., 288*:1318 (1973).
7. R. W. Shepherd, D. G. Butler, E. Cutz, et al: The mucosal lesion in viral enteritis: Extent and dynamics of the epithelial response to virus invasion in transmissible gastroenteritis of piglets, *Gastroenterology, 76*:000 (1979).
8. L. M. Kraft, Studies on the etiology and transmission of epidemic diarrhea of infant mice, *J. Exp. Med., 106*:743 (1957).
9. G. P. Davidson, D. G. Gall, M. Petric, et al: Human rotavirus enteritis induced in conventional piglets, *J. Clin. Invest., 60*:1402 (1977).
10. D. G. Butler, D. G. Gall, M. H. Kelly, et al: Transmissible gastroenteritis. Mechanisms responsible for diarrhea in an acute viral enteritis in piglets, *J. Clin. Invest., 53*:1335 (1974).
11. P. J. Middleton, M. T. Szymanski, G. D. Abbott, et al: Orbivirus acute gastroenteritis of infancy, *Lancet, 1*:1241 (1974).
12. R. F. Bishop, G. P. Davidson, I. H. Holmes, et al: Virus particles in epithelial cells of duodenal mucosa from children with acute non-bacterial gastroenteritis, *Lancet, 2*:1281 (1973).
13. L. Widerlite, J. S. Trier, N. R. Blacklow, et al: Structure of the gastric mucosa in acute infectious nonbacterial gastroenteritis, *Gastroenterology, 68*:425 (1975).
14. S. Tallet, C. MacKenzie, P. Middleton, et al: Clinical, laboratory and epidemiologic features of a viral gastroenteritis in infants and children, *Pediatrics, 60*:217 (1977).

15. M. Kelly, D. G. Butler, and J. R. Hamilton, Transmissible gastroenteritis of piglets: A model of infantile viral diarrhea, *J. Pediatr, 80*:925 (1972).

16. H. J. McClung, D. G. Butler, B. Kerzner, et al: Transmissible gastroenteritis Mucosal ion transport in acute viral enteritis, *Gastroenterology, 70*:1091 (1976).

17. J. Telch, R. W. Shepherd, D. G. Butler, et al: Jejunal glucose transport in acute invasive viral enteritis, *Clin. Res., 26*:852A (1978).

18. B. Kerzner, M. H. Kelly, D. G. Gall, et al: Transmissible gastroenteritis: Sodium transport and the intestinal epithelium during the course of viral enteritis, *Gastroenterology, 72*:457 (1977).

19. W. C. Heird, J. M. Driscoll, Jr., J. N. Schullinger, et al: Intravenous alimentation in pediatric patients, *J. Pediatr., 80*:351 (1972).

20. M. Pensaert, E. O. Haelterman, and T. Bernstein, Transmissible gastroenteritis of swine. 1. Immunofluorescence, histopathology and virus production in the small intestine through the course of infection, *Arch. Ges. Virusforsch., 31*:321 (1970).

21. R. Torres-Pinedo, M. Lavastida, H. Rodriquez, et al: Studies on infant diarrhea. 1. A comparison of the effects of milk feeding and intravenous therapy upon the composition and volume of the stool and urine, *J. Clin. Invest., 45*:469 (1966).

22. B. M. Totterdell, I. L. Chrystie, and J. E. Banatvala, Rotavirus infections in a maternity unit, *Arch. Dis. Child., 51*:924 (1976).

23. A. M. Murphy, M. B. Albrey, and E. B. Creive, Rotavirus infections of neonates, *Lancet, 2*:1149 (1977).

24. D. J. S. Cameron, R. F. Bishop, A. A. Veenstra, and G. L. Barnes, Noncultivable viruses and neonatal diarrhea: Fifteen-month survey in a newborn special care nursery, *J. Clin. Microbiol., 8*:93–98 (1978).

25. N. R. Blacklow, P. Echeverria, and D. H. Smith, Serologic studies with reovirus-like enteritis agent, *Infect. Immun., 13*:1563 (1976).

26. A. Simhon and L. Mata, Anti-rotavirus antibody in human colostrum, *Lancet, 1*:39 (1978).

27. J. A. K. Carlson, P. J. Middleton, M. T. Szymanski, et al: Fatal rotavirus gastroenteritis: Analysis of 21 cases, *Am. J. Dis. Child., 132*:477 (1978).

28. R. H. Yolken, R. G. Wyatt, G. Zissis, et al: Epidemiology of human rotavirus types 1 and 2 as studied by enzyme-linked immunosorbent assay, *N. Engl. J. Med., 299*:1156 (1978).

29. R. G. Wyatt, R. Dolin, N. R. Blacklow, et al: Comparison of three agents of acute infectious non-bacterial gastroenteritis by cross-challenge in volunteers, *J. Infect. Dis., 129*:709 (1974).

30. R. Dolin, N. R. Blacklow, H. Du Pont, et al: Transmission of acute infectious nonbacterial gastroenteritis to volunteers by oral administration of stool biltrates, *J. Infect. Dis., 123*:307 (1971).

31. P. J. Middleton, M. T. Szymanski, and M. Petric, Viruses associated with acute gastroenteritis in young children, *Am. J. Dis. Child., 131*:733 (1977).

14

Acute Diarrheal Diseases in Humans Caused by Bacteria

R. Bradley Sack The Johns Hopkins University School of Medicine and Baltimore City Hospitals, Baltimore, Maryland

The inclusion of this chapter will serve to make the reader generally aware of another large body of knowledge regarding a different group of etiologic agents. In no sense will this be an exhaustive treatise of the field; for that another book would be necessary. Rather, this chapter will give an overview, bringing into perspective our present understanding and particularly highlighting the newer developments in this rapidly expanding field. The reader is referred to several recent review articles for more exhaustive treatment of selected aspects [1-9].

Only when the importance of each of the diarrheogenic agents, including the viruses, is examined in many diverse places in the developing and developed countries can we come to a true perspective of these agents and how they influence the health and nutrition of the world.

One can, however, be optimistic about the prospects for control of these diseases. As agents are defined and understood clinically, immunologically, and ecologically, there follows the possibility for control through specific environmental interventions, therapeutic improvements and simplifications, and the development of effective vaccines. All these seem reasonable possibilities in the near future.

Historical Information

Until about the past decade, our understanding of bacterial etiologies of diarrhea included only a few species: *Vibrio cholerae, Shigella, Salmonella* (nontyphoid species), *Staphylococcus aureus,* certain "pathogenic" serotypes of *Escherichia coli,* and *Vibrio parahaemolyticus.* All these organisms could be cultured relatively easily; unfortunately, except in outbreak situations, these organisms usually accounted for less than 20% of diarrheal episodes studied. The remaining 80% were often designated "viral," since no bacterial etiology could be demonstrated. Although, as this book amply illustrates, the real viral diarrheas were eventually characterized, new bacterial etiologies were also discovered and their etiologic relationship to diarrhea confirmed: Enterotoxigenic *E. coli, V. cholerae,* non-0 group 1 (previously called nonagglutinating vibrios or noncholera vibrios), *Yersinia enterocolitica, Campylobacter jejuni, Bacillus cereus, Aeromonas hydrophila, Clostridium perfringens,* and most recently, *Clostridium difficile.* With this expansion of agents has come the expanded need for laboratory capabilities for isolating them. Unfortunately, at present, relatively few laboratories in the world can isolate all these organisms.

Ecology of the Gastrointestinal Tract

The bacterial flora of the gastrointestinal tract is established within several weeks after birth, and except for intrusions by pathogens or antibiotics, the ecosystem remains relatively stable for the life of the individual [10,11]. The stomach and proximal small bowel are kept relatively free of significant microbial flora. Ingested organisms are killed efficiently by the low pH of the gastric contents; those that survive passage through the stomach are rapidly propulsed through the small bowel by normal peristalsis. Toward the distal small bowel, there is a gradual increase in microbial flora, mainly of coliforms; distal to the ileocecal valve there is an abrupt increase in numbers and types of bacteria, now dominated heavily by anaerobic species, representative of the fecal flora. We are now only beginning to understand the importance of other regulatory mechanisms of the intestine, including the secretory immune system, the microenvironment such as mucous secretion, oxidation-reduction potentials, and bacterial factors such as production of colicins, chemotaxis, and utilization of nutrients. Rather drastic changes are needed to disturb this ecosystem significantly; these include the loss of gastric acid production, the impairment of normal peristalsis, the creation of blind, nondraining loops of intestine, severe abnormalities in the immune system or the administration of antibiotics.

Unlike many animal species, the proximal small bowel of humans has a scant microbial flora, and therefore would seem particularly vulnerable to bacterial pathogens, assuming that bacterial competition is a major factor in excluding newly introduced organisms. Indeed, most bacterial enteric pathogens either primarily attack the small bowel, or at least have a phase in pathogenesis which involves the small bowel.

Etiologic Agents

The presently recognized bacterial etiologic agents are listed in Table 1, along with information regarding their virulence mechanisms and methods for recognition of the diseases they produce. Although many of these organisms grow on ordinary bacteriologic media, species identification alone may not be sufficient for designating them as pathogenic.

Pathogenesis and Pathophysiology

At present there are only two well-recognized virulence mechanisms: enterotoxin production and invasion of mucosal cells. Although these are usually thought of as mutually exclusive mechanisms, there are some organisms in which both have been described in experimental models, i.e., *Shigella, Salmonella, Yersinia,* and *V. parahaemolyticus.*

We know much more about the events that occur in enterotoxic diseases than in invasive disease, as will become evident from the discussion to follow. Mechanisms which affect colonization will first be reviewed, followed in turn by a more detailed review of the enterotoxic and invasive processes.

Inoculum

In all these illnesses, with the exception of the enterotoxic disease caused by *S. aureus* (and possibly *B. cereus*), the causative organisms are ingested. In staphylococcal food poisoning, the enterotoxin which is produced in food products is ingested intact. Althouth this mechanism could theoretically occur in other enterotoxic diseases, such as cholera [12,13], it has never been documented to occur in nature.

The size of the bacterial inoculum needed to establish clinical disease in natural populations is unknown. Under laboratory conditions in which graded inocula are administered to healthy volunteers, attack rates between 25 and 50% have been produced with *V. cholerae* [14], *E. coli* [15], *Shigella* [16], and *Salmonella* [17]. In natural populations, in which the attack rates are considerably lower (usually less than 1%), the infecting dose is undoubedly also less and more variable, depending on the characteristics of the host and the vehicle of ingestion.

Under experimental conditions in humans large inocula of approximately 10^8-10^{10} *V. cholerae* are needed to produce clinical illness; when gastric acidity has been neutralized, however, 10^4-10^6 organisms are sufficient [14]. For clinical disease to occur with enterotoxigenic *E. coli,* also approximately 10^8

Table 1 Currently Recognized Bacterial Causes of Acute Diarrheal Disease

Organism	Site of colonization		Mechanism of pathogenesis		Methods of diagnosis			
	Small bowel	Large bowel	Enterotoxin production	Invasion	Direct stool examination	Isolation from stool selective media	Serologic diagnosis[a]	
							Antitoxin	Antibacterial
V. cholerae, 0 group 1	+		+	-	+b,c,d	+ (TCBS agar)	+	+
V. cholerae, non-0 group 1	+		+	-	-	+ (TCBS agar)	NTe	-
V. parahaemolyticus	+		+f	+	-	+ (TCBS agar)	-	-
E. coli								
Enterotoxigenic (EPEC)	+		+	-	+d	-	+	-
Invasive		+	-	+	+g	-	-	-
Classic enteropatho-genic serotypes (ETEC)	+		Probable	-	+b	-	-	+ Type specific
Shigella		+	+f	+k	+f,g	+	+	+ Type specific
Salmonella	+	+	+f	+	-	+	-	+ Type specific
Aeromonas hydrophila	Unknown		+f	?	-	+	NTe	-
Yersinia enterocolitica		+	+f	+	-	+ (Cold enrichment)	-	+
Campylobacter jejuni		+	-	+l	-	+ (Antibiotic-containing media)	-	+ Type specific

S. aureus						
Food-poisoning strains	Do not colonize	+	-	-[h]	NT[e]	-
Enterocolitis strains	+	-	+[i]	+	-	-
C. perfringens						
Type A—food poisoning strains	+	+	+[d]	-[h]	+	-
Type C—pig-bel strains	+	+[j]	-	+	+	-
B. cereus	+	+	-	-[h]	NT[e]	-
C. difficile	+	+	+[d,g]	+	NT[e]	-

[a] Fourfold or greater serum antibody rise to enterotoxin or 0 antigen.
[b] Darkfield microscopy, immobilization test
[c] Fluorescent antibody identification possible.
[d] Toxin detectable in stool.
[e] Extensive testing has not been done.
[f] Role of enterotoxin in pathogenesis not established.
[g] Presence of polymorphonuclear exudate helpful.
[h] Isolation from food necessary to establish etiologic role.
[i] Gram stain may be helpful.
[j] *C. perfringens* beta toxin, not classified as enterotoxin.
[k] From Ref. 223.
[l] From Ref. 224.

organisms given without antacids are necessary [15]. For *Salmonella* infections, approximately 10^6–10^8 organisms are necessary to produce a 25% clinical attack rate [17]. *Shigella* infection requires the lowest inoculum, and as few as 10-100 organisms can produce clinical disease [16,18]. It should also be pointed out that in some animal models, as few as 10 *V. cholerae* organisms can initiate the typical disease [19].

Factors that determine why more of one bacterial species than another are needed to initiate infection are poorly understood, the only exception being the obvious pH effect of the stomach which allows relatively few acid-sensitive organisms to reach the duodenum.

Colonization

The early phase of colonization is largely obscured by our inability to visualize small concentrations of bacteria. We know, however, that the bacteria must overcome or coexist in the normal microenvironment, which includes an unstirred water layer, a blanket of mucus which covers the mucosal cells, intraluminal enzymes, bile salts and secretory antibodies, and in the large bowel a

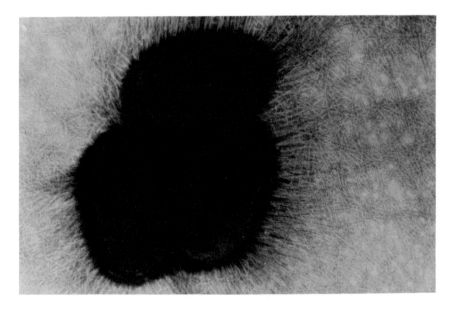

Figure 1 Negative stain preparation of human *E. coli* strain PB-200, showing colonization factor antigen. (Courtesy of Drs. Dolores and Doyle Evans, from Ref. 22.)

heavy concentration of resident microbes. The newly colonizing bacteria may be equipped with flagella and fimbria (which aid in locomotion and attachment), and the ability to produce hydrolytic enzymes (mucinases, lecithinases, and other proteases) and colicins, and may possess appropriate chemotactic receptors, all of which aid in penetrating this microenvironment.

The best understood of these colonization virulence factors are surface fimbria or pili. In *E. coli* these are plasmid-mediated, antigenic, structural proteins which aid in adherence and thus colonization of the small bowel. Although these structures have been most extensively studied as K88 and K99 pili in animal strains of *E. coli* [20,21], they have also been recognized and characterized in certain human strains of enterotoxigenic *E. coli,* as CFAI and CFAII [22,23] (Fig. 1). Undoubtedly, additional colonization factors in human strains are yet to be discovered. Since both the mucosal epithelial cells and the bacteria possess a covering glycocalyx, and each may produce lectins (specific proteins which recognize carbohydrate binding sites) or closely related substances, binding of bacteria to mucosae may occur through these mechanisms [24]. *V. cholerae* has been shown to possess a lectin-like material [25], which could specifically bind to the glycocalyx of the epithelial cells, but has not been shown to possess adherence pili. Conversely, *V. cholerae* [26] and *V. parahaemolyticus* [27] have also been shown to produce a carbohydrate slime (capsular-like) material, which may represent the glycocalyx of the bacterial cell, which could bind to lectins produced by the mucosal cells.

In some strains of pigs, the mucosal receptor sites for K88 fimbria are genetically inherited as autosomal dominants, and resistance to colonization, and thus infection, is complete in animals that are homozygous for the recessive genes [28,29]. It is possible that analogous receptor sites could occur in human epithelial cells, although none have yet been identified.

The importance of the resident microbial flora in providing a protective barrier in humans can best be illustrated in the antibiotic-associated diarrheal disease. Only after the resident, largely anaerobic flora has been eliminated by antibiotics, can the toxin-producing *C. difficile* grow sufficiently to produce the toxin responsible for the clinical illness [9].

In animal models, it has been conclusively demonstrated that the resident anaerobic flora of the small and large bowel protect against infection with salmonella. Removing this flora with antibiotics lowers the infecting dose from 10^6 to 10^1 [30]. A comparable situation, however, has not been conclusively demonstrated in humans. Since salmonella primarily invade the small bowel which normally has a sparse flora in humans, compared to a heavy flora in mice, the analogy breaks down. It has, however, been demonstrated that the normal flora may be helpful in excluding salmonella from the large bowel following illness, since treatment with antibiotics prolongs the time necessary for this clearance of salmonella to occur [31,32].

In shigellosis, the organisms traverse the small bowel, without invading the mucosa, and enter the large bowel where invasion of mucosal cells does occur. It is thought that multiplication of the inoculum may take place in the small bowel during transit, although this has not been well documented.

The entire process of colonization in all these diseases must take at least 12-48 h, which is the usual incubation period for volunteer experiments with these organisms.

Once colonization has begun the organizms grow to large population densities. In the small bowel, concentrations of 10^6-10^9 per milliliter *V. Cholerae* [33] or *E. coli* [34] are found; in salmonellosis [17,35] and shigellosis [26,36] fecal concentrations of 10^6-10^9 per milliliter have been found. The organisms growing in either the small or large bowel are washed distally into the fecal effluent, resulting in large fecal concentrations of the organisms.

Enterotoxin-Mediated Diarrheas

Production of Enterotoxins

When actively growing in the small intestine, and for *C. difficile* and *S. aureus* which grow in the large intestine, the organisms produce the entero-toxins which are mediators of the disease process. The nutrient and physical requirements for some organisms to produce and release enterotoxins have been well defined in vitro (*V. cholerae* and *E. coli*) [37-40], but these do not resemble the microenvironment of the small intestine. Although it would seem that organisms growing in close proximity to the mucosa would most efficiently deliver the toxin to its site of action, it is also true that intralumi-nal toxin (as introduced into the luminal space) can penetrate the normal physical barriers of the small bowel.

Enterotoxins

Enterotoxins have now been described from a number of bacteria caus-ing diarrheal disease. Only in certain instances, however, is it clear that the enterotoxin is important in mediating clinical disease. Furthermore, entero-toxins have often been loosely defined; in the strictest sense, an "enterotoxin" must produce secretory effects in an enteric model system. Enterotoxins can also be described as "cytotonic" or "cytotoxic" depending upon whether destructive morphologic effects are produced in the target cell [41]. Substances which have been shown to be toxic only in systems other than the intestine may not be true enterotoxins.

The best studied and best characterized are the enterotoxins of *V. cholerae* and *E. coli*. In *V. cholerae* the genetic control of enterotoxin production resides in the chromosome [42] and is closely related to the genes for "0" antigen production, since nearly all naturally occurring *V. cholerae* 0 group 1 strains produce enterotoxin. (The only possible exceptions to this have been described recently in isolates from the Western hemisphere in which toxin production could not be demonstrated in the usual model systems [43].) Some vibrios devoid of the 0 group 1 antigen have also been shown to produce cholera-like enterotoxins [44].

In *E. coli*, enterotoxin production resides perhaps exclusively in plasmids [45], and the genetic material involved has been cloned [46,47]. In this species, 0 antigen and enterotoxin production, though clearly related, are not uniformly associated.

A comparison of the enterotoxins which have been described from all these enteric pathogens is given in Table 2. Also included in the table are the methods currently used for the demonstration of these enterotoxins. The original rabbit ileal loop model, although cumbersome, still remains the standard assay against which new techniques are compared [48]. As can be noted, most of the assays measure biologic activity rather than antigenic determinants; as the enterotoxins are purified, serologic identification will undoubtedly replace many of the unwieldy biologic assays.

Cholera enterotoxin (CT) was the first of the enterotoxins to be highly purified; each molecule consists of five binding (B) subunits to one active (A) subunit [2,3,5,49,50]. The configuration of the molecule is schematically shown in Fig. 2; amino acid sequencing has been completed on the B chain [51, 52]. The heat-labile enterotoxin (LT) of *E. coli* also shares many of the properties of CT, including a similar molecular weight, subunit structure, and immunologic cross-reactions [47,53-55]. Whereas there is only one cholera enterotoxin, produced by either of the two serotypes of *V. cholerae* (Inaba and Ogawa), there may also be only a single LT molecule, produced by the large number of enterotoxigenic *E. coli* serotypes [56]. By way of contrast, the heat-stable enterotoxin (ST) of *E. coli* is a nonantigenic, small molecular weight polypeptide, which has now been purified in several laboratories [57,58]. There may, indeed, be several different ST molecules produced by different *E. coli* species [59].

Enterotoxin Binding to Mucosal Cells

The enterotoxins elaborated by the colonizing bacteria must interact with the epithelial cells to bring about the characteristic secretory effects. Specific substances have been identified which bind the enterotoxins of *V. cholerae* and *E. coli* LT. These are membrane-bound gangliosides, specifically G_{M1} for cholera toxin [60,61] and for LT [62,63], although the specificity of the latter is not as well established. The binding is rapid and tenacious; as little as 1 min of contact is necessary for complete binding to occur, which cannot then be reversed by extensive washing [64,65].

Table 2 Enterotoxins Produced by Bacteria Causing Acute Diarrheal Disease

Organism	Ileal loop	Skin permeability	Tissue[a] culture	Infant mouse	ELISA and/or RIA	Rat ileal perfusion model	Molecular weight	Subunit structure
V. cholerae, 0 group 1	+	+	A,C	-	+	+	83,000	Binding and active
V. cholerae, non-0 group 1	+	+	A,C	-	+		-	
V. parahaemolyticus[b]	-	-	C	-	-		-	
E. coli								
LT producing	+	+	A,C	-	+	+	73,000	Binding and active
ST producing	+	-	-	+	-	+	~3,000	No
Enteropathogenic serotype	-	-	-	-	-	+[b]	-	No
Shigella[b]	+	-	H,F,C	-	-		55,000	
Salmonella[b]	+	+	-	-	-		-	
Aeromonas hydrophila[b]	+	-	A,H	-	-		-	
Yersinia enterocolitica[b]	-	-	H	+[d]	-	-	-	
*S. aureus**								
Delta toxin[b]	-	+	H	-	-	+	-	
Enterotoxins (A → E)	-	-	-	-	+	-	28-34,000	
S. perfringens								
Type A, enterotoxin	+	+	-	-			35,000	
Type C, beta toxin	-	-						
B. cereus								
Enterotoxin	+	+					~50,000	
Emetic toxin	-	-	-	-			< 5,000	
C. difficile	+	+	A,H,F	-	-		~107,000	

V. cholerae, 0 group 1	L	+	G_{M1}	With NAG,[e] LT	↑ cAMP	225–227
V. cholerae, non-0 group 1	L	+	G_{M1}	With CT, LT	Probably ↑ cAMP	228–231
V. parahaemolyticus[b]	L		–	–		232–236
E. coli						
LT producing	L	+	G_{M1}	With CT[c]	↑ cAMP	237–239
ST producing	S	–	–	–	↑ cGMP	240
Enteropathogenic serotype	L		–			–
Shigella[b]	S	+	DGlcNAc		Cytotoxic, neurotoxic	241–248
Salmonella[b]	L	+	–	With CT	Cytotonic	249–253
Aeromonas hydrophila[b]	L	+	–		Cytotoxic	254–256
Yersinia enterocolitica[b]	S	+			Cytotonic	257–260
S. aureus*						
Delta toxin[b]					Cytotonic	261–263
Enteroxins (A → E)	S	+			Cytotoxic, CNS effect	264–266
S. perfringens						
Type A, enterotoxin	L	+			Cytotoxic	267–269
Type C, beta toxin		+			Cytotoxic	270–271
B. cereus						
Enterotoxin	L	+			↑ cAMP	272–273
Emetic toxin	S				CNS effect	274,275
C. difficile	L	+		With C. sordelli	Cytotoxic	276–277

[a] A = adrenal cell, C = Chinese hamster ovarian cells, F = fibroblasts, H = Hela cells.
[b] Role in pathogenesis speculative at present.
[c] All LT preparations cross-react among themselves, regardless of serotype of strain.
[d] Produced only at 25°C.
[e] NAG refer to V. cholerae non-0 group 1.

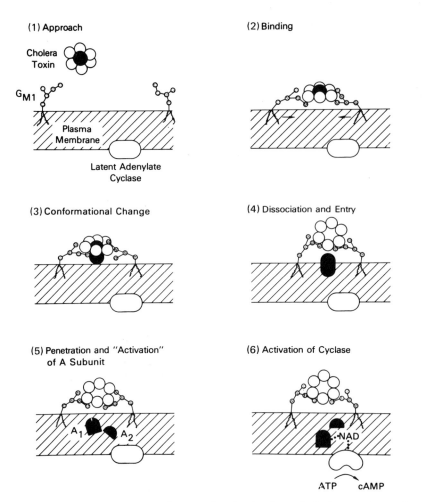

Figure 2 Hypothetical mechanism for the binding of cholera toxin to the cell surface and subsequent activation of adenylate cyclase. This figure which shows six B subunits was originally published prior to the establishment of the five B-subunit structure as described in the text. [From P. H. Fishman and O. R. Brady, Biosynthesis and function of gangliosides, *Science, 194*:906-915 (1976), American Association for the Advancement of Science.]

No specific receptors have been identified for ST or most of the other enterotoxins. ST can be easily rinsed away, thereby abruptly terminating the secretory response [66].

The only other enterotoxin in which a mucosal binding substance has been postulated is that of *Shigella dysenteriae* 1. Evidence has been presented

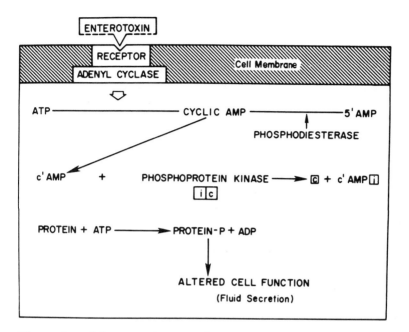

Figure 3 Schematic diagram of a postulated interaction between cholera enterotoxin and the mucosal cell. (Courtesy of Dr. John Banwell, from Ref. 281.)

for membrane receptors in Hela cells and rat liver cells involving $B_1 \rightarrow 4$-linked N-acetyl-d-glucosamine oligomers [67].

Secretory Effects of Enterotoxins on Mucosal Cells

Once binding of CT and LT has occurred through the B subunits, the A subunits are transported into the cytoplasm where a series of biochemical events is set in motion; this results in the activation of adenylate cyclase, increases in intracellular cAMP, and finally active secretion of chloride (Fig. 3) [3,5,68-79]. The enzymatic nature of this process has been extensively studied, and NAD and ATPase are necessary for this reaction to occur [3,5]. Adenylate cyclase can be activated without the binding subunits, if broken cell preparations are used [3,5,71]. Furthermore, the activation is nonspecific, in that other body cells in addition to intestinal mucosal cells will also respond to CT. This property has resulted in many widely diverse biologic systems being studied with the aid of the cholera toxin [3,5,65,72,73].

E. coli ST has been shown to activate guanylate cyclase [74,75]. In contrast, however, this activation is specific to mucosal cells of the small intestine; other body cells fail to respond to the action of ST [74].

The cellular events that occur following the application of the other enterotoxins are less well understood. The cytotoxins all produce obvious morphologic changes in intestinal mucosal cells, which may result in the death of these cells. How this inflammatory and destructive lesion relates to the secretory events that follow is not understood. cAMP increases have been described following exposure to the delta toxin of *S. aureus* [76], and for shigella toxins [77, 78], although whether this is the cause or a result of the toxic effect is not known.

Secretory Cells

The mucosal cells primarily involved in the secretory process have not been conclusively identified. Some evidence suggests that crypt cells are primarily and selectively involved [79,80], whereas other data implicate primarily the villous cells [81,82]. Since the intestine is quite heterogeneous, and since mucosal cells may change in function, as they migrate up the villus in the normal process of cell turnover, these differences in experimental data may be difficult to reconcile. What seems clear is that in most instances there is a prolonged, perhaps irreversible, binding of the toxin to the cells, which probably explains the prolonged action of CT and LT, and the inability of most pharmacologic agents to reverse the action of these toxins, once they are bound.

Gross Secretory Effects

The secretory response to CT and probably LT is greatest per unit length in the most proximal part of the small bowel and decreases distally [83]. (The stomach is not involved in this toxin-mediated secretory response; there is some evidence that the large bowel may be minimally involved [84].)

The time course of action of these enterotoxins is shown in Fig. 4 [1]. The actions of CT and LT are indistinguishable in animal models [66]. Both have a well-defined lag period during which the described intracellular biochemical events are occurring, and a prolonged period of effect, lasting between 18 and 24 h. By way of contrast, ST produces an immediate response, without a lag period, which terminates as soon as it is removed from the mucosa. The composition of the secreted fluid is characteristic for the part of the bowel from which it comes. Thus, enterotoxin-induced secretion is an exaggeration of the normal secretory processes of the small bowel. The protein content is uniformly low (less than 100 mg per 100 ml). The sodium concentration is nearly isotonic in all parts of the small bowel; however, bicarbonate secretion is lowest in the proximal small bowel and increases distally. In the large bowel, there is a steroid-regulated exchange of potassium for sodium. The final result of these processes is a watery diarrheal fluid which has a predictable electrolyte content, which varies depending on the stool rate (Table 3). As the stool rate decreases, the sodium concentration decreases and the potassium concentration increases [85].

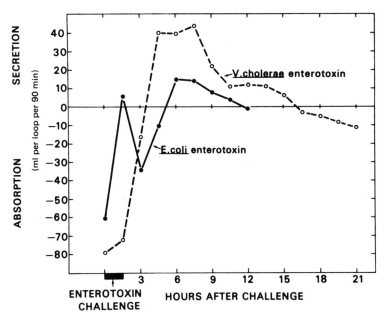

Figure 4 Enterotoxin-mediated secretory responses in approximately 70 cm canine jejunal Thiry-Vella loops. The values given are means of eight dogs for crude cholera enterotoxin and five dogs for *E. coli* 408-3 (078:H12) lyophilized filtrate, containing both heat-labile and heat-stable enterotoxins. For both preparations the challenge dose consisted of 500 ED_{50} units as measured in the rabbit ileal loop. The enterotoxin was perfused over 90 min, followed by fluid measurements at 90 min intervals. (Reproduced with permission from the Annual Review of Microbiology *29*:333–353 © 1975 by Annual Reviews, Inc.)

In small children the stool contains less sodium and more potassium, presumably because of a more effective sodium-potassium exchange in the large bowel [86]. The composition of the enterotoxin-induced diarrheal stool is the same, regardless of the bacterial etiologic agents [87].

In spite of this massive loss of fluid from the small bowel, other absorptive and transport functions remain intact, such as absorption of glucose and amino acids [88]. There is, however, a transient decrease in disaccharidases (particularly lactase) in the epithelial brush borders during the acute illness and early convalescence, again regardless of the etiologic agent involved [89,90].

Pathology

There is no evidence to suggest that the enterotoxins of *V. cholerae* or *E. coli* produce any structural lesions, as seen by either light or electron microscopy [91]. The small bowel pathology in human cholera has been described

Table 3 Electrolyte Composition of Stool in Acute Diarrheal
Disease in Adults and Children

Etiologic agent	Age of patients	mEq1/L			
		Na$^+$	K$^+$	HCO$_3$-	Cl-
V. cholerae[a]	Adults (n = 15)	140	13	44	104
	Children (< 5 years) (n = 32)	101	27	32	92
Noncholera diarrhea[b]	Children (< 5 years) (n = 16)	56	25	14	55
V. cholerae non 0 group 1[c]	Adults (n = 10)	124	14	36	82
Enterotoxigenic E. coli[d]	Adults (n = 88)	110	26	40	76
Rotavirus[e]	Children (< 2½ years) (n = 44)	32	34	5	22

[a]From Ref. 86.
[b]Noncholera diarrheas, a designation used prior to the recognition of enterotoxigenic E. coli and rotavirus. From Ref. 86.
[c]From Ref. 278.
[d]From Ref. 87.
[e]From Ref. 131.

fully in endemic situations [92] and in sporadic and epidemic [93] cases, whereas only a few humans infected with any of the other enterotoxigenic organisms have had small bowel biopsies. In cholera and in enterotoxigenic E. coli diarrhea, the epithelial lining is intact, there is edema of the submucosa, dilated crypts, and minimal numbers of inflammatory cells in the lamina propria; the intercellular tight junctions and capillary endothelial cells are also normal (Fig. 5).

By way of contrast, in animal models and tissue culture assays, the cytotoxic enterotoxins produce destructive changes in epithelial cells with an accompanying inflammatory response which is easily visualized.

Invasive Diarrheas

The invasive diarrheas include those produced by a number of organisms (Table 2), the best characterized being those due to shigella and salmonella. With both

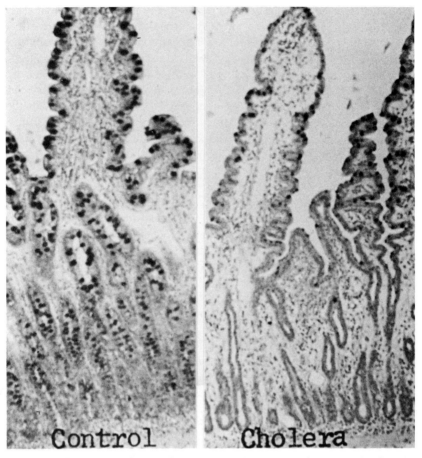

Figure 5 Photomicrographs of canine jejunal mucosa before and 6 h after intra-luminal administration of cholera enterotoxin. The stain is alcian blue, which stains the mucous in the goblet cells. Alterations seen after enterotoxin administration include marked discharge of mucus for the goblet cells, and moderate dilatation of the lumen of the crypts and of the villous capillaries (X 80). (From *Cholera and Other Enterotoxin-Related Diarrheal Diseases,* Charles C. J. Carpenter, ed., *126*:, © 1972. University of Chicago Press, Ref. 98.)

these organisms, the invasion of intestinal mucosa by the organism is essential for the disease process to occur. And yet invasion alone may not be enough; other factors, such as enterotoxin, may then be released by the organisms and mediate the secretory response [35,36].

In the large bowel, shigella and invasive *E. coli* invade the mucosal cells, either as a result of colonization or as an integral part of it. The organisms multiply within epithelial cells, enter the lamina propria but rarely invade the bloodstream. Although this sequence of events is readily observable, the mechanisms whereby this occurs are not well understood. Several factors can be identified in shigella that correlate with invasiveness, and thus virulence of the organisms: colony morphology, lipopolysaccharide structure, and the ability to multiply in mucosal cells [7]. Mutations in any of these characteristics render the organisms avirulent; thus the feature of invasiveness is thought to be under polygenetic control [7]. The properties of the large bowel which allow the invasion to occur are not known. These properties must be absent from the small bowel epithelial cells, since these are not invaded by shigella.

Salmonella, on the other hand, are capable of invading the mucosal cells of both the ileum and the colon (they do not seem to invade the jejunum), and more frequently enter the bloodstream, producing sepsis [35]; virulence seems to be related primarily to 0 antigen structure.

The pathophysiologic events in diarrheal fluid production in the invasive diarrheas are only poorly understood. Following invasion of the large bowel mucosa, and the appearance of destructive lesions in the mucosa, there appears an exudative diarrheal fluid, in small volumes, that contain mucus and blood with a high protein content, and many polymorphonuclear inflammatory cells.

In addition, however, a watery diarrheic phase of illness with both shigella and salmonella has been described clinically in humans and more exactly in the primate model, which often precedes and/or accompanies the symptoms of colitis, characteristic of enterotoxin-mediated small bowel hypersecretion [35,36]. No jejunal histopathology has been found in the primate model, although the jejunum is hypersecreting, and it is postulated that this may represent the effects of enterotoxin(s) produced as these organisms transit this area of the small bowel [35,36]. These findings remain unexplained, however, since there are no cytotoxic effects on small bowel biopsy (which is the characteristic lesion of one of the shigella enterotoxins).

Pathology

The proctoscopic lesions in shigellosis have been well described and range from hyperemia alone, to diffuse ulcerative lesions with or without pseudomembrane formation in the most severe cases [16,18,94]. Histologically, the damage seen correlates with the gross appearance. Similarly, mild colitis has been described proctoscopically in the majority of patients with salmonellosis in whom the procedure has been done [95,96]. The pathologic lesions seen in severe postantibiotic pseudomembranous colitis are similar to those seen with severe shigellosis (Fig. 6).

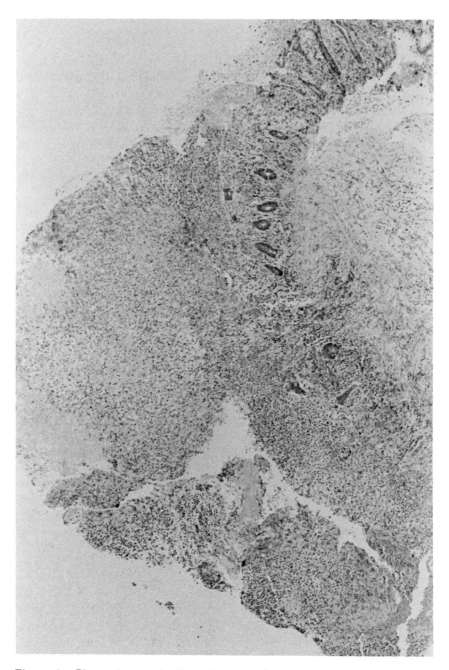

Figure 6 Photomicrograph of rectal mucosa in patient with severe dysentery due to *Shigella dysenteriae* type 1, showing severe mucosal damage and pseudomembrane formation. (Courtesy of Drs. Frederick Koster and Robert Gilman.)

Clinical Disease

Infections with any of these organisms may either cause a spectrum of illness ranging from no disease (i.e., asymptomatic infection) to mild to moderate diarrhea, or severe diarrheal illness such as cholera and severe dysentery, both of which may be associated with significant mortality. In their most characteristic form, two clinically distinct pictures can be readily identified: the small bowel, enterotoxic, or cholera syndrome, and the large bowel, invasive, or dysentery syndrome. Milder forms of each may result in illness not easily distinguishable on clinical grounds alone.

Cholera Syndrome

This is most often caused by *V. cholerae* and enterotoxigenic *E. coli*, but may occasionally be produced by salmonella infection [97]. The clinical events are the results of the physiologic effects of the enterotoxins which cause an outpouring of electrolyte-rich fluid from the small bowel in amounts which overwhelm the absorptive capacity of the large bowel, thereby resulting in massive diarrhea [98]. Therefore, the hallmark of this syndrome is the passing of large volumes of watery diarrhea, resulting in saline depletion, acidosis, and potassium depletion. Vomiting often follows the onset of diarrhea, and there may be a low-grade fever and mild abdominal discomfort. The stool, which is effortlessly passed, is watery in consistency and in its most severe form consists only of clear watery fluid containing flecks of mucus. As the diarrhea continues, the extracellular fluid volume is diminished and signs of saline depletion occur: rapid, weak pulse, poor skin turgor, sunken eyelids, muscle cramps in the extremities, and eventually shock. In cholera this may occur within 8-12 h of the onset of the disease. The serum sodium remains normal, since the diarrheal fluid is isotonic, but the blood pH and bicarbonate drop indicating a base-deficit acidosis, and the serum potassium, which may be normal in the presence of the acidosis, drops rapidly when this is corrected. In the severe cholera syndrome, mortality rates over 50% have been reported. Secondary clinical problems include hypoglycemia in undernourished children [99], third trimester abortions [100], and acute renal failure [101].

All signs and symptoms are easily corrected with appropriate fluid and electrolyte replacement. Vomiting usually stops shortly after shock and acidosis are corrected, although the diarrhea continues for a variable length of time. Diarrhea due to enterotoxigenic *E. coli* often lasts only 1-3 days, whereas that due to *V. cholerae* may last 3-7 days, without antibiotic treatment. Whether these differences are due primarily to the organism or to the host is not known. Cholera patients who are malnourished have diarrhea which lasts longer than that of well-nourished patients; this is thought to be due to the slower intestinal mucosal cell turnover rate in malnutrition [102]. In persons living in cholera-endemic areas, enterotoxigenic E. coli may produce a disease indistinguishable clinically from cholera, though of shorter duration [87]. In travelers to developing countries, however, E. coli typically produce a milder diarrhea but of longer duration, often 2-4 days [103,104].

Following a clinical recovery, the pathogenic organisms are usually no longer found in the intestinal tract. Some patients who continue to excrete pathogens for only a few days after recovery have been termed short-term carriers. However, in a few cholera patients who have not been treated with antibiotics, the gall bladder is colonized by V. cholerae. This colonization may or may not be associated with cholecystitis, and in rare cases may persist for several years [105]. Presumably, the vibrios migrate from the heavily colonized small bowel into the gall bladder through the patent bile ducts. What role this carrier state plays in the spread of cholera is not known. No other enteric pathogens, other than salmonella, have been found to inhabit the gall bladder, although no extensive searches have been made.

Dysentery Syndrome

This is most frequently caused by shigella, but may also be caused by invasive E. coli, V. parahaemolyticus, and Campylobacter jejuni. A similar clinical syndrome indistinguishable from these caused by bacteria may also be caused by Entamoeba histolytica. Fever, cramping abdominal pains, and the frequent passage of small volumes of liquid stool containing blood and mucus are the characteristic features of this syndrome. The patient may appear quite toxic, but usually without evidence of severe saline depletion. Proctoscopic examination reveals inflammation of the rectal mucosa, as described above.

The disease characteristically lasts longer than the enterotoxic disease, usually from 4 to 10 days. Malnutrition is frequently seen in association with dysentery. Therapy consists of supportive care, including fluid replacement, and the administration of an appropriate antibiotic. An hemolytic-uremic syndrome, thought to be secondary to circulating endotoxin, has been described following severe dysentery due to S. dysenteriae 1 [106]. Reiter's syndrome has also been associated with shigellosis, occuring in a small percentage of Caucasian adults following recovery from dysentery. The syndrome may result from an immunologic attack mediated by immune response genes, but the connection with shigellosis is unexplained [107]. Severe malnutrition, especially kwashiorkor, may follow clinical shigellosis; marked protein excretion from the gut, as much as 10 g/day, certainly contributes, and has prompted some to include shigellosis among the "protein-wasting enteropathies."

Diagnosis

In many cases the clinical picture will serve to differentiate the category of disease present. In milder cases, however, there is much overlap in clinical presentation, making the clinical distinction almost impossible, particularly in small children. An etiologic diagnosis can be established through the selective use of several laboratory procedures, including a direct light microscopic examination of the stool, culture of the stool for bacteriologic diagnosis, or determination of serum antibody titers.

Direct Microscopic Stool Examination

Methylene Blue Stain
Methylene blue stain for the detection of fecal leukocytes may be of help in distinguishing "invasive" from "enterotoxic" diarrhea [108]. The examination is most helpful when there are many polymorphonuclear leukocytes present (strongly positive) or none present (clearly negative). Small numbers of fecal leukocytes can be seen in noninvasive diarrheas, and in mixed infections.

Darkfield Examination
A direct darkfield examination of watery stool can be used to make the presumptive diagnosis of cholera rapidly. When specific *V. cholerae* antisera are mixed with stool containing *V. cholerae,* the characteristic darting motility of the vibrios will cease [109].

Fluorescent Antibody
Fluorescent antibody techniques have been used successfully to detect *V. cholerae* and certain serotypes of enteropathogenic *E. coli* and salmonella in direct stool smears [110-112]. Because of the many technical limitations, however, these methods have not been widely used.

Gram Stain
Except to the very experienced eye, a gram stain of stool is rarely of any use diagnostically. The obvious exception is in staphylococcal enterocolitis, where large numbers of clumps of gram-positive cocci may be seen.

Detection of Enterotoxins in Stool

The enterotoxins of *V. cholerae* [113-115], *E. coli* LT [115,116], *C. perfringens* [117], and *C. difficile* [118,119] can be identified directly in stool, either by their characteristic biologic activities, or their antigenic specificity by enzyme-linked immunosorbent assay (ELISA) [116]. These assays are now research tools, but hold promise of widespread application when the methods are further refined.

The detection of the enterotoxin of *C. difficile* in stool is at present the preferred way to establish that diagnosis [9].

Bacteriologic Diagnosis

In most cases, the etiologic agent must be grown from the stool. The exceptions to this are those illnesses caused by ingestion of preformed staphylococcal enterotoxin, or the ingestion of large numbers of *C. perfringens* or *B. cereus* in food. In such instances the organisms or the toxin must be detected in the implicated food. The standard bacteriologic procedures developed for the detection of salmonella and shigella are not adequate for the isolation of some of the newly described pathogens. The selective methods needed are given in Table 1.

Serologic Diagnosis

Paired acute and convalescent sera may show diagnostic (fourfold or greater) rises in antibody titer. Such antibody responses against somatic antigen [120, 121] or enterotoxin [122] may be useful in cholera; similarly, such responses to anti-enterotoxins may be useful in detecting *E. coli* LT disease in endemic areas [123]. Antibody rises against somatic antigen may also be useful in diagnosis of diarrheas due to campylobacter [8], shigella (particularly *S. dysenteriae* type 1) [124], and yersinia [125]. Antitoxins may be found following infection with *C. perfringens* [117] or shigella [126], although these are not widely used diagnostically.

Therapy

The therapy of all the diarrheal diseases, regardless of etiology, is similar, and consists of: (1) replacement of the fluids and electrolytes lost in the stool, (2) treating the specific etiologic agent when that therapy is known to be effective, and (3) providing nutritional support during the diarrheal episode.

Fluid Replacement Therapy

This can be accomplished either parenterally or orally. In patients who are hypotensive or comatose or who have severe vomiting, the initial replacement must be by the intravenous route. A number of fluids can be used for this purpose; they should be isotonic, contain potassium and some form of base, and have a sodium chloride concentration of about 120 mEq/L. Guidelines for the practical use of this therapy are given elsewhere [127]. In treating hypovolemic shock, the intravenous fluids must be given rapidly to restore blood pressure to normal; this is infrequently necessary except in the cholera syndrome.

Of more general use and applicability is the replacement of diarrheal losses by the oral route. This therapy, initially developed for the treatment of cholera, has been shown to be effective for therapy of all diarrheal diseases, regardless of etiology, and in all age groups (Table 4) [128,129]. The rationale for using this glucose-electrolyte solution is based on the observation that the small bowel glucose-coupled sodium transport mechanism is sufficiently intact

Table 4 Composition of Oral Glucose-
Electrolyte Solution Used for Therapy
of Acute Diarrheal Diseases*

Electrolyte	mEq/L
Sodium	90
Potassium	20
Chloride	80
Bicarbonate	30
Glucose	111

*One liter contains sodium chloride,
3.5 g; sodium bicarbonate, 2.5g; Potassium chloride, 1.5 g; Glucose, 20.0 g;
or Sucrose, 40.0 g.
Source Compiled from Refs. 127 and 128.

in all diarrheas to promote adequate sodium absorption even in the presence of diarrhea. Bicarbonate and potassium absorption also occurs adequately during diarrhea. Although glucose is the preferred sugar to use in this fluid, sucrose can also be successfully substituted in areas where glucose is not available [130, 131]. This is possible because the disaccharidase sucrase is largely unimpaired in most patients with diarrheal disease [90]. Detailed guidelines for use of oral therapy in diarrheal disease treatment are given elsewhere [128].

Antimicrobial Therapy

There are three diarrheal diseases in which antimicrobial therapy is clearly indicated: cholera, shigellosis, and antibiotic-associated pseudomembranous enterocolitis.

Cholera

In cholera, tetracycline is clearly the drug of choice. When given as 500 mg every 6 h for 2 days to adults, the disease is predictably shortened to about 36 h, and vibrio excretion ceases after 1–2 days [132]. No clinical effect is seen during the first 24 h, presumably due to the continuing action of mucosal-bound enterotoxin. *V. cholerae* have remained uniformly sensitive to tetracyclines, with few exceptions [133,134], in spite of their widespread use over the past 15 or so years.

Other antimicrobials which are effective are: doxycycline, given either as a single large dose [135] or as multiple doses [136], furazolidone [137], chloramphenicol [138], or trimethoprim-sulfamethoxazole [139]. Interestingly, ampicillin is not uniformly effective.

Shigellosis

The course of shigellosis is also markedly shortened with antibiotics; fever rapidly declines, dysenteric stools diminish, and the excretion of shigella organisms ceases. The antibiotic of choice, however, depends on the sensitivity patterns of the shigella. Tetracycline, though effective against sensitive strains, is rarely used since most strains are now resistant in vitro. There is, however, evidence to suggest that disease due to these resistant strains can be successfully treated with tetracycline, presumably because of the high intraintestinal concentrations of the drug achieved [140]. Ampicillin is the drug of choice in most parts of the world; it is given as 50 mg/kg per day for 5 days in adults [94]; recent evidence suggests that a single large dose may also be adequate therapy [141]. In areas where resistance is found, trimethoprim-sulfamethoxazole has also been found effective [142,143]. Small children under 3 years of age often require larger doses of antibiotics (100 mg ampicillin per kg per day) to prevent clinical and bacteriologic relapses [94].

Antibiotic-Associated Pseudomembranous Enterocolitis

In this disease, antibiotic therapy is clearly indicated. Clinically the disease is terminated within 1-2 days after institution of therapy, and mortality, which is significant in untreated cases, is therefore prevented [144-146]. Vancomycin, given orally, 2 g/day in adults, is effective against both etiologic agents: *S. aureus* and *C. difficile.*

Other Diarrheal Diseases

The one diarrheal disease in which antibiotic therapy is usually contraindicated is salmonellosis. In the simple acute diarrheal disease caused by these organisms, antibiotics do not alter the clinical course of disease or eradicate the organism. Indeed, they often prolong the length of time the patient excretes the organism following recovery [31,32]. It should be stressed, however, that in those cases in which the salmonella are thought to have invaded the bloodstream, as evidenced by high fever, toxicity, or positive blood cultures, antibiotics are clearly indicated. Ampicillin or chloramphenicol are the drugs of choice for this indication.

The role of antibiotics in the treatment of the remaining diarrheal diseases is unclear. In diarrhea due to enterotoxigenic *E. coli,* which is already of short duration, there seems to be little effect of tetracycline in further shortening of the disease [87]. Controlled trials of antibiotics in the other bacterial diarrheal illnesses have not been done, although erythromycin is felt to be the drug of choice for the treatment of campylobacter diarrheas [8].

Nutritional Support

Malnutrition is commonly associated with recurrent and/or prolonged bouts of diarrhea in children living in the developing world. If food is withheld during the illness, the nutritional state of the child further deteriorates. To prevent this, food should be given as soon as the child can accept it, this interval is usually no longer than 12 h after fluid and electrolyte replacement have begun [147,148]. Breast milk should be continued if the child is breast feeding. In children with severe lactose intolerance during and shortly after the diarrheal episode, a lactose-poor diet may be temporarily given.

Antisecretory Agents

Since the recognition of the role of cholera enterotoxin in the pathophysiology of that disease, attempts have been directed toward pharmacologic agents which would block the action of the toxin. A number of agents have been found that, when administered before the toxin, will prevent the expected effects: charcoal [149], aspirin [150], amphotericin B [151], indomethacin [152], polymyxin [153], propanolol [154], and bismuth subsalicylate [155]. Of these, bismuth subsalicylate has been shown to improve the symptoms of the diarrhea of travelers [156]. None of the other have demonstrated clinical usefulness. A number of agents have been found that are effective in animal models, but are not useful clinically: cyclohexamide [157], ethacrynic acid [158], and steroids [159]. Only three have been found that can effectively reverse the action of the toxin once it is bound: nicotinic acid [160], chlorpromazine [161], and berberine [162,163]. Clinical studies have confirmed the antisecretory effect of chlorpromazine in patients with severe cholera [164]. At this time, however, there is no clear indication for its place in the treatment of cholera; only further studies will clarify its general usefulness.

On the other hand, cholestyramine, a cationic exchange resin, has been found to be effective in cases of antibiotic-associated enterocolitis [165]. This agent binds the enterotoxin produced by *C. difficile*, thus interrupting the pathologic process. This drug is not effective in other acute diarrheal syndromes of bacterial etiology.

Other Therapeutic Measures

No other measures are of proven value in the treatment of acute diarrheal diseases. Absorptive agents, such as kaolin and pectin, do not appreciably change the course of illness [166]. Agents which slow intestinal motility, such as diphenoxylate (Lomotil), may be used as temporizing symptomatic treatment in adults, but there is no evidence that they shorten the course of illness. Furthermore, there is a potential hazard in their use; invasive organisms such as shigella may produce more severe clinical illness when these agents are used [167].

Epidemiology

Geographic Distribution

Where extensive studies have been done, most of the etiologic agents causing acute diarrheas have been found worldwide. Some organisms, however, such as Shigella and toxigenic *E. coli*, are clearly more common in the developing world [168-172]. The one agent that has a restricted distribution is *V. cholerae* 0 group 1, the only cause of pandemic disease. With intensive surveillance, however, even this organism is now being found in sewage and aquatic environments in areas in which clincal cholera has not been found, such as in Japan [173], the United States (Chesapeake Bay) [174], and areas of South America [43].

Seasonal Occurrences

In temperate climates, most acute bacterial diarrheas occur during the warm season [168]. In tropical climates, cases occur throughout the year, again often reaching a peak incidence during the hottest seasons. Cholera often occurs seasonally, though the cycle, for unknown reasons, is characteristic of the geographic area [175].

Patterns of Disease

These diseases can occur in several different patterns, which can be characterized as: pandemic, epidemic, endemic, common-source outbreaks, the diarrhea of travelers, and antibiotic-associated diarrheas (Table 5).

Pandemic
Pandemic disease has been caused only by *V. cholerae*. We are presently in the seventh pandemic of cholera; the disease has extended throughout Southeast Asia and the Far East, to the Middle East, Russia, Southern Europe, Africa, and now threatens South America [177]. It is of interest that *V. cholerae* of a different type has caused cholera in the United States [176].

Epidemic
Epidemics of disease have been caused by shigella, *V. cholerae, E. coli,* and salmonella. Large epidemics of dysentery due to *S. dysenteriae* 1 carrying plasmids conferring multiple antibiotic resistance have appeared and disappeared simultaneously in Central America [178] and Bangladesh [179]. Annual epidemics of cholera often occur regularly in cholera-endemic areas of Southeast Asia. Outbreaks of shigellosis and salmonellosis have occurred in custodial institutions and nursing homes where sanitary conditions were suboptimal; nursery outbreaks of *E. coli*-mediated diarrheal disease are well documented.

Table 5 Recognized Epidemiologic Patterns of Acute Diarrheal Disease

Pandemic	Epidemic	Endemic[a]	Common-source outbreaks	Travelers' diarrhea	Antibiotic-associated entercolitis
V. cholerae	*V. cholerae*	*V. cholerae*	*V. cholerae*	*E. coli*-ETEC[b]	*S. aureus*
	E. coli-ETEC[b]	*V. cholerae* non-0 group 1[b]	*V. cholerae* non-0 group 1[b]	*E. coli*-invasive	*C. difficile*
	E. coli-EPEC	*V. parahaemolyticus*	*V. parahaemolyticus*	Shigella	
	Shigella	*E. coli*-ETEC[b]	*E. coli*-ETEC[b]	Salmonella[c]	
	Salmonella[c]	*E. coli*-invasive	*E. coli*-invasive		
		Shigella	Shigella		
		Salmonella[c]	Salmonella[c]		
		Campylobacter[b]	Yersinia[b]		
		Aeromonas	Campylobacter[b]		
			S. aureus-food poisoning		
			C. perfringens-food poisoning		
			C. perfringens[c]-pig-bel		
			B. cereus		

[a]Sporadic cases of food poisoning almost impossible to identify.
[b]Known animal reservoirs, although transmission from animals to humans only speculative.
[c]Known animal reservoir, with known animal-to-human transmission.

Endemic

Endemic disease undoubtedly accounts for the vast majority of diarrheal disease worldwide. Furthermore, of all the bacterial pathogens, enterotoxigenic *E. coli* probably accounts for the majority of endemic diarrheal disease of bacterial origin, particularly in small children [169]. The developing world and areas where sanitation is poor are the geographic areas where endemic diarrheal diseases flourish.

In Bangladesh, the endemic patterns of diarrheal disease have been studied. Enterotoxigenic *E. coli* and rotavirus occur primarily in children between 6 and 24 months of age, whereas *V. cholerae* occurs primarily in older children, aged 3-4 years [169]. No such systematic studies have been carried out elsewhere in the developing world.

Sporadic cases of diarrhea in these areas are also caused by shigella and salmonella, although the infection rate is much less than for *E. coli*. The age of highest incidence also is under 3 years. In South Africa and Belgium, *Campylobacter jejuni* has been isolated from as high as 7-10% of sporadic cases [8, 180].

Common-Source Outbreaks

There have been common-source outbreaks due to practically all these recognized pathogens. Water, milk, and a wide variety of foods have been known to be responsible for large outbreaks. In fact, the occurrence of outbreaks has facilitated the recognition of some of these organisms as pathogens, particularly *V. cholerae* non-0 group 1 [181], *Yersinia enterocolitica* [182], and *C. jejuni* [183].

Travelers' Diarrhea

Travelers' diarrhea is a special category of disease which occurs primarily in persons from the developed world who visit developing areas. Attack rates may be as high as 50-70% within the first 2-3 weeks of arriving in the area [103,104,184-186]. Although a number of bacterial and viral agents can occasionally be responsible for this syndrome, the most common cause is enterotoxigenic *E. coli,* which can be detected in 40-70% of episodes [103,104,184]. It is postulated that the immunologically inexperienced traveler acquires the organisms endemic to these developing areas, which are the same organisms responsible for diarrhea in small children living there.

Since in many parts of the world these organisms are unusually sensitive to antibiotics, such as tetracycline, it has been possible to protect travelers against the disease by the prophylactic administration of doxycycline, a long-acting tetracycline (given as 100 mg once a day) for periods of up to 3 weeks [187,188].

Antibiotic-Associated Entercolitis

Antibiotic-associated enterocolitis occurs mainly in those persons taking broad-spectrum antibiotics, particularly clindamycin. The symptoms may develop while the patient is taking the drug or up to 2 weeks after it has been discontinued. The primary organism responsible, *C. difficile,* though found in only a small percentage of normal stools (1-2%), is able to grow to large concentrations because of the antibiotic-induced suppression of the remainder of the anaerobic large bowel flora [9]. There is also evidence that this organism may be nosocomially spread [189].

Transmission

Transmission usually occurs through contaminated water and food, with the notable exception of shigella, which may be spread by person-to-person contact. Humans are the only known reservoirs for many of these pathogens; the clear exceptions to this are salmonella, *V. cholerae* non-0 group 1, yersinia, and campylobacter, which are found widespread in many animal species. *V. cholerae* [105], salmonella [190], and shigella [191] occasionally may be carried by humans for months or years. Probably of more importance in transmission, however, are short-term convalescent carriers and persons with asymptomatic infection, as well as those with clinical disease [192].

Immunology

Recovery from clinical cholera is known to produce substantial immunity that lasts at least 1-2 years [193]. Likewise, infection with shigella confers some degree of immunity against reinfection with the same species [16], but not against the other shigella species. Little is known, however, about the specific protective mechanisms that account for this protection. Likewise little is known about the protective immunity that develops following diarrheal disease to the other bacterial pathogens.

At present there are no highly effective vaccines against any of these pathogens, with the possible exception of a *C. perfringens* toxoid vaccine shown to be effective in reducing the incidence of pig-bel in Papua, New Guinea [194]. Cholera vaccine, the only widely used vaccine against human diarrheal disease, provides only limited protection (60% for up to 6 months) in endemic areas [195]. This may be improved by using adjuvanted vaccines [196,197]. No studies of effectiveness in other settings have been performed. Live attenuated oral vaccines for the prevention of shigellosis, which produce species-specific immunity, have been studied under controlled conditions but are not yet at the stage of being practically useful [198].

The secretory immune system of the gastrointestinal tract and its role in promoting recovery from illness and in the prevention of illness is only now beginning to be investigated. Clearly, serum antibodies generally correlate poorly with protection [193], although their titers often rise during convalescence, making them useful as diagnostic markers. Secretory immunoglobulins primarily of the IgA class, have been identified as antitoxins [199], and have been found to protect against clinical cholera in animal model systems [200-202]. Large amounts of antitoxic serum antibody of the IgG type can also protect against clinical cholera in these models; presumably in this situation serum antibody is transported across the mucosal epithelial lining [203]. It is presumed that secretory immunoglobulins directed against surface antigens of the bacteria (0 antigens and colonization factor antigens) may be important in preventing colonization in the small bowel, although this has yet to be clearly shown experimentally. An antibody-mediated effect on the selective growth of the two serotypes of *V. cholerae* has been demonstrated in germ-free mice immunized parenterally with type-specific antigens [204].

What seems feasible in the near future, based on the expanding knowledge of the secretory immune system, is the development of oral vaccines, preferably replicating ones, that contain the appropriate antigens, i.e., enterotoxin, somatic antigens, and colonization factors, that will optimally stimulate local antibody production and thus provide high levels of protection. This could obviously be of major importance in the control of a number of diarrheal illnesses, including cholera, enterotoxigenic *E. coli* diarrhea, and shigellosis.

Discussion of Specific Problems

Serotyping as a Virulence Marker for *E. coli*

Prior to the discovery of enterotoxins, several serotypes of *E. coli*, then designated enteropathogenic serotypes (EPEC) were incriminated epidemiologically as etiologic agents in nursery outbreaks of diarrheal disease. The illness they produced was severe, and mortality rates of 40-50% were reported [205,206]. Autopsy reports showed only a hyperemic, intact, small bowel, without evidence of invasion or inflammation. Several isolates of EPEC, when fed to volunteers, reproduced the clinical diarrheal picture [207]. Because these *E. coli* could only be recognized by their serotypes (no other virulence factors were then known) it was generally assumed that these serotypes were pathogenic when isolated from small children under any circumstances. Several prospective studies, however, failed to show any difference in isolation rates between cases and controls [208], while a few studies did show a higher rate of isolation from cases [209]. When EPEC were tested for enterotoxin production they were uniformly negative, regardless of whether the strains were epidemic or were isolated from sporadic cases [210-212]. Two of these EPEC strains, however, isolated from nursery outbreaks in England, produced diarrheal disease

Table 6 Most Common Serotypes of Enterotoxigenic and Classic Enteropathogenic *Escherichia coli*[a]

Enterotoxigenic strains[b]	Classic enteropathogenic strains[c]
06:K15:H16	026:K60:H11,NM[d]
08:K40:H9	055:K59:H6,7,NM
015:H11	0111:K58:H2,12,NM
025:K7:H42	0119:K69:H6,NM
078:H11,12,NM	0125:K70:H21
0115:H21,40	0126:K71:H27,NM
0128:H7	0127:K63:NM
0149:H10	0128:K67:H12
0159:H4,34	

[a]The frequency of isolation varies with geographic location.
[b]From Ref. 215.
[c]From Ref. 279.
[d]NM = nonmotile strains.

when fed to adult volunteers [213]. These same strains were later shown to produce enterotoxin by the use of a rat ileal perfusion model [214]. At present, then, it seems that some EPEC are probably enterotoxigenic, although the toxin(s) are clearly different from LT and ST. Furthermore, there is no evidence that all isolates of any given EPEC are necessarily toxigenic or even diarrheogenic.

Serotyping may also prove to be a useful marker for enterotoxigenic *E. coli,* particularly those that produce both LT and ST [215,216]. These ETEC have been found to fall into a rather limited number of 0:K:H serotype patterns and biotypes, regardless of their geographic origin [217]. These serotypes are clearly different, however, from the EPEC (Table 6). These ETEC have also been responsible for several nursery outbreaks of diarrhea. Thus, there is a correlation between serotype, biotype, and enterotoxin plasmids in these strains, the nature of which is yet to be explained. Whether serotyping will become a useful tool for recognition of enterotoxigenic *E. coli* is yet to be determined.

Other Bacterial Species as Pathogens

Klebsiella

Klebsiella have been isolated in high concentrations from the small bowel of patients with tropical sprue [218]. They have not been implicated, however, as etiologic agents in acute diarrheal disease. By the rat ileal perfusion technique these organisms can be shown to produce enterotoxins, which have some of the same properties as *E. coli* enterotoxins [219]. These enterotoxins do not give reproducibly positive results, however, in any of the other standard enterotoxin assays. It is postulated that these enterotoxins may be important in mediating the symptoms of tropical sprue. It should be pointed out, however, that many patients with this disease do not harbor these organisms in their small bowel [220].

Pseudomonas *and* Pleisiomonas

Pseudomonas has been shown to produce a skin permeability factor [221], but has never been incriminated in acute diarrheal disease. *Pleisiomonas* has been tentatively linked to acute diarrheal disease in several reports [222].

Acknowledgments

I would like to thank those persons who supplied figures used in the text, those in the Division of Geographic Medicine for their helpful review of the manuscript—Drs. Bob Gilman, Fred Koster, Nate Pierce, and Bill Spira—and Mrs. Vivian Buehler for typing and assembling the manuscript.

References

1. R. B. Sack, Human diarrheal disease caused by enterotoxigenic *Escherichia coli, Ann. Rev. Microbiol., 29*:333–353 (1975).
2. R. A. Finkelstein, Progress in the study of cholera and related enterotoxins. In *Mechanisms in Bacterial Toxicology* (A. W. Bernheimer, ed.), Wiley, New York, 1976, pp. 53–84.
3. D. M. Gill, Mechanism of action of cholera toxin. In *Advances in Cyclic Nucleotide Research*, Vol. 8 (P. Greengard and G. A. Robison, eds.), Raven, New York, 1977, pp. 85-118.
4. T. R. Hendrix and H. T. Paulk, Intestinal secretion. In *International Review of Physiology, Gastrointestinal Physiology, II,* Vol. 12 (R. K. Crane, ed.), University Park Press, Baltimore, 1977, pp. 257–284.
5. M. Vaughan and J. Moss, Mechanism of action of choleragen, *J. Supramol. Struct., 8*:473-488 (1978).
6. G. R. Plotkin, R. M. Luge, and R. H. Waldman, Gastroenteritis: Etiology, pathophysiology and clinical manifestations, *Medicine, 58*:95-114 (1979).
7. A. D. O'Brien, M. K. Gentry, M. R. Thompson, P. Doctor, P. Gemski, and S. B. Formal, Shigellosis and *Escherichia coli* diarrhea; Relative importance of invasive and toxigenic mechanisms, *Am. J. Clin. Nutr., 32*: 229-233 (1979).
8. J. P. Butzler and M. B. Skirrow, Campylobacter enteritis, *Clin. Gastroenterol. 8*:737-765 (1979).
9. J. G. Bartlett, Antibiotic-associated pseudomembranous colitis, *Rev. Infect. Dis., 1*:530-539 (1979).

10. D. C. Savage, Microbial ecology of the gastrointestinal tract, *Ann. Rev. Microbiol., 31*:107-133 (1977).

11. S. L. Gorbach, Intestinal microflora, *Gastroenterology, 60*:1110-1129 (1970).

12. C. Benyajati, Experimental cholera in humans, *Br. Med. J., 1*:140-142 (1966).

13. R. B. Sack and C. C. J. Carpenter, Experimental canine cholera. II. Production by cell-free culture filtrates of *Vibrio cholerae, J. Infect. Dis., 119*:150-157 (1969).

14. R. A. Cash, S. I. Music, J. P. Libonati, M. J. Snyder, R. P. Wenzel, and R. B. Hornick, Response of man to infection with *Vibrio cholerae.* I. Clinical, serologic, and bacteriologic responses to a known inoculum, *J. Infect. Dis., 129*:45-52 (1974).

15. H. L. DuPont, S. B. Formal, R. B. Hornick, M. J. Snyder, J. P. Libonati, D. G. Sheahan, E. H. LaBrec, and J. P. Kalas, Pathogenesis of *Escherichia coli* diarrhea, *N. Engl. J. Med., 285*:1-9 (1971).

16. H. L. DuPont, R. B. Hornick, A. T. Dawkins, M. J. Snyder, and S. B. Formal, The response of man to virulent *Shigella flexneri* 2A, *J. Infect. Dis., 119*:296-299 (1969).

17. N. B. McCullough and C. W. Eisele, Experimental human salmonellosis. I. Pathogenicity of strains of *Salmonella meleagudis* and *Salmonella anatum* obtained from spray-dried whole egg, *J. Infect. Dis., 88*:278-289 (1951).

18. M. M. Levine, H. L. DuPont, S. B. Formal, R. B. Hornick, A. Takeuchi, E. J. Gangarosa, M. J. Snyder, and J. P. Libonati, Pathogenesis of *Shigella dysenteriae* I (Shiga) dysentery, *J. Infect. Dis., 127*:261-270 (1973).

19. J. D. Gillmore, P. M. Versage, and R. A. Phillips, Specific and nonspecific passive immunity in infant rabbit cholera, *J. Infect. Dis., 116*:313-318 (1966).

20. H. W. Smith and M. A. Linggood, Observations on the pathogenic properties of the K88, Hly, and Ent plasmids of *Escherichia coli* with particular reference to porcine diarrhea, *J. Med. Microbiol., 4*:467-485 (1971).

21. I. Ørskov, F. Ørskov, H. W. Smith, and W. J. Sojka, The establishment of K99, a thermolabile, transmissible *Escherichia coli* K antigen, previously called "Kco," possessed by calf and lamb enteropathogenic strains, *Acta Pathol. Microbiol. Scand., 83*:31-36 (1975).

22. D. G. Evans, D. J. Evans, Jr., W. S. Tjoa, and H. L. DuPont, Detection and characterization of the colonization factor of enterotoxigenic *Escherichia coli* isolated from adults with diarrhea, *Infect. Immun., 19*:727-236 (1978).

23. D. G. Evans and D. J. Evans, Jr., New surface associated heat-labile colonization factor antigen (CFA/II) produced by enterotoxigenic *Escherichia coli* of serogroups 06 and 08, *Infect. Immun., 21*:638-647 (1978).

24. J. W. Costerton, G. G. Geesey, and J. J. Cheng, How bacteria stick, *Sci. Am., 238*:86-95 (1978).

25. R. A. Finkelstein, M. Arita, J. D. Clements, and E. T. Nelson, "*Cholera*

lectin": A hemagglutinative adhesive factor from *Vibrio cholerae, Bacteriol. Proc.*, (1978) p. 14.

26. K. N. Neogy and S. N. Sanyal, Adhesive properties and slime formation of vibrios and their relationship to haemagglutination, *Bull. WHO, 40*: 329-330 (1969).

27. B. D. Chatterjee and K. N. Neogy, Detection of capsule in *Vibrio parahaemolyticus, Separatum Experientia, 28*:103-104 (1972).

28. J. M. Rutter, M. R. Burrows, R. Sellwood, and R. A. Gibbons, A genetic basis for resistance to enteric disease caused by *E. coli, Nature, 257*:135-136 (1975).

29. R. A. Gibbons, R. Sellwood, M. Burrows, and P. A. Hunter, Inheritance of resistance to neonatal *E. coli* diarrhoea in the pig: Examination of the genetic system, *Theor. Appl. Genet., 51*:65-70 (1977).

30. M. Bohnhoff, C. P. Miller, and W. R. Martin, Resistance of the mouse's intestinal tract to experimental salmonella infection. I. Factors which interfere with the initiation of infection by oral inoculation, *J. Exp. Med., 120*:805-816 (1964).

31. J. M. S. Dixon, Effect of antibiotic treatment on duration of excretion of *Salmonella typhimurium* by children, *Br. Med. J., 2*:1343-1345 (1965).

32. B. Aserkoff and J. V. Bennett, Effect of antibiotic therapy in acute salmonellosis in the fecal excretion of salmonellae, *N. Engl. J. Med., 281*: 636-640 (1969).

33. S. L. Gorbach, J. G. Banwell, B. Jacobs, B. D. Chatterjee, R. Mitra, K. L. Brigham, and K. N. Neogy, Intestinal microflora in Asiatic cholera. II. The small bowel, *J. Infect. Dis., 121*:38-45 (1970).

34. S. L. Gorbach, J. G. Banwell, B. D. Chatterjee, B. Jacobs, and R. B. Sack, Acute undifferentiated human diarrhea in the tropics. I. Alterations in intestinal microflora, *J. Clin. Invest., 50*:881-889 (1971).

35. W. R. Rout, S. B. Formal, G. J. Dammin, and R. A. Giannella, Pathophysiology of salmonella diarrhea in the Rhesus monkey: Intestinal transport, morphological and bacteriological studies, *Gastroenterology, 67*:59-70 (1974).

36. W. R. Rout, S. B. Formal, R. A. Giannella, and G. J. Dammin, Pathophysiology of shigella diarrhea in the Rhesus monkey: Intestinal transport, morphological and bacteriological studies, *Gastroenterology, 68*: 270-278 (1975).

37. D. J. Evans, Jr. and S. H. Richardson, In vitro production of choleragen and vascular permeability factor by *Vibrio cholerae, J. Bacteriol., 96*: 126-130 (1968).

38. P. B. Fernandez and H. L. Smith, Jr., The effect of anaerobiosis and bile salts on growth and toxin production by *Vibrio cholerae, J. Gen Microbiol., 98*:77-86 (1977).

39. J. F. Alderete and D. C. Robertson, Nutrition and enterotoxin synthesis by enterotoxigenic strains of *Escherichia coli*: Defined medium for production of heat-stable enterotoxin, *Infect, Immun., 15*:781-788 (1977).

40. P. H. Gilligan and D. C. Robertson, Nutritional requirements for synthesis

of heat-labile enterotoxin by enterotoxigenic strains of *Escherichia coli*, *Infect. Immun.*, *23*:99-107 (1979).

41. G. T. Keusch and S. T. Donta, Classification of enterotoxins on the basis of activity in cell culture, *J. Infect. Dis.*, *131*:58-63 (1975).

42. M. L. Vasil, R. K. Holmes, and R. A. Finkelstein, Conjugal transfer of a chromosomal gene determining production of enterotoxin in *Vibrio cholerae, Science, 187*:849-850 (1975).

43. I. K. Wachsmuth, B. R. Davis, J. P. Craig, C. D. Parker, R. B. Sack, T. J. Barrett, H. L. Smith, J. C. Feeley, V. S. Baselski, P. A. Blake, G. Pessoa, E. Hofer, G. A. Costa, E. A. Cosendey, A. S. P. Pinto, and T. M. Martins, *Vibrio cholerae* 01 isolates from sewage in Brazil. Questionable Ogawa, questionable El tor, questionably toxigenic, and questionably pathogenic, *U.S.-Japan Cooperative Medical Science Program*, Bethesda, Md., 1979, p. 83.

44. Y. Zinnaka and C. C. J. Carpenter, Jr., An enterotoxin produced by noncholera vibrios, *Johns Hopkins Med. J.*, *131*:403-411 (1972).

45. H. W. Smith and M. A. Linggood, The transmissible nature of enterotoxin production in a human enteropathogenic strain of *Escherichia coli*, *J. Med. Microbiol.*, *4*:301-305 (1971).

46. M. So, H. W. Boyer, M. Betlach, and S. Falkow, Molecular cloning of an *Escherichia coli* plasmid determinant that encodes for the production of heat-stable enterotoxin, *J. Bacteriol.*, *128*:463-472 (1976).

47. W. S. Dallas and S. Falkow, The molecular nature of heat-labile enterotoxin (LT) of *Escherichia coli*, *Nature, 277*:406-407 (1979).

48. S. N. De and D. N. Chatterjee, An experimental study of the mechanisms of action of *Vibrio cholerae* on the intestinal mucous membrane, *J. Pathol. Bacteriol., 66*:559-562 (1953).

49. I. Lonnroth and J. Holmgren, Subunit structure of cholera toxin, *J. Gen. Microbiol.*, *76*:417-427 (1973).

50. R. A. Finkelstein, M. Boesman, S. H. Neoh, M. K. LaRue, and R. Delaney, Dissociation and recombination of the subunits of the cholera enterotoxin (choleragen), *J. Immunol., 113*:145-150 (1974).

51. Y. Nakashima, P. Napiorkowski, D. E. Schafer, and W. H. Konigsberg, Primary structure of B subunit of cholera enterotoxin. *FEBS Lett., 68*: 275-278 (1976).

52. A. Kurosky, D. E. Markel, J. W. Peterson, and W. M. Fitch, Primary structure of cholera toxin β-chain: A glycoprotein hormone analog? *Science, 195*:299-301 (1977).

53. Z. Dafni, R. B. Sack, and J. P. Craig, Purification of heat-labile enterotoxin from four *Escherichia coli* strains by affinity immunoadsorbent: Evidence for similar subunit structure, *Infect. Immun.*, *22*:852-860 (1978).

54. J. D. Clements and R. A. Finkelstein, Isolation and characterization of homogeneous heat-labile enterotoxins with high specific activity from *Escherichia coli* cultures, *Infect. Immun., 24*:760-769 (1979).

55. S. L. Kunkel and D. C. Robertson, Purification and chemical characterization of the heat-labile enterotoxin produced by enterotoxigenic *Escherichia coli, Infect. Immun., 25*:586-596 (1979).

56. R. B. Sack and J. L. Froehlich, Antigenic similarity of heat-labile entero-toxins from diverse strains of *Escherichia coli, J. Clin. Microbiol., 5*:570-572 (1977).

57. M. Field, W. J. Laird, L. H. Graf, P. L. Smith, and M. Gill, Purification and mode of action of heat-stable enterotoxin of *Escherichia coli. U.S.-Japan Cooperative Medical Science Program,* Atlanta, Ga., 1977, pp. 127-136.

58. J. F. Alderete and D. C. Robertson, Purification and chemical character-ization of the heat-stable enterotoxin produced by porcine strains of enterotoxigenic *Escherichia coli, Infect. Immun., 19*:1021-1030 (1978).

59. R. A. Kapitany, A. Scoot, G. W. Forsyth, S. L. McKenzie, and R. W. Worthington, Evidence for two heat-stable enterotoxins produced by en-terotoxigenic *Escherichia coli, Infect. Immun., 24*:965-966 (1979).

60. W. E. van Heyningen, C. C. J. Carpenter, Jr., N. F. Pierce, and W. B. Greenough, Deactivation of cholera toxin by ganglioside, *J. Infect. Dis., 124*:415-418 (1971).

61. J. Holmgren, I. Lonnroth, J. E. Mansson, and L. Svennerholm, Interaction of cholera toxin and membrane G_{MI} ganglioside of small intestine, *Proc. Natl. Acad. Sci. USA, 72*:2520-2524 (1975).

62. A. M. Svennerholm and J. Holmgren, Identification of *Escherichia coli* heal-labile enterotoxin by means of a ganglioside immunosorbent assay (G_{M1} ELISA) procedure, *Curr. Microbiol., 1*:19-24 (1978).

63. S. T. Donta and J. P. Viner, Inhibition of the steroidogenic effects of cholera and heat-labile *Escherichia coli* enterotoxins by G_{M1} ganglioside: Evidence for a similar receptor site for the two toxins, *Infect. Immun., 11*:982-985 (1975).

64. J. T. Goodgame, J. G. Banwell, and R. R. Hendrix, The relationship be-tween duration of exposure to cholera toxin and the secretory response of rabbit jejunal mucosa, *Johns Hopkins Med. J., 132*:117-126 (1973).

65. S. T. Donta and D. M. Smith, Stimulation of steroidogenesis in tissue culture by enterotoxigenic *Escherichia coli* and its neutralization by spe-cific antiserum, *Infect. Immun., 9*:500-505 (1974).

66. R. B. Sack, J. Johnson, N. F. Pierce, D. F. Keren, and J. H. Yardley, Challenge of dogs with live enterotoxigenic *Escherichia coli* and effects of repeated challenges on fluid secretion in jejunal Thiry-Vella loops, *J. Infect. Dis., 134*:15-24 (1976).

67. G. T. Keusch and M. Jacewicz, Pathogenesis of shigella diarrhea. 7. Evi-dence for a cell-membrane toxin receptor involving beta-1-4 linked N-acetyl-D-glucosamine oligomers, *J. Exp. Med., 146*:535-546 (1977).

68. J. Moss and S. H. Richardson, Activation of adenylate cyclase by heat-labile *Escherichia coli* enterotoxin. Evidence for ADP ribosyltransferase activity similar to that of choleragen, *J. Clin. Invest., 62*:281-285 (1978).

69. D. E. Schafer, W. D. Lust, B. Sircar, and N. D. Goldberg, Elevated con-centration of adenosine $3':5'$-cyclic monophosphate in intestinal mucosa after treatment with cholera toxin, *Proc. Natl. Acad. Sci. USA, 67*:851-856 (1970).

70. D. J. Evans, Jr., L. C. Chen, G. T. Curlin, and D. G. Evans, Stimulation of adenyl cyclase by *Escherichia coli* enterotoxin, *Nature (New Biol.)*, *236*:137-138 (1972).

71. P. D. Zieve, N. F. Pierce, and W. B. Greenough, Stimulation of glycogenolysis by purified cholera exotoxin in disrupted cells, *Johns Hopkins Med. J., 129*:299-303 (1971).

72. W. B. Greenough III, N. F. Pierce, and M. Vaughan, Titration of cholera enterotoxin and antitoxin in isolated fat cells, *J. Infect. Dis., 121*:S111-S113 (1970).

73. R. L. Guerrant, L. L. Brunton, T. C. Schnaitman, L. I. Rebhun, and A. G. Gilman, Cyclic adenosine monophosphate and alteration of Chinese hamster ovary cell morphology: A rapid sensitive in vitro assay for the enterotoxins of *Vibrio cholerae* and *Escherichia coli, Infect. Immun., 10*:320-327 (1974).

74. M. Field, L. H. Graf, W. J. Laird, and P. L. Smith, Heat-stable enterotoxin of *Escherichia coli*; in vitro effects on guanylate cyclase activity, cyclic GMP concentration, and ion transport in small intestine, *Proc. Natl. Acad. Sci. USA, 75*:2800-2804 (1978).

75. J. M. Hughes, F. Murad, B. Chang, and R. L. Guerrant, Role of cyclic GMP in the action of heat-stable enterotoxin of *Escherichia coli, Nature, 271*:755-756 (1978).

76. A. D. O'Brien and F. A. Kapral, Increased cyclic adenosine 3',5'-monophosphate content in guinea pig ileum after exposure to *Staphylococcus aureus* delta-toxin, *Infect. Immun., 13*:152-162 (1976).

77. A. N. Charney, R. E. Gots, S. B. Formal, and R. A. Giannella, Activation of intestinal mucosal adenylate cyclase by *Shigella dysenteriae* 1 enterotoxin, *Gastroenterology, 70*:1085-1090 (1976).

78. Y. Takeda, K. Okamoto, and T. Miwatani, Toxin from the culture filtrate of *Shigella dysenteriae* that causes morphological changes in Chinese hamster ovary cells and is distinct from the neurotoxin, *Infect. Immun., 18*:546-548 (1977).

79. G. M. Roggin, J. G. Banwell, J. H. Yardley, and T. R. Hendrix, Unimpaired response of rabbit jejunum to cholera toxin after selective damage to villus epithelium, *Gastroenterology, 63*:981-989 (1972).

80. H. A. Serebro, F. L. Iber, J. H. Yardley, and T. R. Hendrix, Inhibition of cholera toxin action in the rabbit by cyclohexamide, *Gastroenterology, 56*:506-511 (1969).

81. H. R. de Jonge, The response of small intestinal villous and crypt epithelium to choleratoxin in the rat and guinea pig. Evidence against a specific role of the crypt cells in choleragen-induced secretion, *Biochim. Biophys. Acta, 381*:128-143 (1975).

82. M. M. Weiser and H. Quill, Intestinal villous and crypt cell responses to cholera toxin, *Gastroenterology, 69*:479-482 (1975).

83. C. C. J. Carpenter, R. B. Sack, J. C. Feeley, and R. W. Steenberg, Site and characteristics of electrolyte loss and effect of intraluminal glucose in experimental canine cholera, *J. Clin. Invest., 47*:1210-1220 (1968).

84. M. Donowitz and H. J. Binder, Effect of enterotoxins of *Vibrio cholerae, Escherichia coli,* and *Shigella dysenteriae* type 1 on fluid and electrolyte transport in the colon, *J. Infect. Dis., 134*:135-143 (1976).

85. D. R. Nalin and R. A. Cash, Sodium content in oral therapy for diarrhea, *Lancet, 2*:957 (1976).

86. D. Mahalanabis, C. K. Wallace, R. J. Kallen, A. Mondal, and N. F. Pierce, Water and electrolyte losses due to cholera in infants and small children. A recovery balance study, *Pediatrics, 45*:374-385 (1970).

87. M. H. Merson, R. B. Sack, S. Islam, G. Saklayen, N. Huda, I. Huq, A. W. Zulich, R. H. Yolken, and A. Z. Kapikian, Enterotoxigenic *Escherichia coli* (ETEC) disease in Bangladesh: Clinical aspects and a controlled trial of tetracycline, *J. Infect. Dis., 141*:702-711 (1980).

88. J. E. Rohde and R. A. Cash, Transport of glucose and amino acids in human jejunum during Asiatic cholera, *J. Infect. Dis., 127*:190-192 (1973).

89. N. Hirschhorn and A. Molla, Reversible jejunal disaccharidase deficiency in cholera and other acute diarrheal diseases, *Johns Hopkins Med. J., 125*: 291-300 (1969).

90. A. Chatterjee, D. Mahalanabis, K. N. Jalan, T. K. Maitra, S. K. Agarwal, D. K. Bagchi, and S. Indra, Evaluation of a sucrose-electrolyte solution for oral rehydration in acute infantile diarrhea, *Lancet, 1*:1333-1335 (1977).

91. H. L. Elliott, C. C. J. Carpenter, R. B. Sack, and J. H. Yardley, Small bowel morphology in experimental canine cholera, *Lab. Invest., 22*:112-120 (1970).

92. E. J. Gangarosa, W. R. Beisel, C. Benyajati, H. Sprinz, and P. Piyaratin, The nature of the gastrointestinal lesion in Asiatic cholera and its relation to pathogenesis: A biopsy study, *Am. J. Trop. Med. Hyg., 9*:125-135 (1960).

93. G. Pastore, G. Schiraldi, G. Fera, E. Sforza, and O. Schiraldi, A bioptic study of gastrointestinal mucosa in cholera patients during an epidemic in Southern Italy, *Am. J. Dig. Dis., 21*:613-617 (1976).

94. R. H. Gilman, F. Koster, S. Islam, J. McLaughlin, and M. M. Rahaman, A randomized trial of high and low dose ampicillin therapy for severe dysentery due to *Shigella dysenteriae* type 1, *Antimicrob. Agents Chemother., 17*:402-405 (1980).

95. B. K. Mandal and V. Mani, Colonic involvement in salmonellosis, *Lancet, 1*:887-888 (1976).

96. B. Saffouri, R. S. Bartolomeo, and B. Fuchs, Colonic involvement in salmonellosis, *Am. J. Dig. Dis., 24*:203-208 (1979).

97. R. A. Giannella, S. A. Broitman, and N. Zamcheck, Salmonella enteritis. II. Fulminant diarrhea in the effects on the small intestine, *Am. J. Dig. Dis., 16*:1007-1013 (1971).

98. C. C. J. Carpenter, Cholera and other enterotoxin-related diarrheal diseases, *J. Infect. Dis., 126*:551-564 (1972).

99. N. Hirschhorn, W. B. Greenough III, J. Lindenbaum, and S. M. Alam, Hypoglycemia in children with acute diarrhea, *Lancet, 2*:128-133 (1966).

100. N. Hirschhorn, A. K. M. A. Chowdhury, and J. Lindenbaum, Cholera in pregnant women, *Lancet, 1*:1230-1232 (1969).

101. C. Benyajati, M. Keoplug, W. R. Beisel, E. J. Gangarosa, H. Sprinz, and V. Sitprija, Acute renal failure in Asiatic cholera: Clinicopathologic correlations with acute tubular necrosis and hypokalemic nephropathy, *Ann. Intern. Med., 52*:960-975 (1960).

102. D. L. Palmer, F. T. Koster, A. K. M. J. Alam, and M. R. Islam, Nutritional status: A determinant of severity of diarrhea in patients with cholera, *J. Infect. Dis., 134*:8-14 (1976).

103. M. H. Merson, G. K. Morris, D. A. Sack, J. G. Wells, J. C. Feeley, R. B. Sack, W. B. Creech, A. Z. Kapikian, and E. J. Gangarosa, Travelers' diarrhea in Mexico. A prospective study of physicians and family members attending a congress, *N. Engl. J. Med., 294*:1299-1305 (1976).

104. D. A. Sack, D. C. Kaminsky, R. B. Sack, I. A. Wamola, F. Ørskov, I. Ørskov, R. C. B. Slack, R. R. Arthur, and A. Z. Kapikian, Enterotoxigenic *Escherichia coli* diarrhea of travelers: A prospective study of American Peace Corps Volunteers, *Johns Hopkins Med. J., 141*:63-70 (1977).

105. C. K. Wallace, N. F. Pierce, P. N. Anderson, T. C. Brown, G. W. Lewis, S. N. Sanyal, G. V. Segre, and R. H. Waldman, Probable gallbladder infection in convalescent cholera patients, *Lancet, 1*:865-868 (1967).

106. F. T. Koster, J. Levin, L. Walker, K. S. K. Tung, R. H. Gilman, M. M. Rahaman, M. A. Majid, S. Islam, and R. C. Williams, Jr., Hemolytic-uremic syndrome after shigellosis. Relation to endotoxemia and circulating immune complexes, *N. Engl. J. Med. 298*:927-933 (1978).

107. D. G. Simon, Reiter syndrome following epidemic shigellosis, *E. I. S. Conference* (abstract) p. 47 (1979).

108. J. C. Harris, H. L. DuPont, and R. B. Hornick, Fecal leukocytes in diarrheal illness, *Ann. Intern. Med., 76*:697-703 (1972).

109. A. S. Benenson, M. R. Islam, and W. B. Greenough III, Rapid identification of *Vibrio cholerae* by darkfield microscopy, *Bull. WHO, 30*:827-831 (1964).

110. R. A. Finkelstein and E. H. LaBrec, Rapid identification of cholera vibrios with fluorescent antibody, *J. Bacteriol., 78*:886-891 (1959).

111. H. B. Marsden, W. A. Hyde, and E. Bracegirdle, Immunofluorescence in the diagnosis of enteropathogenic *E. coli* infections, *Lancet, 1*:189-191 (1965).

112. W. B. Cherry and B. M. Thomason, Fluorescent antibody technique for salmonella and other enteric pathogens. A status report, *Public Health Rep., 84*:887 (1969).

113. A. R. Dutt, Enterotoxic activity in cholera stool, *Indian J. Med. Res., 53*:605-609 (1965).

114. J. P. Craig, A permeability factor (toxin) found in cholera stools and culture filtrates and its neutralization by convalescent cholera sera, *Nature (London), 207*:614-616 (1965).

115. P. Echeverria, L. Verheart, C. V. Ulyanco, and L. T. Santiago, Detection of heat-labile enterotoxin-like activity in stools of patients with cholera and *Escherichia coli* diarrhea, *Infect. Immun., 19*:343-344 (1978).

116. M. H. Merson, R. H. Yolken, R. B. Sack, J. L. Froehlich, H. B. Greenberg, I. Huq, and R. W. Black, Detection of *Escherichia coli* enterotoxins in stool, *Infect. Immun., 29*:108-113 (1980).

117. R. Skjelkvale and T. Uemura, Detection of enterotoxin in faeces and antienterotoxin in serum after *Clostridium perfringens* food-poisoning, *J. Appl. Bacteriol., 42*:355-363 (1977).

118. G. D. Rifkin, F. R. Fekety, J. Silva, Jr., and R. B. Sack, Antibiotic-induced colitis implication of a toxin neutralised by *Clostridium sordellii* antitoxin, *Lancet, 2*:1103-1106 (1977).

119. J. G. Bartlett, T. W. Chang, M. Gurwith, S. L. Gorbach, and A. B. Onderdonk, Antibiotic-associated pseudomembranous colitis due to toxin-producing clostridia, *N. Engl. J. Med., 298*:531-534 (1978).

120. R. B. Sack, D. Barua, R. Saxena, and C. C. J. Carpenter, Vibriocidal and agglutinating antibody patterns in cholera patients, *J. Infect. Dis., 116*:630-640 (1966).

121. A. S. Benenson, A. Saad, W. H. Mosley, and A. Ahmed, Serological studies in cholera. 3. Serum toxin neutralization-rise in titer response to infection with *Vibrio cholerae*, and the level in the "normal" population of East Pakistan, *Bull. WHO, 38*:287 (1968).

122. N. F. Pierce, J. G. Banwell, R. B. Sack, R. C. Mitra, and A. Mondal, Magnitude and duration of antitoxic response to human infection with *Vibrio cholerae, J. Infect. Dis., 121*:S31-S35 (1970).

123. R. B. Sack, B. Jacobs, and R. Mitra, Antitoxin responses to infections with enterotoxigenic *Escherichia coli*, J. Infect. Dis., 129:330-335 (1974).

124. A. Caceres and L. J. Mata, Serologic response of patients with Shiga dysentery, *J. Infect. Dis., 129*:439-443 (1974).

125. L. T. Gutman, E. A. Ottesen, T. J. Quan, P. S. Noce, and S. L. Katz, An interfamilial outbreak of *Yersinia enterocolitica* enteritis, *N. Engl. J. Med., 288*:1372-1377 (1973).

126. G. T. Keusch, M. Jacewicz, M. M. Levine, R. B. Hornick, and S. Kochwa, Pathogenesis of shigella diarrhea. Serum anticytotoxin antibody response produced by toxigenic and nontoxigenic *Shigella dysenteriae* 1, *J. Clin. Invest., 57*:194-202 (1976).

127. World Health Organization, *Treatment and Prevention of Dehydration in Diarrheal Diseases.* WHO, Geneva, 1976.

128. N. F. Pierce and N. Hirschhorn, Oral fluid—a simple weapon against dehydration in diarrhoea. How it works and how to use it, *WHO Chronicle, 31*:87-93 (1977).

129. R. B. Sack, N. F. Pierce, and N. Hirschhorn, The current status of oral therapy in the treatment of acute diarrheal illness, *Am. J. Clin. Nutr., 31*:2251-2257 (1978).

130. D. L. Palmer, F. T. Koster, A. F. M. Rafiqul Islam, A. S. M. Mizanur Rahman, and R. B. Sack, Comparison of sucrose and glucose in the oral

electrolyte therapy of cholera and other severe diarrheas, *N. Engl. J. Med.,* *297*:1107-1110 (1977).

131. D. A. Sack, A. Eusof, M. H. Merson, R. E. Black, A. M. A. K. Chowdhury, M. A. Ali, S. Islam, and K. H. Brown, Oral hydration in rotavirus diarrhoea: A double-blind comparison of sucrose with glucose electrolyte solution, *Lancet, 2*:280-283 (1978).

132. C. K. Wallace, P. N. Anderson, T. C. Brown, G. W. Khanra, G. W. Lewis, N. F. Pierce, S. N. Sanyal, G. V. Segre, and R. H. Waldman, Optimal antibiotic therapy in cholera, *Bull. WHO, 39*:239 (1968).

133. F. O'Grady, M. J. Lewis, and N. J. Pearson, Global surveillance of antibiotic sensitivity of *Vibrio cholerae, Bull. WHO, 54*:181-184 (1976).

134. F. S. Mhalu, P. W. Mmari, and J. Ijumba, Rapid emergence of El tor *Vibrio cholerae* resistant to antimicrobial agents during first six months of fourth cholera epidemic in Tanzania, *Lancet, 1*:345-347 (1979).

135. D. A. Sack, S. Islam, H. Rabbani, and A. Islam, Single-dose doxycycline for cholera, *Antimicrob. Agents Chemother., 14*:462-464 (1978).

136. M. M. Rahaman, M. A. Majid, A. K. M. Jamiul, and M. R. Islam, Effects of doxycycline in actively purging cholera patients: A double-blind clinical trial, *Antimicrob. Agents Chemother., 10*:610-612 (1976).

137. N. F. Pierce, J. G. Banwell, R. C. Mitra, G. J. Caranosos, R. I. Keimowitz, J. Thomas, and A. Mondal, Controlled comparison of tetracycline and furazolidone in cholera, *Br. Med. J., 3*:277-280 (1968).

138. J. Lindenbaum, W. B. Greenough, and M. R. Islam, Antibiotic therapy of cholera, *Bull. WHO, 36*:871-883 (1967).

139. R. A. Cash, R. S. Northrup, and A. S. Mizanur Rhaman, Trimethprim and sulfamethoxazole in clinical cholera. Comparison with tetracycline, *J. Infect. Dis., 128*:749-753 (1973).

140. L. K. Pickering, H. L. DuPont, and J. Olarte, Single-dose tetracycline therapy for shigellosis in adults, *JAMA, 239*:853-854 (1978).

141. R. Gilman, W. Spira, H. Rabbani, M. Mahmoud, A. Islam, and M. M. Rahaman, Single dose ampicillin therapy for the treatment of severe shigellosis in Bangladesh, *Johns Hopkins/ICMR Ann. Rep.,* pp. 28-41 (1978).

142. J. D. Nelson, H. Kusmiesz, and L. H. Jackson, Comparison of trimethoprim-sulfamethoxazole and ampicillin therapy for shigellosis in ambulatory patients, *J. Pediatr., 89*:491-493 (1976).

143. M. J. Chang, L. M. Dunkle, D. Vanreken, D. Anderson, M. L. Wong, and R. D. Feigin, Trimethoprim-sulfamethoxazole compared to ampicillin in treatment of shigellosis, *Pediatrics, 59*:726-729 (1977).

144. J. F. Wallace, R. H. Smith, and R. G. Petersdorf, Oral administration of vancomycin in the treatment of staphylococcal enterocolitis, *N. Engl. J. Med., 272*:1014-1015 (1965).

145. F. Tedesco, R. Markham, M. Gurwith, D. Christie, and J. G. Bartlett, Oral vancomycin for antibiotic-associated pseudomembranous colitis, *Lancet, 2*:226-228 (1978).

146. M. R. B. Keighley, D. W. Burdon, Y. Arabi, J. Alexander-Williams, H. Thompson, D. Younge, M. Johnson, S. Bentley, R. H. George, and G. A. G.

Mogg, Randomized controlled trial of vancomycin for pseudomembranous colitis and post-operative diarrhea, *Br. Med. J., 2*:1667-1669 (1978).

147. International Study Group, A positive effect on the nutrition of Philippine children of an oral glucose-electrolyte solution given at home for the treatment of diarrhea, *Bull. WHO, 55*:87-94 (1977).

148. N. Hirschhorn, The treatment of acute diarrhea in children: An historical and physiological perspective, *Am. J. Clin. Nutr., 33*:637-663 (1980).

149. R. B. Sack, J. Cassells, R. Mitra, C. Merritt, R. Butler, J. Thomas, R. Jacobs, A. Chaudhuri, and A. Mondal, The use of oral replacement solutions in the treatment of cholera and other severe diarrhoeal disorders, *Bull WHO, 43*:351-360 (1970).

150. A. D. Finck and R. L. Katz, Prevention of cholera-induced intestinal secretion in the cat by aspirin, *Nature, 238*:273-274 (1972).

151. L. C. Chen, R. L. Guerrant, J. E. Rhode, and A. G. Casper, Effect of amphotericin B on sodium and water movement across normal and cholera toxin-challenged canine jejunum, *Gastroenterology, 65*:252-258 (1973).

152. R. E. Gots, S. B. Formal, and R. A. Giannella, Indomethacin inhibition of *Salmonella typhimurium, Shigella flexneri*, and cholera-mediated rabbit ileal secretion, *J. Infect. Dis., 130*:280-284 (1974).

153. H. N. Maimon, W. E. Mitch, J. G. Banwell, and T. R. Hendrix, Inhibition of enterotoxin-induced intestinal secretion by the polypeptide antibiotic, polymyxin, *Johns Hopkins Med. J., 138*:82-90 (1976).

154. M. Donowitz, A. N. Charney, and R. Hynes, Propranolol prevention of cholera enterotoxin-induced intestinal secretion in the rat, *Gastroenterology, 76*:482-491 (1979).

155. C. D. Ericsson, D. G. Evans, H. L. DuPont, D. J. Evans, Jr., and L. K. Pickering, Bismuth subsalicylate inhibits activity of crude toxins of *Escherichia coli* and *Vibrio cholerae, J. Infect. Dis., 136*:693-696 (1977).

156. H. L. DuPont, P. Sullivan, L. K. Pickering, G. Haynes, and P. B. Ackerman, Symptomatic treatment of diarrhea with bismuth subsalicylate among students attending a Mexican university, *Gastroenterology, 73*: 715-718 (1977).

157. H. A. Serebro, F. L. Iber, J. H. Yardley, and T. R. Hendrix, Inhibition of cholera toxin action in the rabbit by cyclohexamide, *Gastroenterology, 56*:506-511 (1969).

158. C. C. J. Carpenter, G. T. Curlin, and W. B. Greenough III, Response of canine Thiry-Vella jejunal loops to cholera exotoxin and its modification by ethacrynic acid, *J. Infect. Dis., 120*:332-338 (1969).

159. A. N. Charney and M. Donowitz, Prevention and reversal of cholera enterotoxin-induced intestinal secretion by methyl-prednisilone induction of Na-K-ATPase, *J. Clin. Invest., 57*:1590-1599 (1976).

160. N. Turjman, G. S. Gotterer, and T. R. Hendrix, Prevention and reversal of cholera enterotoxin effects in rabbit jejunum by nicotinic acid, *J. Clin. Invest., 61*:1155-1160 (1978).

161. J. Holmgren, S. Lange, and I. Lonnroth, Reversal of cyclic AMP-mediated intestinal secretion in mice by chlorpromazine, *Gastroenterology, 75*: 1103-1108 (1978).

162. M. Sabir, M. H. Akhter, and N. K. Bhide, Antagonism of cholera toxin by berberine in the gastrointestinal tract of adult rats, *Indian J. Med. Res.*, *65*:305-313 (1977).

163. R. B. Sack, J. L. Froehlich, and J. H. Yardley, Berberine inhibits secretory response of cholera enterotoxin and *E. coli* heat-labile enterotoxin, *Clin. Res.*, *28*:78A (1980).

164. G. H. Rabbani, W. B. Greenough III, J. Holmgren, and I. Lonnroth, Chlorpromazine reduces fluid-loss in cholera, *Lancet*, *1*:410-411 (1979).

165. E. W. Kreutzer, and F. D. Milligan, Treatment of antibiotic-associated pseudomembranous colitis with cholestyramine resin, *Johns Hopkins Med. J.*, *143*:67-72 (1978).

166. B. L. Portnoy, H. L. DuPont, D. Pruitt, J. A. Abdo, and J. T. Rodrique, Antidiarrheal agents in treatment of acute diarrhea in children, *JAMA*, *236*:844-846 (1976).

167. H. L. Dupont and R. B. Hornick, Adverse effect of diphenoxylate therapy in shigellosis, *JAMA*, *226*:1525-1528 (1973).

168. W. E. Woodward, N. Hirschhorn, R. B. Sack, R. A. Cash, I. Brownlee, G. H. Chickadonz, L. K. Evans, R. H. Shepard, and R. C. Woodward, Acute diarrhea on an Apache Indian reservation, *Am. J. Epidemiol.*, *99*:281-290 (1974).

169. R. E. Black, M. H. Merson, B. Rowe, P. R. Taylor, A. S. M. M. Rahman, M. A. Haque, A. R. M. A. Aleem, D. A. Sack, and G. Curlin, Epidemiology of enterotoxigenic *Escherichi coli* in rural Bangladesh, *U.S.-Japan Cooperative Medical Science Program*, Karatsu, Japan, 1978, p. 83.

170. P. Echeverria, M. T. Ho, N. R. Blacklow, G. Quinnan, B. Portnoy, J. G. Olson, R. Conklin, H. L. DuPont, and J. H. Cross, Relative importance of viruses and bacteria in the etiology of pediatric diarrhea in Taiwan, *J. Infect. Dis.*, *136*:383-390 (1977).

171. M. J. Gurwith and T. W. Williams, Gastroenteritis in children: A two year review in Manitoba. I. Etiology, *J. Infect. Dis.*, *136*:239-247 (1977).

172. P. Echeverria, N. R. Blacklow, and D. H. Smith, Role of heat-labile toxigenic *Escherichia coli* and reovirus-like agent in diarrhoea in Boston children, *Lancet*, *2*:1113-1116 (1975).

173. H. Fukumi, Brief summary report of cholera happening in Tsurumi River, Kanagawa, Japan, *U. S.-Japan Cooperative Medical Science Program*, Karatsu, Japan, pp. 18-22 (1978).

174. R. R. Colwell, M. J. Voll, L. A. McNicol, J. Kaper, R. Seidler, S. Garges, H. Lockman, E. Remmer, and S. W. Joseph, Isolation of 01 and non-01 *Vibrio cholerae* from estuaries and brackish water environments, *U.S.-Japan Cooperative Medical Science Program*, Bethesda, p. 19 (1979).

175. E. J. Gangarosa and W. H. Mosley, Epidemiology and surveillance of cholera. In *Cholera* (D. Barua and W. Burrows, eds.), W. B. Saunders, Philadelphia, 1974, pp. 381-403.

176. P. A. Blake, D. T. Allegra, J. D. Snyder, T. J. Barrett, N. D. Puhr, and R. A. Feldman, *Vibrio cholerae* 0-group 1 infection in Louisiana, 1978. *U.S.-Japan Cooperative Medical Science Program*, Bethesda, p. 16 (1979).

177. B. Cvjetanovic and D. Barua, The seventh pandemic of cholera, *Nature, 239*:137-138 (1972).

178. L. B. Reller, E. N. Rivas, R. Masferrer, M. Bloch, and E. J. Gangarosa, Epidemic shiga-bacillus dysentery in Central America. Evolution of the outbreak in El Salvador, 1969-70, *Am. J. Trop. Med. Hyg., 20*:934-940 (1971).

179. M. M. Rahaman, A. K. M. Jamiul Alam, M. R. Islam, W. B. Greenough, and J. Lindenbaum, Shiga bacillus dysentery associated with marked leukocytosis and erythrocyte fragmentation, *Johns Hopkins Med. J., 136*: 65-70 (1975).

180. M. J. Blaser, I. D. Kerkowitz, F. M. LaForce, J. Cravens, L. B. Reller, and W. L. L. Wang, Campylobacter enteritis: Clinical and epidemiologic features, *Ann. Intern. Med., 91*:179-185 (1979).

181. E. Aldova, K. Laznickova, E. Stepankova, and J. Lietava, Isolation of nonagglutinable vibrios from an enteritis outbreak in Czechoslovakia, *J. Infect. Dis., 118*:25-31 (1968).

182. R. E. Black, R. J. Jackson, T. Tsai, M. Medvesky, M. Shayegani, J. C. Feeley, K. E. MacLeod, and A. M. Wakelee, Epidemic *Yersina enterocolitica* infection due to contaminated chocolate milk, *N. Engl. J. Med., 298*:76-79 (1977).

183. Center for Disease Control, Waterborne campylobacter gastroenteritis—Vermont, *MMWR, 27*:207 (1978).

184. S. L. Gorbach, B. H. Kean, D. G. Evans, D. J. Evans, and D. Bessudo, Traverlers' diarrhea and toxigenic *Escherichia coli*, *N. Engl. J. Med., 292*: 933-936 (1975).

185. B. H. Kean and S. R. Waters, The diarrhea of travelers. III. Drug prophylaxis in Mexico, *N. Engl. J. Med., 261*:71-74 (1959).

186. H. L. Dupont, G. A. Haynes, L. K. Pickering, W. Tjoa, P. Sullivan, and J. Olarte, Diarrhea of travelers to Mexico—relative susceptibility of United States and Latin American students attending a Mexican university, *Am. J. Epidemiol., 105*:37-41 (1977).

187. D. A. Sack, D. C. Kaminsky, R. B. Sack, J. N. Itotia, R. R. Arthur, A. Z. Kapikian, F. Ørskov, and I. Ørskov, Prophylactic doxycycline for travelers' diarrhea. Results of a prospective double-blind study of Peace Corps Volunteers in Kenya, *N. Engl. J. Med., 298*:758-763 (1978).

188. R. B. Sack, J. L. Froehlich, A. W. Zulich, D. Sidi Hidi, A. Z. Kapikian, F. Ørskov, I. Ørskov, and H. B. Greenberg, Prophylactic doxycycline for travelers' diarrhea: Results of a prospective double-blind study of Peace Corps Volunteers in Morocco, *Gastroenterology, 76*:1368-1373 (1979).

189. R. Fekety, J. Silva, R. Toshniwal, M. Allo, J. Armstrong, R. Browne, J. Ebright, and G. Rifkin, Antibiotic-associated colitis: Effects of antibiotics on *Clostridium difficile* and the disease in hamsters, *Rev. Infect. Dis., 1*: 386-397 (1979).

190. D. M. Musher and A. D. Rubenstein, Permanent carriers of nontyphosa salmonellae, *Arch. Intern. Med., 132*:869-872 (1973).

191. M. M. Levine, H. L. DuPont, M. Khodabandelou, and R. B. Hornick, Long-term shigella carrier state, *N. Engl. J. Med., 288*:1169-1171 (1973).

192. R. Sinha, B. C. Deli, S. P. De, B. K. Sirkar, A. H. Abou-Gareeb, and D. L. Shivastava, Role of carriers in the epidemiology of cholera in Calcutta, *Indian J. Med. Res., 56*:964 (1968).

193. R. A. Cash, S. I. Music, J. P. Libonati, J. P. Craig, N. F. Pierce, and R. B. Hornick, Response of man to infection with *Vibrio cholerae*. II. Protection from illness afforded by previous disease and vaccine, *J. Infect. Dis., 130*:325-333 (1974).

194. G. Lawrence, F. Shann, D. S. Freestone, and P. D. Walker, Prevention of necrotising enteritis in Papua New Guinea by active immunisation, *Lancet, 1*:266-267 (1979).

195. W. H. Mosley, K. M. A. Aziz, A. S. M. Mizanur Rahman, A. K. M. Alauddin Chowdhury, A. Ahmed, and M. Fahimuddin, Report of the 1966-67 cholera vaccine trial in rural East Pakistan. 4. Five years of observation with a practical assessment of the role of a cholera vaccine in cholera control programmes, *Bull. WHO, 47*:229-238 (1972).

196. J. S. Saroso, W. Bahrawi, H. Witjaksono, R. L. Budiarso Brotowasisto, Z. Bencic, W. E. Dewitt, and C. Z. Gomes, Controlled field trial of plain and aluminum hydroxide adsorbed cholera vaccines in Surabaya, Indonnesia, during 1973-75, *Bull. WHO, 56*:619-627 (1978).

197. Cholera Research Center, Controlled field trial on the efficacy of aluminum phosphate adjuvant cholera vaccine in Calcutta. (Final Report) *Annual Report of the Cholera Research Center, Calcutta,* pp. 5-6 (1977).

198. D. Mel, E. J. Gangarosa, M. L. Radovanovic, B. L. Arsic, and S. Litvinjenko, Studies on vaccination against bacillary dysentery. 6. Protection of children by oral immunization with streptomycin-dependent *Shigella* strains, *Bull. WHO, 45*:457-464 (1971).

199. N. F. Pierce, Role of antigen form and function in primary and secondary intestinal immune responses to cholera toxin and toxoid in rats, *J. Exp. Med., 148*:195-206 (1978).

200. A. M.Svennerholm, S. Lange, and J. Holmgren, Correlation between intestinal synthesis of specific immunoglobulin A and protection against experimental cholera in mice, *Infect. Immun., 21*:1-6 (1978).

201. N. F. Pierce, W. C. Cray, and B. K. Sircar, Induction of a mucosal antitoxin response and its role in immunity to experimental canine cholera, *Infect. Immun., 21*:185-193 (1978).

202. N. F. Pierce, R. B. Sack, and B. K. Sircar, Immunity to experimental cholera. III. Enhanced duration of protection after sequential parenteral-oral administration of toxoid to dogs, *J. Infect. Dis., 135*:888-896 (1977).

203. N. F. Pierce and H. Y. Reynolds, Immunity to experimental cholera. 1. Protective effect of humoral IgG antitoxin demonstrated by passive immunization, *J. Immunology, 113*:1017-1023 (1974).

204. R. B. Sack and C. E. Miller, Progressive changes of vibrio serotypes in germ-free mice infected with *Vibrio cholerae, J. Bacteriol., 99*:688-695 (1969).

205. J. Bray, Isolation of antigenically homogeneous strains of *Bact. coli neapolitanium* from summer diarrhea of infants, *J. Pathol. Bacteriol., 57*: 239-247 (1945).

206. C. Giles, G. Sangster, and J. Smith, Epidemic gastroenteritis of infants in Aberdeen during 1947, *Arch. Dis. Child., 24*:45-53 (1949).

207. W. W. Ferguson and R. C. June, Experiments on feeding adult volunteers with *Escherichia coli* 111, B_4, a coliform organism associated with infant diarrhea, *Am. J. Hyg., 55*:155-169 (1952).

208. E. J. Gangarosa and M. H. Merson, Epidemiologic assessment of the relevance of the so-called enteropathogenic serogroups of *Escherichia coli* in diarrhea, *N. Engl. J. Med., 296*:1210-1213 (1977).

209. M. Gurwith, D. Hinde, R. Gross, and B. Rowe, A prospective study of enteropathogenic *Escherichia coli* in endemic diarrheal disease, *J. Infect. Dis., 137*:292-297 (1978).

210. R. B. Sack, N. Hirschhorn, I. Brownlee, R. A. Cash, W. E. Woodward, and D. A. Sack, Enterotoxigenic *Escherichia coli*-associated diarrheal disease in Apache children, *N. Engl. J. Med., 292*:1041-1045 (1975).

211. M. C. Goldschmidt and H. L. DuPont, Enteropathogenic *Escherichia coli*: Lack of correlation of serotype with pathogenicity, *J. Infect. Dis., 133*: 153-156 (1976).

212. R. J. Gross, S. M. Scotland, and B. Rowe, Enterotoxin testing of *Escherichia coli* causing epidemic infantile enteritis in the U.K., *Lancet, 1*:629-631 (1976).

213. M. M. Levine, D. R. Nalin, R. B. Hornick, E. J. Bergquist, D. H. Waterman, C. R. Young, and S. Sotman, *Escherichia coli* strains that cause diarrhoea but do not produce heat-labile or heat-stable enterotoxins and are noninvasive, *Lancet, 1*:1119-1122 (1978).

214. F. A. Klipstein, B. Rowe, R. F. Engert, H. B. Short, and R. J. Gross, Enterotoxigenicity of enteropathogenic serotypes of *Escherichia coli* isolated from infants with epidemic diarrhea, *Infect. Immun., 21*:171-178 (1978).

215. F. Ørskov, I. Ørskov, D. J. Evans, Jr., R. B. Sack, and D. A. Sack, Special *E. coli* serotypes among enterotoxigenic strains from diarrhea in adults and children, *Med. Microbiol. Immunol., 162*:73-80 (1976).

216. M. H. Merson, F. Ørskov, I. Ørskov, R. B. Sack, I. Huq., and F. T. Koster, Relationship between enterotoxin production and serotype in enterotoxigenic *Escherichia coli, Infect. Immun., 23*:325-329 (1979).

217. I. Ørskov and F. Ørskov, Special O:K:H serotypes among enterotoxigenic *E. coli* strains from diarrhea in adults and children, *Med. Microbiol. Immunol., 163*:99-110 (1977).

218. F. A. Klipstein, R. F. Engert, and H. B. Short, Enterotoxigenicity of colonising coliform bacteria in tropical sprue and blind-loop syndrome, *Lancet, 2*:342-344 (1978).

219. F. A. Klipstein, I. R. Horowitz, R. F. Engert, and E. A. Schenk, Effect of *Klebsiella pneumoniae* enterotoxin on intestinal transport in rats, *J. Clin. Invest., 56*:799-807 (1975).

220. S. L. Gorbach, Microflora of the gastrointestinal tract in tropical enteritis—a current appraisal, *Am. J. Clin. Nutr., 25*;1127-1133 (1972).

221. H. Kusama and R. H. Suss, Vascular permeability factor of *Pseudomonas aeruginosa, Infect. Immun., 5*:363-369 (1972).

222. T. Tsukamoto, Y. Kinoshita, T. Shimada, and R. Sakazaki, Two epidemics of diarrhoeal disease possibly caused by *Plesiomonas shigelloides, J. Hyg. Camb., 80*:275-280 (1978).

223. B. Sereny, Experimental keratoconjunctivitis shigellosa, *Acta Microbiol. Acad. Sci. Hung., 4*:367-376 (1957).

224. M. Maki, P. Gronroos, and T. Vesikari, In vitro invasiveness of *Yersinia enterocolitica, J. Infect. Dis., 138*:677-680 (1978).

225. K. E. Hejtmancik, J. W. Peterson, D. E. Markel, and A. Kurosky, Radio-immunoassay for the antigenic determinants od cholera toxin and its components, *Infect. Immun., 17*:621-628 (1977).

226. R. L. Richards, J. Moss, C. R. Alving, P. H. Fishman, and R. O. Brady, Choleragen (cholera toxin): A bacterial lectin, *Proc. Natl. Acad. Sci. USA, 76*:1673-1676 (1979).

227. T. Honda and R. A. Finkelstein, Selection and characteristics of a *Vibrio cholerae* mutant lacking the A (ADP-ribosylating) portion of the cholera enterotoxin, *Proc. Natl. Acad. Sci. USA, 76*:2052-2056 (1979).

228. W. M. Spira, R. R. Daniel, Q. S. Ahmed, A. Huq, A. Yusuf, and D. A. Sack, Clinical features and pathogenicity of 0 group 1 nonagglutinating *Vibrio cholerae* and other vibrios isolated from cases of diarrhea in Dacca, Bangladesh. In *Proceedings of the Fourteenth Joint Conference, U.S.-Japan Cooperative Medical Science* Program, Karatsu, Japan, pp. 137-153 (1978).

229. R. R. Daniel and W. M. Spira, Biotype clusters formed on the basis of virulence characters in non-0-group 1 *Vibrio cholerae, U.S.-Japan Cooperative Medical Science Program*, Bethesda, Md., p. 21 (1979).

230. H. L. Smith, Serotyping of noncholera vibrios, *J. Clin. Microbiol., 10*: 85-90 (1979).

231. J. Kaper, H. Lockman, R. R. Colwell, and S. W. Joseph, Ecology, serology, and enterotoxin production of *Vibrio cholerae* in Chesapeake Bay, *Appl. Environ., 37*:91-103 (1979).

232. W. H. Barker, Jr. and E. J. Gangarosa, Food poisoning due to *Vibrio parahaemolyticus, Ann. Rev. Med., 25*:75-81 (1974).

233. D. E. Johnson and F. M. Calia, False-positive rabbit ileal loop reactions attributed to *Vibrio parahaemolyticus* broth filtrates, *J. Infect. Dis., 133*: 436-440 (1976).

234. T. Honda, M. Shimizu, Y. Takeda, and T. Miwatani, Isolation of a factor causing morphological changes of Chinese hamster ovary cells from the culture filtrate of *Vibrio parahaemolyticus, Infect. Immun., 14*:1028-1033 (1976).

235. T. Kaneko and R. R. Colwell, Annual cycle of *Vibrio parahaemolyticus* in Chesapeake Bay, *Microbiol. Ecol., 42*:135-155 (1978).

236. B. K. Boutin, S. F. Townsend, P. V. Scarpino, and R. M. Twedt, Demonstration of invasiveness of *Vibrio parahaemolyticus* in adult rabbits by immunofluorescence, *Appl. Environ., 37*:647-653 (1979).

237. H. B. Greenberg, D. A. Sack, W. Rodriguez, R. B. Sack, R. G. Wyatt, A. R. Kalica, R. L. Horswood, R. M. Chanock, and A. Z. Kapikian, Microtiter solid-phase radioimmunoassay for detection of *Escherichia coli* heat-labile enterotoxin, *Infect. Immun., 17*:541-545 (1977).

238. J. Holmgren and A. M. Svennerholm, Immunological cross-reactivity between *Escherichia coli* heat-labile enterotoxin and cholera toxin-A and toxin-B subunits, *Curr. Microbiol., 2*:55-58 (1979).

239. M. M. Levine, D. R. Nalin, D. L. Hoover, E. J. Bergquist, R. B. Hornick, and C. R. Young, Immunity to enterotoxigenic *Escherichia coli, Infect. Immun., 23*:729-736 (1979).

240. Y. Takeda, T. Takeda, T. Yano, K. Yamamoto, and T. Mitwatani, Purification and partial characterization of heat-stable enterotoxin of enterotoxigenic *Escherichia coli, Infect. Immun., 25*:978-985 (1979).

241. P. Gemski, Jr., A. Takeuchi, O. Washington, and S. B. Formal, Shigellosis due to *Shigella dysenteriae* 1: Relative importance of mucosal invasion versus toxin production in pathogenesis, *J. Infect. Dis., 126*:523-530 (1972).

242. H. L. DuPont, R. B. Hornick, M. Snyder, J. B. Libonati, S. B. Formal, and E. J. Gangarosa, Immunity in shigellosis. II. Protection induced by oral live vaccine or primary infection, *J. Infect. Dis., 125*:12-16 (1972).

243. J. Flores, G. F. Grady, J. McIver, P. Witkum, B. Beckman, and G. W. G. Sharp, Comparison of the effects of enterotoxins of *Shigella dysenteriae* and *Vibrio cholerae* on the adenylate cyclase system of the rabbit intestine, *J. Infect. Dis., 130*:374-379 (1974).

244. G. T. Keusch and M. Jacewicz, The pathogenesis of shigella diarrhea. V. Relationship of shiga enterotoxin, neurotoxin, and cytotoxin, *J. Infect. Dis., 131*:S33-S39 (1975).

245. J. McIver, G. F. Grady, and G. T. Keusch, Production and characterization of exotoxin(s) of *Shigella dysenteriae* type 1, *J. Infect. Dis., 131*:559-566 (1975).

246. S. E. Steinberg, J. G. Banwell, J. H. Yardley, G. T. Keusch, and T. R. Hendrix, Comparison of secretory and histological effects of Shigella and cholera enterotoxins in rabbit jejunum, *Gastroenterology, 68*:309-317 (1975).

247. A. D. O'Brien, M. R. Thompson, P. Gemski, B. P. Doctor, and S. B. Formal, Biological properties of *Shigella flexneri* 2A toxin and its serological relationship to *Shigella dysenteriae* 1 toxin, *Infect. Immun., 15*:796-798 (1977).

248. M. M. Levine, W. E. Woodward, S. B. Formal, P. Gemski, Jr., H. L. DuPont, R. B. Hornick, and M. J. Snyder, Studies with a new generation of oral attenuated shigella vaccine: *Escherichia coli* bearing surface antigens of *Shigella flexneri, J. Infect. Dis., 136*:577-582 (1977).

249. J. P. Duguid, M. R. Darekar, and D. W. F. Wheater, Fimbriae and infectivity in *Salmonella typhimurium*, *J. Med. Microbiol.*, 9:459-473 (1976).

250. P. D. Sandefur and J. W. Peterson, Isolation of skin permeability factors from culture filtrates of *Salmonella typhimurium*, *Infect. Immun.*, 14: 671-679 (1976).

251. P. D. Sandefur and J. W. Peterson, Neutralization of *Salmonella* toxin-induced elongation of Chinese hamster ovary cells by cholera antitoxin, *Infect. Immun.*, 15:988-992 (1977).

252. H. Kuhn, H. Tschape, and H. Rische, Enterotoxigenicity among Salmonellae—a prospective analysis for a surveillance programme, *Zentral. Bakteriol. [Orig. A]*, 240:171-183 (1978).

253. R. H. Deibel, D. M. Sedlock, and L. R. Koupal, Production and partial purification of salmonella enterotoxin, *Infect. Immun.*, 20:375-380 (1978).

254. A. Ljungh, M. Popoff, and T. Wadstrom, *Aeromonas hydrophilia* in acute diarrheal disease: Detection of enterotoxin and biotyping of strains, *J. Clin. Microbiol.*, 6:96-100 (1977).

255. N. Cumberbatch, M. J. Gurwith, C. Langston, R. B. Sack, and J. L. Brunton, Cytotoxic enterotoxin isolates to diarrheal disease, *Infect. Immun.*, 23:829-837 (1979).

256. R. S. Dubey and S. C. Sanyal, Characterization and neutralization of *Aeromonas hydrophila* enterotoxin in the rabbit ileal loop model, *J. Med. Microbiol.*, 12:347-354 (1979).

257. S. Kohl, J. A. Jacobson, and A. Nahmias, *Yersinia enterocolitica* infections in children, *J. Pediatr.*, 89:77-79 (1976).

258. C. H. Pai, V. Mars, and S. Toma, Prevalence of enterotoxigenicity in human and nonhuman isolates of *Yersinia enterocolitica*, *Infect. Immun.*, 22:334-338 (1978).

259. C. H. Pai, S. Sorger, L. Lafleur, L. Lackman, and M. I. Marks, Efficacy of cold enrichment techniques for recovery of *Yersinia enterocolitica* from human stools, *J. Clin. Microbiol.*, 9:712-715 (1979).

260. R. M. Robins-Brown, C. S. Still, M. D. Miliotis, and H. F. Koornhof, Mechanism of action of *Yersinia enterocolitica* enterotoxin, *Infect. Immun.*, 25: 680-684 (1979).

261. F. A. Kapral, A. D. O'Brien, P. D. Ruff, and W. F. Drugan, Jr., Inhibition of water absorption in the intestine by *Staphylococcus aureus* delta toxin, *Infect. Immun.*, 13:140-145 (1976).

262. A. D. O'Brien and F. A. Kapral, Effect of *Staphylococcus aureus* delta toxin on Chinese hamster ovary cell morphology and Y-1 adrenal cell morphology and steroidogenesis, *Infect. Immun.*, 16:812-816 (1977).

263. A. D. O'Brien, H. J. McClung, and F. A. Kapral, Increased tissue conductance and ion transport in guinea pig ileum after exposure to *Staphylococcus aureus* delta toxin in vitro, *Infect. Immun.*, 21:102-113 (1978).

264. T. G. Merrill and H. Spring, The effect of staphylococcal enterotoxin on the fine structure of the monkey jejunum, *Lab. Invest.*, 18:114-123 (1968).

265. A. W. Jarvis, R. C. Lawrence, and G. G. Pritchard, Production of staphylococcal enterotoxins A, B, and C under conditions of controlled pH and aeration, *Infect. Immun., 7*:847-854 (1973).

266. A. Koupal and R. H. Deibel, Rabbit intestinal fluid stimulation by an enterotoxigenic factor of *Staphylococcus aureus, Infect. Immun., 18*:298-303 (1977).

267. D. H. Strong, C. L. Duncan, and G. Perna, *Clostridium perfringens* Type A food poisoning. II. Response of the rabbit ileum as an indication of enteropathogenicity of strains of *Clostridium perfringens* in human beings, *Infect. Immun., 3*:171-178 (1971).

268. R. L. Stark and C. L. Duncan, Purification and biochemical properties of *Clostridium perfringens* type A enterotoxin, *Infect. Immun., 6*:662-673 (1972).

269. R. Skjelkvale and T. Uemura, Experimental diarrhea in human volunteers following oral administration of *Clostridium perfringens* enterotoxins, *J. Appl. Bacteriol., 43*:281-286 (1977).

270. G. Lawrence and P. D. Walker, Pathogenesis of enteritis necrotuans in Papua New Guinea, *Lancet, 1*:125-126 (1976).

271. J. Sakurai and C. L. Duncan, Purification of Beta toxin from *Clostridium perfringens* type C, *Infect. Immun., 18*:741-745 (1977).

272. W. M. Spira and J. M. Goephert, *Bacillus cereus*-induced accumulation in rabbit ileal loops, *Appl. Microbiol., 24*:341-348 (1972).

273. B. A. Glatz, W. M. Spira, and J. M. Goepfert, Alteration of vascular permeability in rabbits by culture filtrates of *Bacillus cereus* and related species, *Infect. Immun., 10*:299-301 (1974).

274. W. Terranova and P. A. Blake, *Bacillus cereus* food poisoning, *N. Engl. J. Med., 298*:143-149 (1977).

275. P. C. Turnbull, J. M. Kramer, K. Jorgensen, R. J. Gilbert, and J. Melling, Properties and production characteristics of vomiting, diarrheal, and necrotizing toxins of *Bacillus cereus, Am. J. Clin. Nutr., 32*:219-228 (1979).

276. C. D. Humphrey, C. W. Condon, J. R. Cantey, and F. E. Pittman, Partial purification of a toxin found in hamsters with antibiotic-associated colitis. Reversible binding of the toxin by cholestyramine, *Gastroenterology, 76*: 468-476 (1979).

277. R. D. Rolfe and S. M. Finegold, Purification and characterization of *Clostridium difficile* toxin, *Infect. Immun., 25*:191-201 (1979).

278. M. H. Merson, R. B. Sack, S. Islam, G. Saklayen, N. Huda, A. K. M. Golam Kibriya, A. Mahamood, Q. S. Ahamed, A. Quder, R. H. Yolken, M. Rahaman, and A. Z. Kapikian, Enterotoxigenic *Escherichia coli* (ETEC) disease in Bangladesh: Clinical therapeutic and laboratory aspects, *U.S.-Japan Cooperative Medical Science Program*, Atlanta, p. 18 (1977).

279. W. J. Martin, Enterobacteriaceae. In *Manual of Clinical Microbiology* (J. E. Blair, E. H. Lennette, and J. P. Truant, eds.), American Society for Microbiology, Bethesda, 1970, pp. 151-174.

280. P. H. Fishman and R. O. Brady, Biosynthesis and function of gangliosides, *Science, 194*:906-915 (1976).
281. J. G. Banwell and H. Sherr, Effect of bacterial enterotoxins on the gastro-intestinal tract, *Gastroenterology, 65*:467-497 (1973).

___ 15 _____

History of the Nebraska Calf Diarrhea Virus

Charles A. Mebus Plum Island Animal Disease Center,
Greenport, New York

In 1965 Nebraska cattle ranchers requested that the Department of Veterinary Science at the University of Nebraska initiate a research project on neonatal calf diarrhea (calf scours). For many ranchers, calf diarrhea was causing monetary losses through deaths, slowed weight gains, or the expense of time and drugs for treatment. In previous years, the newly introduced antibiotics seemed to be of value in treatment; however, the effectiveness of these antibiotics had rapidly decreased.

Most of the literature on calf diarrhea, up to 1965, incriminated *Escherichia coli* as the primary pathogen of neonatal calf diarrhea. Investigations had revealed increased numbers of *E. coli* in the small intestine of diarrheic calves. Thus, the hypothesis was advanced that diarrhea resulted from an overgrowth of *E. coli* from the large into the small intestines.

The initial intent of the research in the Department of Veterinary Science was to evaluate various treatments under controlled conditions to make sound recommendations. This objective required that neonatal calf diarrhea be consistently reproduced in the laboratory. Attempts to produce experimental cases of calf diarrhea were undertaken as follows. Ranches on which neonatal calf diarrhea was occurring were visited, and diarrheal feces were collected as soon as possible after the onset of diarrhea, and frozen. In the laboratory the feces were cultured for *E. coli,* salmonella, and clostridia; antibiotic sensitivity tests were also performed. *E. coli* were essentially the only bacteria isolated. These isolates were of many different serotypes and were resistant to most available antibiotics. Hysterectomy-derived and colostrum-deprived calves were inoculated orally with selected specimens. This type of calf was used to increase the possibility that any illness produced was not from some agent other than that present in the inoculum. The first calf inoculated developed diarrhea. Diarrheal feces from this calf did not cause diarrhea in subsequent calves. Calves inoculated with specimens of diarrheal feces from this and other ranches over the next 9–10 months did not develop diarrhea. These results were very frustrating, for these specimens were collected on ranches where almost every calf developed diarrhea. Again, the literature and observations in the field suggested that the overgrowth of bacteria in the intestinal tract was enhanced by stress; therefore, at the time of inoculation calves were chilled with water and a fan. They still did not develop diarrhea. Since the literature stated that diarrhea was due to a large number of *E. coli* in the upper small intestine, an attempt was made to flood the small intestine by inoculating 1–2 L of 15–18 h broth cultures of fecal bacteria into the duodenum via a cannula two or three times a day. The effect of this was to cause soft feces and a 50% reduction in the circulating leukocyte count for about 24 h.

The next attempt was inoculation of a fecal sample directly into the duodenum via a cannula. The calf developed severe diarrhea 15 h postinoculation and died 6 days after inoculation. Fecal material collected from this calf inoculated via a duodenal cannula caused diarrhea in another calf in 18 h. A culture of a gram-negative bacteria derived from a third calf passage stool was inoculated via a duodenal cannula and caused no diarrhea. A bacteria-free filtrate of experimental calf diarrheal feces inoculated via a duodenal cannula caused severe diarrhea, but the calf survived. Fecal material was then subjected to ultracentrifugation and the pellet sent to the University of Nebraska College of Medicine for electron microscopic examination. The pellet contained a large number of virions which were described as resembling blue tongue virus. Thirty-eight more calves, all housed in isolation rooms, were inoculated with bacteria-free fecal filtrate; they developed diarrhea. However, during the time of diarrhea, in addition to the virus, these calves had a highly resistant *E. coli* in their feces. The isolation rooms were scrubbed and fumigated with formaldehyde gas between experiments; the floor drain and traps, however, could not be sterilized, and it is believed that these drains were the continuous source of *E. coli.* Because of the strong belief that *E. coli* was the cause of calf diarrhea, two gnotobiotic calves were inoculated with filtrate. They developed severe diarrhea and were free of *E. coli* [1].

Cultivation of the virus in cell culture was then attempted. The virus did not grow in fetal bovine kidney (FBK) cells. Fetal bovine thyroid, lung, and choroid plexus cells were then tried. By this time a conjugate had been prepared, so cultures were examined for cytopathic effect (CPE) as well as for immuno-fluorescence. The first cultures to have immunofluorescing cells were choroid plexus, then lung cells. Eventually, with the use of fetal bovine lung cells and serum-free maintenance medium, there was extensive flagging CPE and immuno-fluorescence; however, each subculture had less CPE and fewer immunofluores-cent cells, and by five to six serial passages the virus was lost. Alternating passages between lung cells and calves did not help. Fecal material was then taken to the National Animal Disease Center, Ames, Iowa; the virus was isolated in pig kidney 15 cells. However, this PK 15 cell adapted virus for some unknown reason could not be propagated in Lincoln. The PK 15 propagated virus was inoculated into a calf, and caused diarrhea. The feces were cultured on FBK cells, and the virus isolated caused a flagging CPE, the cells were immunofluorescent positive, and the virus could be subcultured [2].

During these studies a local dairy herd from which colostrum-deprived calves were being purchased developed neonatal calf diarrhea. The disease was reproduced in experimental calves and was shown to be caused by a similar reovirus-like agent. After nearly a year of repeated attempts to propagate the virus on FBK cells, the virus was grown [3].

References

1. C. A. Mebus, N. R. Underdahl, M. B. Rhodes, and M. J. Twiehaus, Calf diarrhea (scours): Reproduced with a virus from a field oubread, *Res. Bull. Univ. Nebraska, 233* (1969).

2. A. L. Fernelius, A. E. Ritchie, L. B. Classick, J. O. Norman, and C. A. Mebus, Cell culture adaptation of a reovirus-like agent of calf diarrhea from a field outbreak in Nebraska, *Arch. Ges. Virusforsh., 37*:114-113 (1972).

3. C. A. Mebus, M. Kono, N. R. Underdahl, and M. J. Twiehaus, Cell culture propagation of neonatal calf diarrhea (scours) virus, *Can. Vet. J. 12*:69-72 (1971).

16

Rotaviruses in Animals

Gerald N. Woode Iowa State University College of Veterinary
Medicine, Ames, Iowa

Rotavirus infections have been identified in several species of mammals, and experimental and epidemiologic evidence has been produced to confirm rotaviruses as potential pathogens, although subclinical infections are common. The disease with which they are associated can be defined as an acute infection of the small intestine, characterized by a short incubation period followed by anorexia, occasional vomiting, and the development of diarrhea. Mortality rate is variable, ranging from 0 to 93% but usually on the order of 3-25%. Most individuals show an acute body weight loss of 5-10% followed by a period of 3-12 days or longer during which they fail to gain weight. Death occurs after 3-7 days of diarrhea, with a 10-30% loss of body weight. No other clinical syndrome has been reported, although some individual animals die with pneumonia after a protracted illness and under inclement weather conditions.

The causes of infantile diarrhea in most mammals are probably legion, and included among the proposed and proven causes are various bacterial species, fungal toxins, and other viruses. It is probable that other infectious causes are yet to be discovered. Most etiologic agents of diarrhea are commonly distributed in the environment, and infection with such agents as *Escherichia coli* and rotavirus can be considered normal. Thus it is not surprising to find some controversy over the relative importance and role of a single agent in the disease. Although one can speculate about the causes of clinical versus subclinical infection,

295

little is known at present concerning the role that rotaviruses play in severe clinical cases of the disease. There are no experimental studies reported with conventionally reared animals which have proved rotavirus to be capable of producing a lethal disease at the age at which the disease occurs naturally; rather, the converse has been suggested by Logan et al. [35] who found that under experimental conditions such infection induced a mild disease. The exception to this rule has been the studies on the weaning of piglets at 2 days of age, when rotavirus infection can produce a lethal disease [31]. Thus it is necessary to define the role of rotavirus in the disease as either: (1) an agent causing mild diarrhea, with other causes being responsible for the occasional case of severe disease which is not related to the rotavirus infection, or (2) that rotavirus infection is only severe under certain environmental, physiological, or other conditions which have not yet been elucidated but which may include severe chilling, the presence of certain other microbes, dose of virus, or virulence of the strain of rotavirus concerned.

History of Rotavirus Isolation

In Chap. 15 the history of the Nebraska calf diarrhea virus (NCDV), later identified as a rotavirus, has been described. The year 1969 [47] markes the commencement of the current era of rotavirus research, but in retrospect it is now known that the work of Light and Hodes [34] on diarrhea induced in calves inoculated with human fecal material and that of Cheever and Mueller [9] on diarrhea in infant mice involved rotaviruses. All subsequent identifications of rotaviruses from humans and animals have been confirmed directly or indirectly by antigenic and morphologic comparison with NCDV. Rotaviruses have been isolated from cases of diarrhea in calves [89], pigs, [32,44,56,87,90], lambs [40,66], foals [17,27,78], deer [75], monkeys [36], rabbits [8,54], pronghorn antelope [55], kittens [63,98], and dogs [14,20], and there is serologic evidence of infection in goats and guinea pigs, dogs, and cats [42,91]. Viruses similar in morphology to rotaviruses have been isolated from turkeys and chickens with diarrhea [3,25,41,43]. The relationship of these viruses to the mammalian rotaviruses has not been fully established, although McNulty et al. [41] reported the presence of antibody to mammalian rotavirus in sera of chickens and turkeys, and McNulty et al. [43] identified an antigen common to both avian and mammalian rotaviruses.

Rotavirus infections of animals have been reported from many countries of the world, and one can conclude that the virus is one of the most widely distributed and common infectious agents.

For further reading on rotavirus infections of animals consult the review articles by Flewett and Woode [19], McNulty [38], and the Colloquium on selected diarrheal diseases of the young [11].

Isolation of Rotavirus and Experimental
Transmission of Disease

Rotaviruses have proved difficult to cultivate in the laboratory, and from the earliest work recorded, experimental animals have been used to demonstrate the presence of the virus. As a consequence of the high frequency of spontaneously occurring diarrhea in young animals, the most recent practice has been to use gnotobiotic animals for experimental infection, as pioneered by Mebus and his colleagues in Nebraska [47]. Diarrheic animals produce virus to high titer in feces, 10^7-10^8 animal infectious doses per gram of feces [90,91]. Inoculation of bacteria-free filtrates orally or intranasally results in anorexia, vomiting in some pigs, and diarrhea within 15 h to 4 days postinfection. The virus appears in the feces at the first sign of diarrhea. Animal inoculation is probably 1000-10,000 times more sensitive for detecting rotavirus in the feces than most of the existing laboratory techniques, and in the pig has been used to identify the presence of pathogenic rotavirus when the laboratory tests were negative [76,90]. The minimal infective dose, defined as that dose capable of causing virus shedding and/or a serologic antibody response, is also the minimal disease dose in gnotobiotic piglets. As the virulence of rotavirus appears to be controlled in part by host factors, the usual practice has been to select, where possible, the part by host factors, the usual practice has been to select, where possible, the species of animal from which the virus was isolated for experimental transmission of infection and disease.

Rotaviruses have been purified by centrifugation through cesium and sucrose density gradients with or without ether-Nonidet P40 treatment followed by serial transmission in gnotobiotic animals. The unique identity of the rotaviruses was first recognized by electron microscopy (EM), but following adaptation to tissue culture, the antigenic and biochemical properties were established [18,19,28,45,53,81,82].

The basic virology of rotaviruses is described in Chap. 7. A new rotavirus from an animal is usually identified by observing the typical morphology and size of the virion by EM studies and demonstrating the presence of the rotavirus group-specific antigen by immunofluorescence (IF), complement fixation (CF), agar gel immunodiffusion (ID), or the enzyme-linked immunosorbent assay (ELISA) [59].

Age of Susceptibility to Rotavirus Infection

Rotaviruses are most commonly associated with diarrhea in animals during the first few weeks of life, at which age the clinical severity of infection is most pronounced [47,87]. However, adult humans, cattle, pigs, and laying hens have all been shown to excrete rotavirus, usually associated with diarrhea [25,41,80, 87]. Adult cows can be seriously affected for 1-3 days, with a pronounced reduction in appetite and milk production. In one study by the author, 20% of diarrheic cows were shown to be excreting rotavirus. Rotavirus has been associated with enteric infection and death in 0 to 9-week-old calves and in yearling cattle [92]. Thus there appears to be no age resistance to infection, which has important epidemiologic significance. Limited studies suggest that susceptibility to reinfection is inversely related to the immune status of the individual, although data from children also demonstrate the probability that reinfection may occur with an antigenically distinct strain unrelated to the previous infection [99].

Clinical Features of Rotavirus Infection

Infection usually occurs as a sudden and rapidly spreading epizootic in young domestic animals [92]. Within 5-10 days following observation of the first case of diarrhea, all susceptible animals, including calves at grass, may be clinically affected. Spread of infection in housed calves or piglets is extremely rapid, and the majority of animals in contact with each other develop diarrhea within 2-3 days. An incubation period of 15-96 h is followed by depression, occasional vomiting in piglets, and shortly afterward by the onset of watery or semisolid diarrhea, profuse in quantity. The incubation period was shown to be dependent on the titer of virus inoculated [90], although the severity of infection under experimental conditions was the same in animals infected with a minimal infectious dose or with 10^7 pig infectious doses. However, under natural conditions, the severity of the disease may be related to the amount of virus ingested during the first few hours, particularly if there is some passively derived immunity present in the form of antibody in the milk and gut contents, or even in the serum [31,38,72,91]. Fever is not a characteristic of the disease in animals, but can occur. If the animal is on a total milk diet the diarrheic feces are frequently brilliant yellow to white, not always putrid, and resemble the classic milk scours. In other calves, the feces may be watery, brown, gray, or light green, with fresh blood from rectal hemorrhages and mucus. The color is dependent on the diet, and in piglets on a solid diet is usually black or gray. There is marked variation between individuals in clinical severity; in some animals body weight declines rapidly by 10-15% and after a variable period they recover and return to a normal rate of weight gain. The period may be 5-28 days, but is usually 5-10 days. Although clinical signs of respiratory disease are usually absent, under inclement weather conditions and severe chilling, calves may die 1-2 weeks later with penumonia, without having recovered from the diarrhea. On other occasions, when death supervenes, it usually occurs after 3-7 days of diarrhea when the animal shows severe loss of body weight (10-30%), dehydration, and sunken eyes. In one study gnotobiotic piglets inoculated with rotavirus at day 0 died on days 3-4 with a 30% decline in birth body weight

[92]. Quantitative observations have been made on experimental infection with rotavirus in 10 colostrum-deprived calves [35]. Two calves remained clinically normal; the remainder developed a mild diarrhea with a minor biochemical disturbance in the blood. These results were less severe than those observed by the author: 12 of 24 colostrum-deprived calves reared under conventional conditions died after spontaneous rotavirus infection, and under experimental conditions, of 4 colostrum-deprived rotavirus-infected calves, 2 were killed for experimental purposes and 2 died [89]. In a later experiment, of 22 conventionally reared calves which were inoculated with rotavirus at 2 days of age, 3 of the calves were unintentionally deprived of colostrum and all 3 died after 4-6 days of diarrhea. All of the remaining 19 colostrum-fed calves developed diarrhea 2-8 days postinfection; some showed severe body weight loss, but all recovered in 5-28 days. Control calves remained free of spontaneous diarrhea during the first 8-10 days of life [92]. In contrast, of those colostrum-deprived calves which were taken immediately at birth, without contamination from the environment, and placed in gnotobiotic isolators, all survived following challenge with rotavirus [87]. Thus it is reasonable to conclude that the most common clinical syndrome associated with rotavirus infection is diarrhea, with a variable effect on body weight and recovery occurring after a few days without treatment. However, under circumstances that are not understood, but including environmental effects such as severe chilling or the presence of other pathogenic agents, the mortality rate can reach 90% (Woode, unpublished data; Bohl, personal communication; Ref. 92).

Subclinical Infection and the Influence of Husbandry

Subclinical infection with rotavirus is probably common, if the high incidence of seropositive humans and animals and the subclinical seroconversion of pigs are considered. Possible explanations for these subclinical infections have been reviewed [92] and include infection in the presence of colostrally derived antibody in the gut lumen, age resistance in some individuals, or infections with low-virulent or avirulent strains.

In contrast to calves, in which species rotavirus-associated diarrhea occurs at all ages and is not apparently dependent on changes in husbandry, the infection in pigs follows the well-recognized patterns of age and husbandry-associated enteric disease. Thus rotavirus has been associated with acute diarrhea of early weaned pigs at 2 days of age [32], in pigs weaned at 3-8 weeks of age and during various stages of the suckling period, but not usually during the first 7-10 days of life when the level of antibody in the milk remains relatively high [4,29, 38,72,90]. A number of authors have explained the occurrence of diarrhea at weaning by the sudden loss of antibody from the diet, even if it is of low titer, and by exposure to virus from older pigs or from some other source. However, diarrhea in suckling piglets has been recorded in herds in which most of the sows were immune, and rotavirus infection at weaning has been reported to occur in 100% of piglets of a litter, although disease may occur in less than 30% of the animals [90,92]. In these latter studies, a rotavirus isolated from a clinically normal, newly weaned pig aged 3.5 weeks caused diarrhea and loss of weight experimentally in gnotobiotic piglets at 7 days of age, but it has proved difficult to cause diarrhea and a clinical syndrome uniformly by inoculating gnotobiotic piglets aged between 3 and 5 weeks [76,92]. In the studies by Lecce and King [29], good evidence was produced that the rotavirus was the cause of diarrhea occurring at 3 weeks of age after weaning; large numbers of virus particles were observed in the feces of diarrheic pigs, but not in normal pigs, and rotaviral antigens were detected in the atrophied villi. However, the authors did not inoculate experimental piglets aged 3 weeks. Other factors may be involved in rotavirus-associated diarrhea in weaned pigs, and Tzipori and his colleagues in Australia have attempted to find these [76]. They studied the effect of diet on the incidence of diarrhea in gnotobiotic piglets aged 28 days caused by porcine rotavirus or by an enteropathogenic strain of E. coli (either singly or in combination), both agents having been isolated from piglets in weaner diarrhea. In these initial experiments the piglets were susceptible to E. coli-induced diarrhea only when fed on milk or immediately following change to a dry food, but were resistant after 4 days on the dry food. In contrast, the severity of rotavirus infection increased in weaning from a milk diet, but as for E. coli, if inoculated with rotavirus after 4 days on the dry food, the piglets remained symptomless. If the piglets were inoculated with rotavirus at weaning followed 4 days later by E. coli, all the piglets died (six of six). Although these data are preliminary and require further experiments, they may prove to be most important in our understanding of the cause of weaner diarrhea in piglets. The hypothesis is that immediately on weaning, the change of diet produced a physiological effect on the intestine which enhances rotavirus and E. coli infections and pathogenicity.

Pathogenic Effects of Mixed Microbial Infections

Probably the majority of normal calves, and certainly the majority of diarrhea epizootics, are characterized by mixed infections with supposed or proven pathogens [1,51,52,88,92]. The agents include strains of E. coli, cryptosporidia, occasionally Salmonella species, commonly bovine rotavirus, bovine coronavirus, and small round viruses (astrovirus and calicivirus-like agents). In attempts to study the pathogenic relationship between E. coli and rotavirus, three laboratories have made limited but interesting studies. Mebus et al. [46] showed that the disease was exacerbated in two calves infected with an apparently nonvirulent strain of E. coli together with bovine rotavirus. In further studies, Gouet et al. [21], inoculated three calves orally at birth with rotavirus and followed this 1 day later with nonlethal inocula of an enterotoxigenic *E. coli* (strain 09:K(A), K99:H⁻ at titers of 3×10^8 to 2×10^9). All three calves died. However, one calf inoculated with this strain of *E. coli* at a titer of 1×10^{10} in the absence of rotavirus also died. These results tend to support the hypothesis that rotavirus infection predisposes calves to bacterial infection and that the bacteria are responsible for the severity of the syndrome [21,51]. In a recent study, Runnels et al. [58] found that gnotobiotic calves inoculated orally with both rotavirus and *E. coli* strain B44 developed more severe diarrhea and more extensive lesions than those that received either rotavirus or B44 alone. However, none of the calves died, and the authors concluded that the differences were not great enough to support the theory of a synergistic interaction between viruses and bacteria. There were differences in the experimental designs of the three studies [21,46,58], and a limited number of experimental animals were used—both these factors may explain the differences reported. Further work is required to finally settle the controversy concerning the role of mixed infections in the pathogenesis of the syndrome.

Since subclinical infection with rotaviruses is common, in both human infants and animals, it is necessary to make a critical study to determine whether a rotavirus multiplying in the intestine is behaving in a pathogenic manner.

Cross-Infection of Animals and Humans and Virulence of Rotaviral Isolates

Studies on rotaviruses inoculated experimentally into animals have demonstrated that most if not all rotavirus isolates, regardless of the mammalian species of origin, will infect pigs, and possibly calves, lambs, and dogs. These animals excrete virus for several days and may or may not develop diarrhea and clinical illness, but all seroconvert. In the United States human rotavirus in calves and pigs caused diarrhea, intestinal lesions were reported [48,49,74], and some gnotobiotic and conventional piglets developed diarrhea [50]. In contrast to these findings, human, ovine, and equine rotavirus (U.K. isolates) infected piglets without the development of diarrhea or body weight loss [6,90,92], and human rotavirus (Australian isolate) infected young dogs but did not cause diarrhea [77]. Bovine rotavirus (U.K. isolate) produced a severe infection and some mortality in piglets (Ref. 23; Tzipori, personal communication), but the U.S. bovine isolate did not clinically affect piglets (Mebus, personal communication). Flewett et al. [18] were not successful in experimentally infecting calves with the human (U.K.) rotavirus. In later studies, Woode et al. [86] successfully infected gnotobiotic calves in the United Kingdom with the human rotavirus (U.S. isolate) which had been passed in gnotobiotic calves [49]. Although this virus caused diarrhea in the U.S. studies in which the intraduodenal inoculation route was used, the calves remained symptomless in the U.K. studies, when the route of inoculation was intranasal. Human virus was also propagated in monkeys (*Macaca mulatta*) by Wyatt et al. [96], and human virus infected lambs with the development of intestinal lesions [62]. Although there is no published evidence that rotavirus strains cross-infect between mammalian species under natural conditions, it is possible that this happens and must be taken into account when attempts are made to control infection. In one report, a human rotavirus isolate appeared to be closely related antigenically to a bovine serotype [6], and in the author's laboratory, one porcine rotavirus was isolated which was also closely related to this bovine serotype.

Reference was made earlier in this chapter to possible explanations for the apparent variation in severity of rotavirus infection. As this varies between subclinical infection and death, it is important to study the reasons. Woode and Crouch [92] reviewed the literature and discussed the probability that rotavirus strains of different virulence exist. Although there are reports of experimental infection with human rotavirus in calves and pigs, these were mild clinically and did not occur in all passes of the viruses or in all animals. Thus it was shown that different rotaviruses in piglets could produce either subclinical infection at any age from 0 to 21 days, or were capable of producing severe illness and death at day 0 or up to day 21, according to the origin of the isolate. On further passages of the viruses in gnotobiotic piglets, the virulence for the host was not significantly altered. Thus, although subclinical infection could be caused by a combination of rotavirus infection and suckled colostrum [32,67,68,93], it is possible that many infections are subclinical due to a rotavirus avirulent for that species of host. Although studies are not possible on the virulence of human rotaviruses for young children, all isolates of rotavirus from calves, lambs, piglets, and foals have proved to be virulent for the species from which they were isolated. However, most of the studies have been made from rotaviruses isolated from cases of diarrhea, and few from viruses isolated from subclinical infection. This is of great importance, for if rotaviruses differ in virulence for different hosts, it is impossible to determine whether a rotavirus is avirulent to all species without extensive animal and human transmission experiments.

The pathogenesis and pathology of rotavirus infections is reviewed in Chaps. 13 and 18. However, the evidence that rotaviruses are potential pathogens is based on the well-proven criteria of Koch's postulates. The virus can be isolated from the feces, purified chemically, physically, or by cell culture, reinoculated into a nonimmune animal, and cause disease and be reisolated. Virus is observed by electron microscopy and viral antigen by immunofluorescence in the damaged cells of the small intestinal villi [19,38,72,84].

Culture of Rotaviruses

Growth of the reovirus-like agent was achieved originally with great difficulty, and for some time only the "0" agent (from cattle or sheep), the SA-11 agent from monkeys, and three isolates of bovine rotavirus were isolated [5,33,36,39, 45]. Apparently rotaviruses infect only kidney cell cultures, but these may be from a variety of animals, including bovine, porcine, ovine, simian, and human. Most viruses produce an abortive infection in kidney cell culture, with the appearance of immunofluorescent cells at 24-72 h postinfection. Infection is usually lost after two to three passes and probably no infectious virus is produced under these conditions. This method has been used for the diagnosis of rotavirus infection [5]. Fetal gut organ culture has not proved better than cell culture [94]. Some bovine isolates were adapted to tissue cultures to produce infectious virus and then were readily subcultured, but this was fortuitous and no explanation has been found. Theil et al. [71] and Babiuk et al. [2] introduced the method of treating rotavirus with trypsin or pancreatin prior to each pass of virus in cell culture. By this means two isolates of porcine rotavirus have been cultured, and several isolates of bovine rotavirus. However, for successful culture, the initial inoculum should have a high titer of infectivity in cell culture. High-titer virus can be produced by this method [10]. Difficulties in culturing human strains and the U.K. (Compton) porcine isolate remain despite this technique. Failure to culture the virus may reflect the in vivo tropism of the virus. Most studies have reported infection only in the villous epithelial cells and not in crypt cells. It is doubtful whether these highly differentiated villus cells multiply in vitro, and thus the virus must be adapted to replicate in kidney cells. The cells of the kidney tubules carry microvilli with similar enzymes to those found in the gut. Perhaps the kidney cells are receptive to infection but are not readily permissive for viral multiplication. Cytopathic effects of the virus have been reported [39] and a plaque assay developed [37].

Characterization of Animal Rotaviruses

On the basis of their morphologic similarity and the double-stranded and segmented nature of the RNA, the reovirus-like agents have been classified in the family reoviridae as the genus rotavirus [13,16]. The morphology, morphogenic, and biochemical and biophysical properties have been reviewed recently [19, 38]. Although all known rotaviruses share a common antigen, demonstrable by a number of techniques, including immunodiffusion, immunofluorescence, complement fixation, immune electron microscopy, and ELISA, they do not share antigens with members of the other two genera, namely, orbivirus or reovirus [5,28].

Antigenic Relationships

An antigenic relationship between bovine and human rotavirus was first demonstrated by immune electron microscopy and immunofluorescence [18]. The common antigen was shown to be present in rotaviruses isolated from humans, calves, pigs, lambs, rabbits, foals, mice, the SA-11 simian virus, 0 agent [28, 73,91], and dogs [20].

Since 1974, however, there have been reports of antigenic differences between rotavirus isolates. Flewett et al. [18] found that not all human sera with antibody to the rotavirus group antigen neutralized the bovine rotavirus, and this was confirmed with isolates of lamb virus, pig virus, some isolates of human virus inoculated into pigs, and with SA-11 virus. These isolates do not show optimal cross-neutralization properties [15,60,66,73,90,91]. Most authors accept the view that various isolates of rotaviruses may show poor or no cross-neutralization. However, full recognition of the antigenic differences between isolates will not be achieved until all strains are cultured. Antisera raised in gnotobiotic animals to a variety of animal and human rotaviruses usually show a 16- to 64-fold difference in the neutralization of cell culture adapted bovine rotavirus when compared with the titer of the homologous system [90,91], but with unadapted rotaviruses these same antisera may only show a 4- to 16-fold difference in the neutralization test [73]. The recognition of these antigenic differences has proved invaluable in the laboratory for identifying various isolates. However, the significance of the differences in terms of immunity has yet to be fully investigated. Woode et al. [86] used three gnotobiotic calves inoculated with each of the human or foal rotavirus, and showed 33% cross-protection when the six calves were challenged with bovine rotavirus. The calves did not produce neutralizing antibody to bovine rotavirus prior to the final challenge, but the two calves that showed cross-protection had developed high heterologous antibody. In contrast to these results, the bovine vaccine rotavirus induced protection to the human type 2 rotavirus in calves [95]. Lecce and King [30] found that the same bovine vaccine did not protect pigs from porcine rotavirus challenge. Similar results were obtained in unpublished work by the author and by Bohl (personal communication).

The presence of antigenically different rotaviruses in one species of animal has not been reported, although the author did isolate from pigs a rotavirus which shared neutralizing antigens with bovine strains. However, it is well established that there are at least two and probably more serotypes of human rotavirus [97]. It would be wise to assume that several serotypes of rotavirus will be discovered eventually in each animal species, some of these shared with other mammals. Blue tongue orbivirus, an infection of sheep and cattle, demonstrates at least 22 antigenic subtypes between which cross-protection is poor.

Differences have been detected between human and animal rotaviruses, using analysis of the viral RNA. However, some but fewer differences were also observed between two closely related bovine rotaviruses, the Nebraska isolate and the U.K. Compton isolate, between two bovine rotaviruses isolated in France [26,79], and between eight bovine rotaviruses isolated in Australia [57].

These viruses show cross-neutralization and cross-protection properties, although the U.K. virus lacks a demonstrable hemagglutinin [70]. Whether these RNA differences have significance in immunity and vaccine development has yet to be determined.

Diagnosis of Rotavirus Infection

In contrast to the difficulties encountered in early studies on rotavirus infection, a number of convenient and sufficiently sensitive tests have been developed for the recognition of rotavirus in fecal samples. With the exception of the fecal smear immunofluorescent technique, in which positive results are only obtained for the first 5 h of diarrhea, the other tests appear to be sufficiently sensitive, largely because of the great number of virus particles produced in diarrheic feces. The methods include electron microscopy, infection in cell culture, immunodiffusion, solid-phase radioimmunoassay, ELISA, complement-fixing antigen, and countercurrent immunoelectroosmorphoresis [19,38]. Most of these tests are dependent on the specificity of the antisera used, and great care must be taken to ensure that the antigen used to produce antisera is free from other viruses. For example, in our laboratory, following the discovery of a contaminating small virus in the standard rotavirus antigen, the author and his colleagues resorted to two unrelated tests for rotavirus diagnosis—electron microscopy and an antigen test, usually immunofluorescence of infected cell cultures.

Epizootiology

The epizootiology of rotavirus infection has been studied to a limited extent only. It has been established that infections can occur at least in some individual animals, at all ages, whether or not clinical disease develops [38,85,87]. The intestinal tract is the site of multiplication of virus which is excreted at high infectious titers in the diarrheic feces for several days. Studies in the pig [90] show that 10^7–10^8 pig infectious doses are produced per gram of feces, probably for at least 4 days. Once an adult or young animal commences excreting rotavirus, the area becomes heavily contaminated and rapid spread of infection occurs. Because rotavirus is stable in feces, can survive for several months at $20°C$ [87,92], and is relatively resistant to commonly used disinfectants [65], it is extremely difficult to prevent heavy contamination of buildings and even of grassland.

There is no evidence that adults act as carriers, and in the author's opinion active infection in adults, either clinical or subclinical, is probably the original source of infection for young or neonatal animals [85]. It has been suggested that rotaviruses may cross the placenta and infect the fetus in utero [38]. Although this situation may occur, it probably does in only a small minority of animals, but would be a very important source of infection for the herd. The data reported appear to be in conflict with the experiences of those studying infection in gnotobiotic animals. There is no report in the literature of gnotobiotic animals being spontaneously infected with rotavirus, possessing antibody, or being resistant to infection, although the dams were drawn from herds in which rotavirus infection was common.

Undoubtedly the greatest problem for an animal species in protecting itself from this very common pathogen is the relative inefficiency of transfer of the herd immunity to the young. If we accept that adults can be clinically infected and that over 90% possess neutralizing antibody in serum and colostrum, the lack of diarrhea in the cows in the average outbreak suggests a high level of adult immunity, in contrast to the young, all of which may be sick. It has been shown that colostrally derived serum antibody does not protect against infection with rotavirus, although the presence of colostral antibody in the gut lumen will prevent disease, if not infection [5,32,48,68,69,93]. In addition, individual cows vary considerably in their titers of serum neutralizing antibody [85], and even after an epizootic, a few show poor levels. It is probable that the level of infection under natural conditions may overwhelm the resistance provided by colostrum, particularly as this declines rapidly in cows after calving (1-2 days) [91] and in sows after farrowing over 7-10 days. In attempts to prolong the secretion in milk of the high levels of neutralizing antibody found in colostrum, Snodgrass et al. [64] vaccinated heifers twice during pregnancy with inactivated rotavirus. This raised the titer of antibody from 1:100 to 1:20,452, and 28 days after calving the mean titer was 1:320. The colostral antibody was primarily of the IgA and IgG_1 classes, whereas at 28 days it consisted almost entirely of IgG_1. On day 7 of age the calves were challenged with virulent rotavirus which had the same isolation history as the vaccine virus, and thus they could be considered homologous antigenically. Diarrhea occurred with equal severity in both groups of calves which were being suckled by either vaccinated or control heifers at the time of challenge. These results confirm the view of other workers that milk possesses poor protective properties against rotavirus infection and disease induction.

Although the source of infection for most animals is direct contact with a rotavirus-excreting animal, the role of contaminated water and food may be important. In recent studies it has been shown that rotaviruses are less effectively removed by conventional sewage treatment processes than enteroviruses, and both survive well in waste water and after adsorption by soil. At low temperatures the enteric viruses can persist for weeks or months in natural waters and marine and river sediment and soils, and enteroviruses have been isolated from wells 100 ft deep. Thus, it is considered probable that in a heavily contaminated area, for instance a farm after an epizootic, rotavirus release into the drinking water supply could follow heavy precipitation of moisture causing desorption of the virus from the soil, perhaps several months after the period of viral contamination [22,24,61].

Other mammalian species may prove to be important sources of infection, carried either clinically or subclinically. In this respect, humans and rodents must be considered likely sources of infection for farm animals, for whichever method of isolating mammalian species is practiced, these species cannot be effectively excluded.

The incidence of human rotavirus infection is seasonal and is greater in winter months [7,12]. However, this may reflect the observation in both humans and animals that the disease is more severe under cold conditions. In one study in calves, no rotavirus-associated diarrhea was recorded for July, August, and September, whereas cases occurred in all the other 9 months. Most cases occurred between October and April, but this largely reflected the calving pattern of cattle [83]. Thus it is probable that infection occurs at all times of the year in animals, but is influenced in severity by weather conditions, and in frequency by the proportion of young in the population.

References

1. S. D. Acres, C. J. Laing, J. R. Saunders, and O. M. Radostits, Acute undifferentiated neonatal diarrhea in beef calves, I. Occurrence and distribution of infectious agents, *Can. J. Com. Med., 39*:116-132 (1975).
2. L. A. Babiuk, K. Mohammed, L. Spence, M. Fauvel, and R. Petro, Rotavirus isolation (first described as the etiological agent of neonatal calf diarrhea) and cultivation in the presence of trypsin, *J. Clin. Microbiol., 6*:610-617 (1977).
3. M. E. Bergeland, J. P. McAdaragh, D. E. Reed, and I. Stotz, A diarrhea syndrome in young turkey poults, *129-130*. Proceedings of the 27th Annual North Central Poultry Disease Conferences, 1976, p. 68.
4. E. H. Bohl, E. M. Kohler, L. J. Saif, R. F. Cross, A. G. Agnes, and K. W. Theil, Rotavirus as a cause of diarrhea in pigs, *J. Am. Vet. Med. Assoc., 172*:458-463 (1978).
5. J. C. Bridger and G. N. Woode, Neonatal calf diarrhoea: Identification of a reovirus-like (rotavirus) agent in faeces by immunofluorescence and immune electron microscopy, *Br. Vet. J., 131*:528-535 (1975).
6. J. C. Bridger, G. N. Woode, J. M. Jones, T. H. Flewett, A. S. Bryden, and H. Davies, Transmission of human rotaviruses to gnotobiotic piglets, *J. Med. Microbiol., 8*:565-569 (1975).
7. A. S. Bryden, H. A. Davies, R. E. Hadley, T. H. Flewett, C. A. Morris, and P. Oliver, Rotavirus enteritis in the West Midlands during 1974, *Lancet, 2*:241-243 (1975).
8. A. S. Bryden, M. E. Thouless, and T. H. Flewett, A rabbit rotavirus, *Vet. Rec., 99*:323 (1976).

9. F. S. Cheever and J. H. Mueller, Epidemic diarrheal disease of suckling mice. I. Manifestation, epidemiology, and attempts to transmit the disease, *J. Exp. Med., 85*:405-416 (1947).

10. S. M. Clark, B. B. Barnett, and R. S. Spendlove, Production of high-titer bovine rotavirus with trypsin, *J. Clin. Microbiol., 9*:413-417 (1979).

11. Colloquium on selected diarrheal diseases of the young, *J. Am. Vet. Med. Assoc., 173*:511-583 (1978).

12. G. P. Davidson, R. F. Bishop, R. R. W. Rownley, I. H. Holmes, and B. J. Ruck, Importance of a new virus in acute sporadic enteritis in children, *Lancet, 1*:242-246 (1975).

13. J. B. Derbyshire and G. N. Woode, Classification of rotaviruses: Report from the World Health Organization/Food and Agriculture Organization Comparative Virology Program, *J. Am. Vet. Med. Assoc., 173*:519-521 (1978).

14. J. J. England and R. P. Poston, Electron microscopic identification and subsequent isolation of a rotavirus from a dog with fatal neonatal diarrhea, *Am. J. Vet. Res., 41*:782-783 (1980).

15. M. K. Estes and D. Y. Graham, Identification of rotavirus of different origins by the plaque-reduction test, *Am. J. Vet. Res., 41*:151-152 (1980).

16. F. Fenner, Classification and nomenclature of viruses. Second report of the International Committee on Taxonomy of Viruses, *Intervirology, 7*: 1-116 (1976).

17. T. H. Flewett, A. S. Bryden, and H. Davies, Virus diarrhoea in foals and other animals, *Vet. Rec., 96*:477 (1975).

18. T. H. Flewett, A. S. Bryden, H. Davies, G. N. Woode, J. C. Bridger, and J. M. Derrick, Relation between viruses from acute gastroenteritis of children and new born calves, *Lancet, 2*:61-63 (1974).

19. T. H. Flewett and G. N. Woode, The rotaviruses, *Arch. Virol., 57*:1-23 (1978).

20. R. W. Fulton, C. A. Johnson, N. J. Pearson, and G. N. Woode, Isolation of rotavirus from a newborn dog with diarrhea, *Am. J. Vet. Res.,* (In press) (1981).

21. P. Gouet, M. Contrepois, H. C. Dubourgier, Y. Riou, R. Scherrer, J. Laporte, J. F. Vautherot, J. Cohen, and R. L'Haridon, The experimental production of diarrhoea in colostrum deprived axenic and gnotoxenic calves with enteropathogenic *Escherichia coli*, rotavirus, coronavirus and in a combined infection of rotavirus and *E. coli, Ann. Rec. Vet., 9:* 433-440 (1978).

22. S. M. Goyal and C. P. Gerba, Comparative adsorption of human enteroviruses, simian rotaviruses and selected bacteriophages to soils, *Appl. Environ. Microbiol., 38*:241-247 (1979).

23. G. A. Hall, J. C. Bridger, R. L. Chandler, and G. N. Woode, Gnotobiotic piglets experimentally infected with neonatal calf diarrhoea reovirus-like agent (rotavirus), *Vet. Pathol., 13*:197-210 (1976).

24. C. J. Hurst and C. P. Gerba, Stability of simian rotavirus in fresh and estuarine water, *Appl. Environ. Microbiol., 39*:1-5 (1980).

25. R. C. Jones, C. S. Hughes, and R. R. Henry, Rotavirus infection in commercial laying hens, *Vet. Rec., 104*:22 (1979).
26. A. R. Kalica, M. M. Sereno, R. G. Wyatt, C. A. Mebus, R. M. Chanock, and A. Z. Kapikian, Comparison of human and animal rotavirus strains by gel-electrophoresis of viral-RNA, *Virology, 87*:247-255 (1978).
27. C. L. Kanitz, Identification of an equine rotavirus as a cause of neonatal foal diarrhea, *Proc. Ann. Conv. Am. Assoc. Equine Pract., 220*:155-165 (1977).
28. A. Z. Kapikian, W. L. Cline, C. A. Mebus, R. G. Wyatt, A. R. Kalica, H. D. James, D. Vankirk, R. M. Chanock, and H. W. Kim, New complement-fixation test for the human reovirus-like agent of infantile gastroenteritis, *Lancet, 1*:1056-1061 (1975).
29. J. G. Lecce and M. W. King, Role of rotavirus (reo-like) in weanling diarrhea of pigs, *J. Clin. Microbiol., 8*:454-458 (1978).
30. J. G. Lecce and M. W. King, the calf reo-like virus (rotavirus) vaccine: An ineffective immunization agent for rotaviral diarrhea of piglets, *Can. Com. Med., 43*:90-93 (1979).
31. J. G. Lecce, M. W. King, and W. E. Dorsey, Rearing regimen producing piglet diarrhea (rotavirus) and its relevance to acute infantile diarrhea, *Science, 199*:776-778 (1978).
32. J. G. Lecce, M. W. King, and R. Mock, Reovirus-like agent associated with fatal diarrhea in neonatal pigs, *Infect. Immun., 14*:816-825 (1976).
33. R. L'Haridon and R. Scherrer, In vitro culture of a rotavirus associated with neonatal calf scours, *Ann. Rec. Vet., 7*:373-381 (1976).
34. J. S. Light and H. L. Hodes, Studies on epidemic diarrhoea in the newborn: Isolation of filterable agent causing diarrhoes in calves, *Am. J. Public Health, 33*:1451-1454 (1943).
35. E. F. Logan, G. R. Pearson, and M. S. McNulty, Quantitative observations on experimental reo-like virus (rotavirus) infection in colostrum deprived calves, *Vet. Rec., 104*:206-209 (1979).
36. H. H. Malherbe and M. Strickland-Cholmley, Simian virus S. A. II and the related 0 agent, *Arch. Ges. Virusforsch, 22*:235-245 (1967).
37. S. Matsuno, S. Inouye, and R. Kono, Plaque assay of neonatal calf diarrhea virus and the neutralizing antibody in human sera, *J. Clin. Microbiol., 5*:1-4 (1977).
38. M. S. McNulty, Rotavirus, *J. Gen. Virol., 40*:1-8 (1978).
39. M. S. McNulty, G. M. Allan, and J. B. McFerran, Isolation of a cytopathic calf rotavirus, *Res. Vet. Sci., 21*:114-115 (1976).
40. M. S. McNulty, G. M. Allan, G. R. Pearson, J. B. McFerran, W. L. Curran, and R. M. McCracken, Reovirus-like agent (rotavirus) from lambs, *Infect. Immun., 14*:1332-1338 (1976).
41. M. S. McNulty, G. M. Allan, and J. C. Stuart, Rotavirus infection in avian species, *Vet. Rec., 103*:319-320 (1978).
42. M. S. McNulty, G. M. Allan, D. J. Thompson, and J. D. O'Boyle, Antibody to rotavirus in dogs and cats, *Vet. Rec., 102*:534-535 (1978).

43. M. S. McNulty, G. M. Allan, D. Todd, and J. B. McFerran, Isolation and cell culture propagation of rotaviruses from turkeys and chickens, *Arch. Virol., 61*:13-21 (1979).

44. M. S. McNulty, G. R. Pearson, J. B. McFerran, D. S. Collins, and G. M. Allan, A reovirus-like agent (rotavirus) associated with diarrhea in neonatal pigs, *Vet. Microbiol., 1*:55-63 (1976).

45. C. A. Mebus, M. Dono, N. R. Underdahl, and M. J. Twiehaus, Cell culture porpagation of neonatal calf diarrhea (scours) virus, *Can. Vet. J. 12*:69-72 (1971).

46. C. A. Mebus, E. L. Stair, N. R. Underdahl, and M. J. Twiehaus, Pathology of neonatal calf diarrhea induced by a reo-like virus, *Vet. Pathol., 8*:490-505 (1971).

47. C. A. Mebus, N. R. Underdahl, M. B. Rhodes, and M. J. Twiehaus, Calf diarrhea (scours): Reproduced with a virus from a field outbreak. University of Nebraska Agricultural Experiment Station Research Bulletin No. 233 (1969).

48. C. A. Mebus, R. G. White, E. P. Bass, and M. J. Twiehaus, Immunity to neonatal calf diarrhea virus, *J. Am. Vet. Med. Assoc., 163*:880-883 (1973).

49. C. A. Mebus, R. G. Wyatt, R. L. Sharpee, M. M. Sereno, A. R. Kalica, A. Z. Kapikian, and M. J. Twiehaus, Diarrhea in gnotobiotic calves caused by the reovirus-like agent of human infantile gastroenteritis, *Infect. Immun., 14*:471-474 (1976).

50. P. J. Middleton, M. Petric, and M. T. Szymanski, Propagation of infantile gastroenteritis virus (orbi-group) in conventional and germ free piglets, *Infect. Immun., 12*:1276-1280 (1975).

51. H. W. Moon, A. W. McClurkin, R. E. Isaacson, J. Pohlenz, S. M. Skartved, and K. G. Gillette, Pathogenic relationships of rotavirus, *Escherichia coli,* and other agents in mixed infections in calves, *J. Am. Vet. Med. Assoc., 173*:577-583 (1978).

52. M. Morin, S. Lariviere, and R. Lallier, Pathological and Microbiological observations made on spontaneous cases of acute neonatal calf diarrhea, *Can. Com. Med., 40*:228-240 (1976).

53. J. F. E. Newman, F. Brown, J. C. Bridger, and G. N. Woode, Characterization of a rotavirus, *Nature, 258*:631-633 (1975).

54. M. Petric, P. J. Middleton, C. Grant, J. S. Tam, C. M. Hewitt, Lapine rotavirus—preliminary studies on epizoology and transmission, *Can. Com. Med., 42*:143-147 (1978).

55. D. E. Reed, C. A. Daley, and H. J. Shane, Reovirus-like agent associated with neonatal diarrhea in pronghorn antelope, *J. Wildl. Dis., 12*:488-491 (1976).

56. S. M. Rodger, J. A. Craven, and I. Williams, Demonstration of reovirus-like particles in intestinal contents of piglets with diarrhoea, *Aust. Vet. J., 51*:536 (1975).

57. S. M. Rodger and I. H. Holmes, Comparison of the genomes of simian, bovine and human rotaviruses by gel electrophoresis and detection of genomic variation among bovine isolates, *J. Virol., 30*:839-846 (1979).

58. L. P. Runnels, H. W. Moon, S. C. Whipp, P. J. Matthews, and G. N. Woode, Effects on rotavirus and enterotoxigenic *Escherichia coli* (ETC) in gnotobiotic calves. Proceedings, Third International Symposium on Neonatal Diarrhea, Vido. University of Saskatchewan, Saskatoon, Canada, 1980 (in press).

59. R. Scherrer and S. Bernard, Application of enzyme-linked immunosorbent assay (ELISA) to the detection of calf rotavirus and rotavirus antibodies, *Ann. Microbiol., 128*:499-510 (1977).

60. B. D. Schoub, G. Lecatsas, and O. W. Prozesky, Antigenic relationship between human and simian rotaviruses, *J. Med. Microbiol., 10*:1-6 (1977).

61. E. M. Smith and C. P. Gerba, Survival and detection of rotaviruses in the environment. Proceedings, Third International Symposium on Neonatal diarrhea. Vido. University of Saskatchewan, Saskatoon, Canada, 1980 (in press).

62. R. D. Snodgrass, K. W. Angus, and E. W. Gray, Rotavirus infection in lambs: Pathogenesis and pathology, *Arch. Virol., 55*:263-274 (1977).

63. D. R. Snodgrass, K. W. Angus, and E. W. Gray, A rotavirus from kittens, *Vet. Rec., 104*:222-223 (1979).

64. D. R. Snodgrass, K. J. Fahey, and P. W. Wells, Rotavirus infections in calves from vaccinated and normal cows. Viral enteritis in humans and animals. Colloquium-INRA. Thiverval-Grignom, France, 4–7 September 1979 (1979).

65. D. R. Snodgrass and J. A. Herring, The action of disinfectants on lamb rotavirus, *Vet. Rec., 101*:81 (1977).

66. D. R. Snodgrass, J. A. Herring, and E. W. Gray, Experimental rotavirus infection in lambs, *J. Comp. Pathol., 86*:637-642 (1976).

67. D. R. Snodgrass, C. R. Madeley, P. W. Wells, and K. W. Angus, Human rotavirus in lambs: Infection and passive protection, *Infect. Immun., 16*: 268-270 (1977).

68. D. R. Snodgrass and P. W. Wells, Rotavirus infection in lambs: Studies on passive protection, *Arch. Virol., 52*:201-205 (1976).

69. D. R. Snodgrass and P. W. Wells, The immunoprophylaxis of rotavirus infections in lambs, *Vet. Rec., 102*:146-148 (1978).

70. L. Spence, M. Fauvel, R. Petro, and L. A. Babiuk, Comparison of rotavirus strains by hemagglutination inhibition, *Can. J. Microbiol., 24*:353-356 (1978).

71. K. W. Theil, E. H. Bohl, and A. G. Agnes, Cell culture propagation of porcine rotavirus (reovirus-like agent), *Am. J. Vet. Res., 38*:1765-1768 (1977).

72. K. W. Theil, E. H. Bohl, R. F. Cross, E. M. Kohler, and A. G. Agnes, Pathogenisis of porcine rotaviral infection in experimentally inoculated gnotobiotic pigs, *Am. J. Vet. Res., 39*:213-220 (1978).

73. M. E. Thouless, A. S. Bryden, T. H. Flewett, G. N. Woode, J. C. Bridger, D. R. Snodgrass, and J. A. Herring, Serological relationships between rotaviruses from different species as studied by complement-fixation and neutralization, *Arch. Virol.*, *53*:287-294 (1977).

74. A. Torres-Medina, R. G. Wyatt, C. A. Mebus, N. R. Underdahl, and A. Z. Kapikian, Diarrhea caused in gnotobiotic piglets by the reovirus-like agent of human infantile gastroenteritis, *J. Infect. Dis.*, *133*:22-27 (1976).

75. S. Tzipori, I. W. Caple, and R. Butler, Isolation of a rotavirus from deer, *Vet. Rec.*, *99*:398 (1976).

76. S. Tzipori, D. Chandler, T. Makin, and M. Smith, *Escherichia coli* and rotavirus infection in 4-week-old gnotobiotic piglets fed milk or dry food, *Aust. Vet. J.*, *56*:279-284 (1980).

77. S. Tzipori and T. Makin, Propagation of human rotavirus (from gnotobiotic pigs) in young dogs, *Vet. Microbiol.*, *3*:55-63 (1978).

78. S. Tzipori and M. Walker, Isolation of rotavirus from foals with diarrhoea, *Aust. J. Exp. Biol. Med. Sci.*, *56*:453-457 (1978).

79. E. Verly and J. Cohen, Demonstration of size variation of RNA segments between different isolates of calf rotavirus, *J. Gen. Virol.*, *35*:1-4 (1977).

80. C. H. Von Bonsdorff, T. Hovi, P. Makela, L. Hovi, and M. Tevalvoto-Aarnio, Rotavirus associated with acute gastroenteritis in adults, *Lancet*, *2*:423 (1976).

81. A. B. Welch, Purification, morphology and partial characterization of a reovirus-like agent associated with neonatal calf diarrhea, *Can. Com. Med.*, *35*:195-202 (1971).

82. A. B. Welch and T. L. Thompson, Physicochemical characterization of a neonatal calf diarrhea virus, *Can. Com. Med.*, *37*:295-301 (1973).

83. G. N. Woode, Viral diarrhoea in calves, *Vet. Ann.*, *16*:30-34 (1976).

84. G. N. Woode, Pathogenic rotaviruses isolated from pigs and calves. In *Acute Diarrhoea in Childhood*, Ciba Symposium No. 42 (K. Elliott and J. Knight, eds.), Elsevier, Amsterdam, 1976.

85. G. N. Woode, Epizootiology of bovine rotavirus infection, *Vet. Rec.*, *103*:44-46 (1978).

86. G. N. Woode, M. E. Bew, and M. J. Dennis, Studies on cross protection induced in calves by rotaviruses of calves, children and foals, *Vet. Rec.*, *103*:32-34 (1978).

87. G. N. Woode and J. C. Bridger, Viral enteritis of calves, *Vet. Rec.*, *96*:85-88 (1975).

88. G. N. Woode and J. C. Bridger, Isolation of small viruses resembling astroviruses and caliciviruses from acute enteritis of calves, *J. Med. Microbiol.*, *11*:441-452 (1978).

89. G. N. Woode, J. C. Bridger, G. A. Hall, and M. J. Dennis, The isolation of a reovirus-like agent associated with diarrhoea in colostrum deprived calves in Great Britain, *Res. Vet. Sci.*, *16*:102-104 (1974).

90. G. N. Woode, J. Bridger, G. A. Hall, J. M. Jones, and G. Jackson, The isolation of reovirus-like agents (rotavirus) from acute gastroenteritis of piglets, *J. Med. Microbiol.*, *9*:203-209 (1976).

91. G. N. Woode, J. C. Bridger, J. M. Jones, T. H. Flewett, A. S. Bryden, H. A. Davies, and G. B. B. White, Morphological and antigenic relationships between viruses (rotaviruses) from acute gastroenteritis of children, calves, piglets, mice and foals, *Infect. Immun.*, *14*:804-810 (1976).

92. G. N. Woode and C. F. Crouch, Naturally occurring and experimentally induced rotaviral infections of domestic and laboratory animals. Colloquium on selected diarrheal diseases of the young, *J. Am. Vet. Med. Assoc.*, *173*:522-526 (1978).

93. G. N. Woode, J. Jones, and J. C. Bridger, Levels of colostral antibodies against neonatal calf diarrhoea virus, *Vet. Rec.*, *97*:148-149 (1975).

94. R. G. Wyatt, A. Z. Kapikian, T. S. Thornhill, M. M. Sereno, H. Y. Kim, and R. M. Chanock, In vitro cultivation in human foetal intestinal organ-culture of a reovirus-like agent associated with non-bacterial gastroenteritis in infants and children, *J. Infect. Dis.*, *130*:523-528 (1974).

95. R. G. Wyatt, C. A. Mebus, R. H. Yolken, A. R. Kalica, H. D. James, A. Z. Kapikian, and R. M. Chanock, Rotaviral immunity in gnotobiotic calves: Heterologous resistance to human virus induced by bovine virus, *Science*, *203*:548-550 (1979).

96. R. G. Wyatt, D. L. Sly, W. T. London, A. E. Palmer, A. R. Kalica, D. H. Van Kirk, R. M. Chanock, and A. Z. Kapikian, Induction of diarrhea in colostrum-deprived newborn rhesus monkeys with the human reovirus-like agent of infantile gastroenteritis, *Arch. Virol.*, *50*:17-27 (1976).

97. G. Zissis and J. P. Lambert, Different serotypes of human rotaviruses, *Lancet, 1*:38-39 (1978).

98. Y. Hoshino, C. A. Baldwin, and F. W. Scott, Isolation and characterization of feline rotavirus, *J. Gen. Virol., 54*:313-323 (1981).

99. R. H. Yolken, R. G. Wyatt, G. Zissis, C. D. Brandt, W. J. Rodriguez, H. W. Kim, R. H. Parrott, J. J. Urrutia, L. Mata, H. B. Greenberg, A. Z. Kapikian, and R. M. Chanock, Epidemiology of human rotavirus types 1 and 2 as studied by enzyme-linked immunosorbent assay, *N. Engl. J. Med., 299*: 1156-1161 (1978).

17

Coronaviruses in Animals

David J. Garwes Argricultural Research Council Institute for
Research on Animal Diseases, Compton, Newbury, Berkshire, England

The family Coronaviridae cómprises a single genus, *Coronavirus,* that is characterized by enveloped virions, 80-120 nm in diameter, surrounded by club-shaped
surface projections 14-26 nm long. The viral genome is composed of single-
stranded RNA having positive polarity [1]. The name *coronavirus* was introduced in 1968 [2] to describe those viruses with a morphology resembling
that of avian infectious bronchitis virus. Negatively stained preparations showed
a characteristic "halo" or "corona" by electron microscopy, formed by the
club-shaped surface projections surrounding the body of the virus (Fig. 1).
Initially the only viruses included in the group were avian infectious bronchitis
virus, mouse hepatitis virus, and several human strains, including 229E and
B814. However, a series of reports followed that allocated other viruses to the
group, including transmissible gastroenteritis virus of swine [3], the pneumotropic rat coronavirus [4], and hemagglutinating encephalomyelitis virus, causing vomiting-and-wasting disease of swine [5]. A second coronavirus of rats
was identified by Bhatt and co-workers [6], the sialodacryoadenitis virus which,
while serologically related to the pneumotropic strain, caused disease of lachry-
mal and salivary glands. At the same time, a group working in Nebraska [7]
reported that coronavirus particles could be recovered from neonatal calf diarrhea, and shortly after this, coronavirus particles were shown to be associated

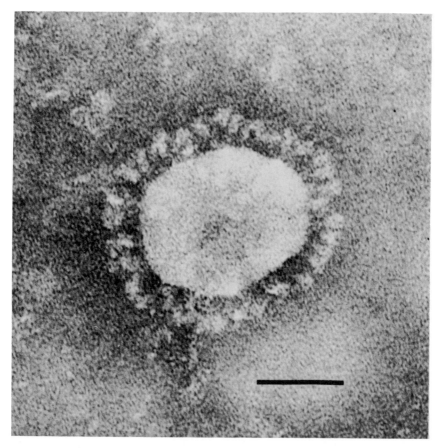

Figure 1 Electron micrograph of transmissible gastroenteritis virus negatively stained with potassium phosphotungstate. The bar represents 50 nm.

with gastroenteritis in turkeys—blue comb disease [8]. Research into the etiology of gastroenteritis was intensified during this period, and several groups were successful in demonstrating coronavirus in cases of diarrhea from dogs [9], foals [10], mice [11,12], and most recently, a form of epidemic diarrhea of older pigs distinct from transmissible gastroenteritis [13,14].

During the 10 years since the coronavirus achieved the status of a taxonomic group, there has been an increasing amount of research devoted to investigating the characteristics of the virion, its antigens, and the way in which it replicates within its host cell. The object of this chapter is to outline what is known about the enteric coronaviruses of pigs, dogs, calves, mice, and turkeys in the areas of the diseases they cause, their spread between hosts, their serology, their isolation and cultivation, and finally, the characteristics of the virions.

Transmissible Gastroenteritis Virus of Swine

Disease

Transmissible gastroenteritis of swine (TGE) was first demonstrated to have a viral etiology by Doyle and Hutchings [15] in the United States, although there were reports of a similar disease in 1935 and 1937 [16]. They showed that the virus could be transmitted to young pigs, in which it caused severe diarrhea and vomiting, with high mortality. Subsequent work by other groups between 1946 and 1950 confirmed the role of a virus in TGE, and during the next 20 years there were reports of the disease from Canada, the United Kingdom, Europe, Japan, and Taiwan (for details of these publications see the review by Woode, Ref. 17).

In piglets under 2 weeks of age, the first clinical sign is usually vomiting 18-24 h after infection. This is rapidly followed by profuse yellow or greenish diarrhea, resulting in loss of weight and dehydration. Death occurs after 2-5 days in most of the animals infected at this age. In animals over 14 days of age, however, the mortality rate drops but morbidity remains high (80-100%). There is no evidence to suggest that some pigs are less susceptible genetically. The clinical signs in weaned and adult pigs are similar to those shown by the neonate: profuse diarrhea after 1-2 days and weakness, incoordination, and some vomiting lasting up to 1 week, followed by recovery. There is generally no rise in rectal temperature associated with the disease.

Virus can be isolated from many organs of the infected pig [18,19], but the small intestine is the major site of replication. The virus grows in the columnar epithelium covering the villi and can be detected with fluorescent antibody within 24 h of infection. Antigen is first demonstrated in the cells at the tip of the villus, followed by involvement of the cells further down the villus and loss of those initially infected. Cell replacement takes place by multiplication of cells within the crypt and migration from the base of the villus, thereby covering the denuded area [20], and during this time there is a marked shortening of the infected villi [21,22]. Virus fails to infect the new cells moving from the crypt, as indicated by an inability to demonstrate antigen in villous epithelium 5-7 days after infection. The reason for the failure of TGE to infect the cells that repopulate the damaged villi is not known. It may be associated with the onset of the immune response or as suggested by several authors, the inability of the regenerating cells to support virus growth [23], perhaps because they are incompletely differentiated [20].

Although virus antigen has been detected in the duodenal epithelium, the jejunum and ileum are the areas in which pathology is most marked, and this is consistent with the physiological changes that lead to diarrhea. An early hypothesis that diarrhea resulted from malabsorption caused by an increase in osmotic pressure due to undigested milk lactose [24] was supported by studies that showed that iron absorption was impaired following infection of 3-week-old pigs with TGE [25]. Further work, however, suggested that the cells that migrate from the crypt to repopulate the virus-damaged villi have a secretory function, resulting in increased sodium secretion [26] and associated with loss of albumin from the blood to the intestinal lumen [27]. The ultimate cause of death in the piglet, however, is probably dehydration and metabolic acidosis coupled with hyperkalemia affecting cardiac function [28].

There is increasing evidence that the higher mortality rates in young piglets infected with TGE is coupled with a higher susceptibility to infection. The degree of villous atrophy was greater in piglets aged 3 days as compared with those aged 21 days [29], and the titer of infectious virus recovered from the small intestines of both groups of pigs was higher in the younger animals [30]. These differences did not correlate with the levels of virus-neutralizing antibody. The susceptibility of the target cell to infection was examined by Ristic's group, who demonstrated TGE in association with the microcanalicular-vesicular system characteristic of piglets under 2 weeks of age [31]. They postulate that the ability of the absorptive epithelial cell to form deep cytoplasmic tubular invaginations is temporally related to the pathogenesis of the disease. Witte and Walther [32] demonstrated that the infectious dose of TGE needed to infect a pig of slaughter weight (about 6 months old) was 10,000 times that required to infect a 2-day-old piglet.

Although virus has been isolated from several organs of the infected piglet, the only organ (other than the small intestine) that has received any attention has been the respiratory tract. Underdahl and his associates [33,34] isolated TGE from the lungs of market-weight swine showing gross pulmonary lesions and from lungs of pigs between 40 and 104 days after intranasal-oral infection with the virus. They described macroscopic pulmonary lesions in 56% of the pigs infected by this route, consisting of reddened and abnormally depressed areas on the lung. Kemeny et al. [35] also isolated virus for up to 11 days from nasal swabs of lactating sows following contact exposure with infected piglets, while Fisher (personal communication) was able to isolate virus from both upper and lower respiratory tracts 24–48 h after infection, with highest titers recorded in the lungs. Immunofluorescence showed viral antigen in the cytoplasm of bronchiolar epithelial cells and alveolar cells. Infection of the respiratory tract does not appear to be associated with respiratory disease but may be important in the epizootiology of the disease, as discussed below.

Epizootiology

Transmission of TGE within a pig herd can be partly explained by exposure of uninfected animals to fecal virus. As little as 2×10^{-7} ml of intestinal content from an infected animal [32] can infect 2-day-old piglets, and the spread among the animals of a herd is characteristically rapid [36]. There is evidence that virus may be shed in feces for up to 8 weeks after infection [37]. Infectious virus has also been isolated from small intestine and lung material from pigs 104 days after infection [34], suggesting that convalescent pigs are also a potential source of infection within the herd. Transmission of infection over short distances in aerosols generated in the respiratory tract may also be important, particularly in animals housed in intensive rearing houses where the atmospheric conditions are most suitable for aerial transfer. This may lead to infection of the respiratory tract of susceptible pigs, followed by infection of the small intestine. In addition, TGE virus is shed in the milk of infected sows over the first 6 days of lactation [38], and this may explain the rapidity with which a litter of piglets becomes infected. In summary, TGE spreads very rapidly within a herd following its introduction, uninfected animals being exposed to infectious virus in excrement, aerosols, and milk.

The spread of disease from one herd to another and the incidence of TGE outbreaks throughout the year introduce other factors that are less clearly understood. Apart from the more obvious forms of direct transmission, such as carriage of contaminated feces or sewage on vehicles traveling between farms, there is now a lot of evidence pointing to the role of the carrier animal. The findings that TGE could be recovered from intestine and lung of apparently healthy pigs several months after they had recovered from TGE suggests that new stock introduced into a susceptible herd could initiate an epizootic. The converse is equally true, that stock bought in from a TGE-free herd may succumb to infection when added to a herd that has experienced TGE in the past. Movement of pigs on a national basis may play a very important role in the spread of TGE. In this context it is interesting to speculate whether the marked reduction in the incidence of TGE in the United Kingdom since 1970 is attributable to the measures taken to restrict pig movement between areas, introduced to control the spread of swine vesicular disease.

Several groups of workers have noted a seasonal incidence in TGE, summarized by Ferris [39], with little or no disease reported between late spring and mid-autumn and increasing numbers of outbreaks from November on. The peak of incidence occurs in January, and subsequently the number of cases declines to the low level seen from May through the summer. Several explanations have been offered for this phenomenon, including (1) better survival of the virus in colder weather, (2) changes in management associated with seasonal changes, (3) hormonal changes in the stock resulting in the activation of quiescent virus, and (4) exposure of herds to animals, other than the pig, carrying the virus.

There are few or no data on the first three suggestions, but evidence is accumulating to support the potential role of alternative hosts. Pilchard [40] showed that infectious virus could be detected in the droppings of starlings 32 h after they were fed TGE. Since transit through the starling's alimentary tract takes only an hour, it was suggested that the virus was probably replicating in the bird. Starlings tend to flock to pig farms to feed when winter weather reduces their normal food supply, and several authors [41,42] have related these findings to the seasonal variation of the disease.

The first demonstration of a nonporcine host for TGE was in 1962, when Haelterman [43] showed that TGE was present in dog feces for up to 1 week after they were fed the virus. This was verified by Norman et al. [44], who were able to feed TGE to specific pathogen-free beagles and then transmit the disease to pigs. There were several reports of neutralizing antibodies to TGE in dog serum during this period, but the significance of these findings was questioned following the identification of a canine coronavirus serologically related to TGE but nonpathogenic for pigs [9]. This virus will be dealt with in detail later in the chapter. Recent work, however, has investigated further the growth of TGE in the dog and has confirmed its replication in the jejunal epithelium of puppies aged 4–11 days without inducing clinical signs of disease but yielding virus that can cause TGE in piglets [45]. Multiple passage of TGE in puppies caused a decrease in virulence for the pig after 17 passes [46]. Pregnant gilts exposed to pass 36 in puppies developed no clinical signs of TGE; neutralizing antibody to the virus was detected in serum and colostral whey, but the animals were unable to protect their piglets against challenge with virulent TGE. It would appear, therefore, that the dog can act as a carrier for TGE, harboring the virus in a replicating, fully infectious form while showing no clinical signs of infection. The significance of the domestic dog in transmission of the virus over large areas is probably low, but a greater potential hazard is presented by the fox which ranges widely and whose young migrate to new areas. Haelterman [43] showed that infectious virus could be isolated from intestines of foxes 2 weeks after they had been fed TGE, so the potential of the fox for transmission of the disease would appear to be high.

Ferris and Abou-Youssef tested the sera from 10 species of animals a month or more after exposure to TGE and demonstrated that neutralizing antibodies had been produced in puppies, kittens, skunks, and opossums that had been experimentally infected [9]. They also found neutralizing antibody in muskrats that had been trapped near a lagoon containing sewage from a TGE-infected pig herd and in the sera from two laboratory workers frequently exposed to the virus. There was no detectable seroconversion in the four laboratory rodent species exposed to TGE, namely, mice, gerbils, guinea pigs, and rats. While the data from controlled experimental exposure to TGE would be expected to give unequivocal results, the detection of neutralizing antibodies in humans and muskrats that may have been exposed to the virus by chance must be considered with reservation. Detection of TGE-neutralizing antibodies in dogs, discussed above, and in cats [47] that had never been exposed to TGE suggests that coronaviruses serologically related to TGE exist in domestic animals.

The potential of the cat as a carrier of TGE was first suggested by Witte and co-workers [48], who found that domestic cats exposed to virulent porcine TGE developed moderate titers of serum neutralizing antibody to the virus but showed no clinical symptoms. The presence of TGE-neutralizing antibodies in cats, however, has been attributed to infection with the coronavirus causing feline infectious peritonitis [47,48], and this inevitably raises doubts about the specificity of the antibody formed in the cats after exposure to TGE. Recent work by Reynolds and Garwes [49] showing formation of serum antibodies by neutralization and indirect immunofluorescence tests, and excretion of TGE in feces for up to 35 days in specific pathogen-free cats fed virulent TGE, provides evidence, however, that TGE can replicate in the cat and continue to be excreted for several weeks in the absence of any clinical signs.

Serology

The serologic aspects of TGE are best dealt with in two sections: (1) antigens of the virion and (2) serologic relationships with other viruses.

Viral Antigens

Strains of TGE have been isolated in the United States, Great Britain, Japan, and several European countries, but no antigenic diversity has been demonstrated. The most recently published study by Kemeny [50] compared eight American isolates, one British isolate, and one Japanese isolate by reciprocal plaque reduction neutralization and found them to be indistinguishable. The single serotype appears to be very stable not only geographically but also under conditions of laboratory cultivation. Comparison of the antigenic properties of intestinal, high-virulence TGE with a strain that had been passed through cell culture 100 times, resulting in reduced virulence for the pig, showed no detectable antigenic differences by immunofluorescence and immune electron microscopy [51].

Immunodiffusion tests on alkaline extracts from TGE-infected intestine revealed two viral antigen lines [52] which were further separable into three antigenic components when subjected to immunoelectrophoresis and counter-immunoelectrophoresis [53], but there was no evidence to suggest which components of the virus were being detected. Stone et al. [54] examined soluble antigens produced in TGE-infected swine testis cells and demonstrated two components. They established the protein nature of the antigen, its buoyant density in sucrose gradients at 1.19 g/cm^3, and its ability to stimulate the formation of TGE-neutralizing antibodies when injected into rabbits. This last finding indicated to the authors that the soluble antigen was directly associated with the virion, but they did not carry out the immune electron microscopy which, they suggested, would establish the relationship.

Studies on the dissociation of TGE virus into its structural components has provided indirect evidence of the nature of the soluble antigen reported by Stone et al. [54]. Removal of the lipid from the viral envelope resulted in the liberation of the surface projections, or peplomers, and their separation from the proteins of the envelope and nucleocapsid [55]. Injection of the recovered viral components into pigs and rabbits [56] resulted in the formation of virus-neutralizing antibodies only in those animals that received the surface projections but not in those that were exposed to the other viral proteins. This suggests, therefore, that the soluble antigens of the strains used by Stone and his co-workers contain two viral components, one of which at least may be identified with the surface projections. A similar picture is emerging from work on another porcine coronavirus, hemaggluting encephalomyelitis virus (Pocock, personal communication), in which the principal soluble antigen comprises a polypeptide associated with the peplomers. Antibody made against this purified antigen neutralizes the virus and inhibits hemagglutination.

Serologic Cross-Reactions

As a generalization, the members of the genus *Coronavirus* exhibit many and frequently confusing antigenic cross-reactions [57]. Until quite recently, however, TGE was considered to be exceptional in its lack of serologic cross-reactivity with other members of the family. Sibinovic and others [58] developed a bentonite agglutination test for the detection of antibody to TGE and assessed the specificity of the test with antisera to 21 other animal pathogens. Of those tested, the only antiserum which registered a positive reaction was chicken serum raised against the avian coronavirus causing infectious bronchitis. This cross-relationship could not be repeated by other tests in other laboratories, however, until 1975, when Romano et al. [59], working in Mexico, published evidence which demonstrated a clear relationship between the Mexican FMVZ 69 strain of TGE and the Massachusetts strain of avian infectious bronchitis virus using neutralization, complement fixation, and immunodiffusion tests. Whether this finding suggests an unusual antigenic composition for the FMVZ strain of TGE or will be repeated for other strains remains to be determined. The British isolate of TGE could not be shown to cross-react with any of the standard reference antisera to the major serotypes of infectious bronchitis virus by neutralization tests (Pocock, personal communication).

Another tenuous relationship was suggested by Phillip et al. [5], who observed a cross-reaction between TGE and hemagglutinating encephalomyelitis virus of pigs (HEV) by immunodiffusion. This observation, however, was not repeated by these authors, and recently studies in our laboratory have not shown any cross-reaction between TGE and HEV by neutralization tests, radioimmunoassay, immunofluorescence, or immunodiffusion (Pocock and Reynolds, personal communication).

The detection of anti-TGE activity in the serum of dogs [44] suggested that dogs may become infected with TGE even though several of the animals examined had not been exposed to pigs. Following the study and isolation of the canine coronavirus [9,60] it became clear by neutralization and immunofluorescence tests that the canine virus was antigenically related to TGE. Detailed serology on this relationship has not been published, and it is not known how closely related the two viruses are, but work in progress on the structure of the canine coronavirus may help to elucidate the similarities.

In the course of an investigation into the presence of complement-fixing antibodies in the sera from many animal species [61], it was noted that the serum from a domestic cat contained heat-stable neutralizing activity against TGE. This phenomenon was studied in more detail [47]. It was established that a high proportion of domestic cats had serum neutralizing antibody to TGE and that the incidence and titer of this antibody was particularly high in closed cat colonies in which feline infectious peritonitis (FIP) was a disease problem. Further evidence was presented by Witte et al. [48], who demonstrated TGE-neutralizing antibody in cats naturally and experimentally infected with FIP and in a leopard naturally infected with FIP; this antibody also detected TGE antigen by immunofluorescence. A similar finding of TGE-neutralizing antibody in sera from domestic cats from Munich has been made by Bachmann (personal communication). Two other groups working on FIP, however, have reported feline antibody that reacts with TGE by immunofluorescence but not by neutralization [63,63]. That these differences are not just reflections of differing techniques has been ruled out by collaborative work among the British, Dutch, American, and German groups, and it is clear that while sera from all cats exposed to FIP react with TGE antigen by immunofluorescence, only sera of cases from Britain and Germany neutralize the porcine virus. This may imply that more than one serotype of FIP virus exists, but until more isolates of the feline coronavirus have been studied this is only conjecture.

Table 1 Antigenic Relationships among Eight Coronaviruses Demonstrated by Immunofluorescence[a]

Antiserum to	MHV3	CDCV	HCV OC43	HEV	TGEV	FIPV	HCV 229E	CCV
MHV3	3+[b]	2+	3+	3+	−	−	−	−
CDCV	±	3+	2+	3+	−	−	−	−
HCV OC43	3+	2+	3+	3+	−	−	−	−
HEV	±	2+	2+	3+	−	−	−	−
TGEV	−	−	−	−	3+	3+	+	3+
FIPV	−	−	−	−	3+	3+	±	3+
HCV 229E	−	−	−	−	2+	+	3+	−
CCV	−	−	−	−	−	−	−	3+

[a]MHV3: Mouse hepatitis virus type 3. CDCV: Bovine enteric coronavirus. HCV OC43: Human coronavirus strain OC43. HEV: Hemagglutinating encephalomyelitis virus of swine. TGEV: Transmissible gastroenteritis virus of swine. FIPV: Feline infectious peritonitis virus. HCV 229E: Human coronavirus strain 229E. CCV: Canine coronavirus.
[b]Immunofluorescence intensity: − , negative; ±, barely detectable; +, weak; 2+ moderate; 3+, strong, equal to homogous reaction.
Source: From Ref. 63.

In an extensive study on the antigenic relationships among eight different coronaviruses by immunofluorescence, Pedersen and his associates [63] demonstrated a clear interaction between TGE and the 229E strain of human respiratory coronavirus. This was the first evidence that the coronaviruses fall into possibly two broad serologic groups and establishes that 229E is related to the TGE-like group which includes the canine and feline coronaviruses, while the other human respiratory coronavirus, serotype OC43, is antigenically related to mouse hepatitis virus, calf enteric coronavirus, and HEV (see Table 1). The detection of cross-reacting antigens in infected cells does not necessarily imply that the viruses are related at the level of their structural antigens. Indeed, the published data on the polypeptide compositions of TGE virus [64] and human coronavirus strain 229E [65,66] suggest that the two viruses are quite unrelated. It is possible, however, that fluorescent antibody could be detecting a nonstructural antigen synthesized by both viruses during infection, such as constituent polypeptides or amino acid sequences of the viral RNA polymerase. Further work on the structure and replication mechanisms of coronaviruses will be required before the characteristics of these antigens can be fully understood.

Isolation, Cultivation, and Diagnosis

TGE can be isolated most reliably from field outbreaks by oral administration of samples to newborn piglets [67], this method has been used recently in experimental studies of virus isolation from small intestine and lung [33,34] and from the milk of infected or convalescent pigs [68]. The use of piglets is unsatisfactory from an economic point of view, however, and primary cultures of pig cells have been used since 1956, when Lee established TEG cultivation in pig kidney cells. Since then, isolation in cell culture has become routine for many diagnostic laboratories, utilizing primary pig kidney cell, secondary adult pig thyroid cells [67,69], or swine testis cells [70,71]. Growth of the virus on primary isolation may not be associated with clear cytopathic changes, but following subculture into fresh cells virus replication usually reaches a level at which the cells round up and detach from the substrate.

Cultivation of TGE has been achieved in other cells, including porcine salivary gland cells [72] and organ cultures from porcine esophagus, ileum, cecum, and colon [73], and intestinal tract [53]. There have been few reports of the growth of the virus in nonporcine tissue, with the major exception of replication in canine kidney cells [74].

The growth of TGE in porcine cells has been shown to be affected by the pH of the growth medium [75]. Not only was the yield of virus from infected cultures lower at $pH > 7$ than at the optimum of pH 6.5, but the virus produced was more unstable at alkaline pH and was rapidly inactivated. The authors recommended the use of an efficient pH buffer, such as HEPES, to prevent the pH increase found in bicarbonate-buffered medium following cell death.

The age of the cell was also shown to be important for reliable demonstration of TGE growth [76]. Plaques of both pig-derived and cell culture-adapted TGE strains were more numerous on swine testis cells that were 5-6 days old than on cultures used within 2 days of reaching confluency. The reason for this phenomenon was not investigated, and whether it applies to cells other than swine testis continuous cultures remains to be determined.

The diagnosis of TGE infections in pig herds showing a rapid spread of diarrhea and enteritis is usually accomplished by isolating the virus in cell cultures and identifying it by immunofluorescence of infected cells [77]. However, immunofluorescent staining of sections of small intestine of affected pigs has been used successfully [78-80], as has the demonstration of rising antibody titers in sera from pigs of the infected herd [81]. Direct electron microscopy has been used to identify TGE [82], although immune electron microscopy adds sensitivity and specificity to the technique [83]. A variety of other procedures have been reported, including indirect hemagglutination [82], immunoperoxidase staining of infected tissue [77,83], and a leukocyte aggregation test [85] , but none of these has been used as extensively as have isolation and immunofluorescence. It is quite clear, however, that observations such as villous atrophy and reduced levels of lactase in the intestine are inadequate unless they are backed up by a more specific diagnostic test [86] .

Virion Characteristics

First estimates of the size of TGE virus were reported by Young and co-workers [87] as 200 nm in diameter, determined by gradocol filtration, although recalculation of their data applying the correction factor of Black [88] gives a figure of 128 nm [17] . Several other reports during the 1960s confirmed that the virus was in the size range 75-150 nm in diameter, showed considerable pleomorphism, and was surrounded by surface projections that were estimated to be 12-24 nm long. It remained for Tajima [3] to confirm these data and recognize that TGE was a member of the recently named coronavirus group. In thin sections of infected cells, Caletti and co-workers [89] observed a doughnut shaped nucleoid surrounded by a double membrane. This and several reports during the 1960s that the infectivity of TGE was sensitive to detergents and organic solvents pointed to the fact that the virion was bounded by a lipid bilayer. Such a structure is consistent with the buoyant density of the virus in sucrose saline of 1.19 g/cm^3 [90] and of 1.21 g/cm^3 in $CsSO_4$ solution, values that reflect a large contribution of lipid. The sedimentation constant of purified TGE virus through sucrose solution was 495S [55] .

Many of the early reports on virus stability were conflicting. Cartwright and co-workers [91] found no change in titer at pH 3 at 37°C for 3 h, whereas McClurkin and Norman [92] showed that five isolates of TGE lost 2-3 log in titer after 1 h at 37°C, pH 3. This may reflect a major difference between the U.K. isolate and the North American strains, but it is quite possible that the conditions during incubation, for example, ionic strength and soluble protein concentration, were dissimilar in the two studies. More recently, Pocock and Garwes [75] reported that the stability of TGE at various temperatures was markedly affected by the pH of the suspending medium. This makes the early reports of temperature stability in which pH was not controlled or specified difficult to interpret. The virus is, as expected, sensitive to ultraviolet radiation, and studies [51] showed that there was no significant difference in inactivation rate between an intestinal (virulent) and cell-culture-adapted strain of the virus.

TGE has been reported to be resistant to trypsin [91] , although this appears to vary between isolates or strains. Furuuchi and his associates [93] , for example, demonstrated that a virulent isolate of TGE was significantly resistant to trypsin and pepsin, whereas an attenuated variant of the same isolate was rapidly inactivated by these enzymes. More recently, however, Laude and

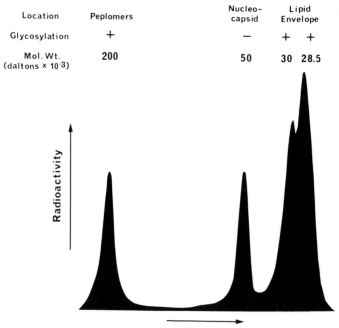

Location	Peplomers		Nucleo-capsid	Lipid Envelope	
Glycosylation	+		−	+	+
Mol. Wt. (daltons × 10⁻³)	200		50	30	28.5

Figure 2 The polypeptide structure of TGE virus. The viral proteins, labeled with [³H] leucine, were dissociated and electrophoresed in polyacrylamide gel.

his associates [94] have examined a larger number of virulent and attenuated strains of TGE and have shown that the differences that occur in trypsin sensitivity do not correlate with the in vivo virulence of the strain. Whether sensitivity to proteolytic enzymes is only one of the characteristics that may confer lowered virulence on TGE, affecting the ability of the virus to replicate and survive in the environment of the anterior small intestine, or only reflects changes in the amino acid sequences of the structural proteins, is not known. It should not be assumed that resistance to trypsin presupposes resistance to all proteolytic enzymes. Our studies on TGE structure [64] revealed that the surface projections of the FS772/70 isolate of the virus, although resistant to the action of trypsin and pepsin, are digested from the surface of the virion by the enzyme bromelain.

   Garwes and Pocock examined the structural polypeptides of TGE [64]. There were only four major polypeptides, of which three were glycosylated, gp 200, gp 30, and gp 28.5, with apparent molecular weights of 200,000, 30,000 and 28,500 daltons, respectively, and one was not, p 50, with an apparent molecular weight of 50,000 daltons (Fig. 2). The location of the polypeptides was examined by bromelain digestion, and gp 200 was found to be associated with the surface projections. Subsequent studies suggested that gp 30 and gp 28.5 were located in the lipid envelope, probably bridging the internal and external surfaces of the lipid bilayer. The nonglycosylated polypeptide p 50 was shown to be rich in basic amino acids and was probably bound to the RNA genome to form the ribonucleoprotein complex [55]. Treatment of the virion with detergents such as Nonidet P40 dissolved the membrane lipid and liberated the surface projections. These could be recovered by centrifugation and subsequent precipitation and were used to raise neutralizing antibodies in pigs and rabbits [56], confirming their role as receptors for attachment to host cell membranes.

The lipids that comprise the viral envelope are derived from the endoplasmic reticulum of the host cell during virus budding and maturation. It was possible that the physicochemical nature of the virion structural proteins could influence the composition of the lipid bilayer, but this was not found in our experiments [95]. Comparison of the lipids of two porcine cell types and purified TGE grown in them showed that the lipid composition of the virus reflects that of the host membrane. The only lipids present in the cell membranes but absent from purified virus were the esters of cholesterol and fatty acids, lipids involved in transport across membranes. It would appear, then, that the lipid membrane may be of antigenic importance if the porcine glycolipids are introduced into a host other than the pig but that the lipid bilayer does not contribute to the quality or quantity of the immune response in the normal host animal [61].

The genome of TGE was reported to be RNA in 1968, when Clarke [96] showed that virus replication was not profoundly affected by actinomycin D, an inhibitor of DNA-dependent RNA synthesis. Further evidence came from Caletti and co-workers [89], who deduced that the RNA was single stranded from its response to nucleases and change in temperature. Mishra and Ryan [97] attempted to further characterize the genome by labeling RNA with radioactive uridine, but they extracted a heterogeneous range of molecules of 18S-28S size. We suggested that the molecular weight of RNA isolated from TGE depended on the temperature used for extraction [98]. At $20°C$ the molecules formed a complex of $6\text{-}9 \times 10^6$ daltons, and as the temperature was raised above $60°C$ the RNA electrophoresed as a broad band of about 3×10^6 daltons. Superficially, this behavior resembled that of oncornavirus RNA in which the genome forms a complex with transfer RNA. No further data on the nature of the TGE RNA molecules have yet been reported, except for the presence of polyadenylic acid. Pocock (reported in Ref. 99) used oligo (dT)cellulose to bind 50-90% of the virion RNA extracted at $20°C$, suggesting that more than half the complexes have polyadenylic acid sequences. Following heat denaturation, approxi-

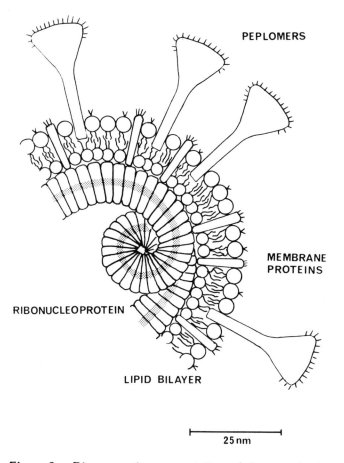

PEPLOMERS

MEMBRANE
PROTEINS

RIBONUCLEOPROTEIN

LIPID BILAYER

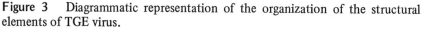

25 nm

Figure 3   Diagrammatic representation of the organization of the structural elements of TGE virus.

mately 50% of the RNA was still able to bind to the oligo(dT) cellulose. Polyadenylation is a characteristic that has been associated with messenger function in RNA and confirms that the TGE genome is positive stranded and able to code for viral proteins.

The organization of the structural elements within the virion has already been mentioned, but in summary the RNA forms a high molecular weight complex which is bound to a 50,000 dalton polypeptide to form the nucleoprotein. This is probably coiled within the virion in contact with the inner surface of the envelope, perhaps associated with the gp 30 and gp 28.5 membrane glycoproteins. The surface projections, composed of a single species of glycopolypeptide, gp 200, appear to be loosely associated with the lipid bilayer on the outer surface, and the resulting structure has little to maintain its shape, perhaps accounting for the variation in size and shape that has been reported. Figure 3 presents these conclusions in a diagrammatic form.

Other Porcine Coronaviruses

It is not my intention to discuss the vomiting-and-wasting disease caused by hemagglutinating encephalomyelitis virus (HEV) in detail in this chapter, since it is not a cause of enteritis. Following infection, probably via the respiratory route, HEV replicates in the pharyngeal tonsils and upper respiratory tract and is soon found in the central nervous system where, it is thought, virus growth causes a nervous syndrome that results in vomiting. Recent studies by Andries et al. [100] suggest that HEV grows in peripheral nerves and that the stomach wall may be a major replication site. Growth in the stomach epithelium, however, has not been reported.

Of greater interest, however, is a coronavirus identified in Belgium [14] and in the United Kingdom [13]. The virus is associated with outbreaks of epidemic diarrhea in young and older pigs, and while the clinical signs resemble those caused by TGE, infected small intestine sections were negative by immunofluorescence using anti-TGE serum. Serum neutralizing antibody to TGE was not produced in convalescent animals; neither was antibody raised against HEV. The infection could be transmitted experimentally to pigs ranging in age between 3 days and 8 weeks. All the pigs developed clinical signs between 1 and 3 days after infection; watery diarrhea was common to almost all the animals, and in addition there was pyrexia, anorexia, and frequently acute depression. Coronavirus particles were seen by electron microscopy in negatively stained samples of feces and intestinal contents and in thin sections of infected small intestine. As yet, the virus has not been cultivated in vitro, so detailed study has not been possible. The identity of this virus may eventually be shown to be a second previously unrecognized serotype of TGE, an enteropathogen from a different host that has mutated and crossed the species barrier, or perhaps a coronavirus unrelated to those described to date. It is intriguing that during the 35 years of research into TGE this agent has not been recognized before, suggesting that the infection is a recent event or that in the past TGE diagnosis was less efficient.

Canine Coronavirus Enteritis

The first suggestion that there might be a "TGE-associated virus" capable of causing gastroenteritis in dogs came from Norman et al. in 1970 [44]. Earlier, Haelterman [43] had demonstrated that exposure of dogs and foxes to porcine TGE virus led to the production of serum neutralizing antibodies and excretion of TGE in feces. Norman and co-workers [44], however, found a wide distribution of TGE-neutralizing antibodies in dogs, including dogs that had never been in contact with pigs and would therefore be unlikely to be infected with porcine TGE. Two years later, Cartwright and Lucas [60] described an outbreak of vomiting and diarrhea in a breeding kennel containing 40 dogs aged from 10 days to 11 years. Adult dogs showed anorexia, vomiting, and scouring for up to 5 days. The youngest puppies were affected with watery yellow diarrhea but showed no vomiting, while the older puppies had some diarrhea and occasional vomiting. No pathogenic bacteria or viruses were isolated, but all the adult dogs showed rising titers of neutralizing antibodies to porcine TGE in their serum. Cartwright and Lucas concluded that a virus similar or identical to porcine TGE was involved, but they could not determine whether the two dogs that had been introduced into the kennel, bringing the virus with them, had been in contact with pigs.

During a similar outbreak of diarrhea in military dogs in 1971, Binn and his associates [9] isolated a virus (1-71) in cultures of primary dog kidney cells and canine thymus 8156 cell line. Electron microscopy of thin sections of infected cell cultures showed particles budding into cytoplasmic vacuoles and resembling coronaviruses. Sera against several established coronaviruses were tested in an in vitro virus neutralization test, and only anti-TGE serum had any activity, although to a significantly lower titer than to the homologous TGE virus. The virus could be transmitted experimentally to puppies, in which it caused acute gastroenteritis and dehydration, but not to piglets. Following inoculation of 5-day-old and 2.5-month-old pigs with the canine isolate, there were no clinical signs, virus could not be recovered, and no neutralizing antibody was formed. Furthermore, the piglets were not protected against TGE when challenged 3 weeks after inoculation with 1-71 virus. This suggested, therefore, that the canine isolate could be differentiated from porcine TGE, to which it was closely related antigenically.

In a detailed study of the virus, Keenan and others [101] showed that enteritis was characterized by atrophy and fusion of intestinal villi, deepening of crypts, and an increase in cellularity of the lamina propria. The epithelial cells on the villi became cuboidal and vacuolated and the goblet cells were almost totally discharged. Cellular enzymes were generally depressed. Viral antigen could be detected by immunofluorescence, starting in the duodenum at 2 days after inoculation and spreading to the ileum by day 4. Unlike TGE of pigs the canine disease is rarely fatal; diarrhea stops in 1-2 weeks and animals recover health rapidly.

The differentiation between this disease and TGE of pigs is not altogether clear. Albrecht and Lupcke [102] reported outbreaks of gastroenteritis in three kennels in Germany. Feces from infected dogs produced typical TGE when fed to piglets, and both dogs and pigs developed TGE-neutralizing antibodies during convalescence. Whether this disease was canine coronavirus that could be transmitted to pigs, was porcine TGE that had become established in dogs, or was even noncoronaviral was not established, but it is clear that the relationship between canine and porcine gastroenteritis requires further study.

A further complication was introduced by the finding of Schnagl and Holmes [103] of particles resembling the human enteric coronavirus in feces of dogs in an Australian aboriginal settlement. These particles, described in a previous chapter, are fringed by surface projections that have been described as "lollypop-shaped" rather than the characteristic "club-shaped." It may be that a coronavirus other than that isolated by Binn [9] exists in dogs, although the possibility cannot be excluded that the particles seen in the Australian dogs may have been ingested with human feces and passed through the canine gut without replication or infection. The humans in these settlements were shown to be producing these particles, and the low nutritional status of the dogs results in their eating excrement. As yet the Australian virus particles have not been cultivated or experimentally transmitted.

Epizootiology

As described above, the disease appears to be highly infectious, affecting dogs of all ages and causing clinical signs within 24–48 h after exposure. The only report that suggested how a kennel had become infected was that of Cartwright and Lucas [60], in which two recently acquired animals had been the first to show signs of disease, indicating that they had been exposed before joining the kennel. Dogs can be infected easily by oral administration of fecal suspension, and this probably represents the usual route of transmission.

The confusion over the ability of the canine enteritis coronavirus to grow in pigs, described above, makes it impossible to say whether transmission could occur via the pig. Haelterman [43] showed that foxes had neutralizing antibodies to TGE and would support the growth of TGE virus if experimentally infected. The antibodies found in the fox population could have been stimulated by a canine coronavirus and thus the fox may be a natural host for the canine coronavirus. This line of reasoning raises the question of whether the TGE-neutralizing antibodies found in serum from muskrats [39] might not have resulted from infection with canine coronavirus or a virus from some other species, rather than TGE as suggested at that time. It seems unlikely that the canine coronavirus was involved, but it does draw attention to the fact that viruses other than porcine TGE can evoke an immune response to produce TGE-neutralizing antibodies. A case in point is our report of TGE-neutralizing antibodies in cats [47]. A possible explanation for this activity is subclinical infection of the cats with feline infectious peritonitis, a disease that several groups have shown to be caused by a coronavirus serologically related to TGE and the canine enteric coronavirus.

Serology

Only one serotype of canine coronavirus has been described to date, and this is serologically related to TGE [9,60] and feline infectious peritonitis virus [63]. In the latter study, however, the relationship appeared to be one-way, in that antiserum raised against the dog virus did not react in an immunofluorescence test with TGE-infected swine testis cells or feline infectious peritonitis-infected liver slices, whereas specific antisera to TGE and feline infectious peritonitis cross-reacted with canine coronavirus-infected cells. More recently, however, we have examined the cross-relationship with TGE in more detail using a virus neutralization test and have established that the relationship is reciprocal although the homologous titer of the antiserum is significantly higher than the heterologous titer (unpublished observation).

Isolation, Cultivation, and Diagnosis

The original isolation by Binn [9] in 1971 was in primary dog kidney cells and a continuous line of canine thymus cells. Appel and associates [104] have also used primary dog kidney cell cultures to isolate the virus from disease outbreaks in North America.

Binn and his associates tested a number of commercially available cell types for cultivation of the 1–71 isolate, using cytopathic effect as the criterion of growth. They found that canine embryo cells and canine synovium DEN cells showed signs of virus growth, whereas the following cells showed no cytopathic changes: Walter Reed canine cell line, primary swine kidney, pig kidney PK15, primary bovine embryonic kidney, primary feline kidney, human embryonic lung WI-38, primary rhesus monkey kidney, primary African green monkey kidney, and VERO cell line. We have shown that 1–71 will not replicate in secondary adult pig thyroid cells, as judged by infectivity titration, cytopathic changes, and immunofluorescence (Reynolds, personal communication).

Diagnosis of canine coronavirus enteritis is based on clinical signs and postmortem findings where highly infectious gastroenteritis is reported. Immunofluorescence of cultures of primary dog kidney cells exposed to fecal suspensions is likely to be the most reliable method, together with detection of rising titers of serum antibodies to the virus later in the course of the disease. Appel and others [104] have highlighted the need for specific serologic tests in diagnosis of this disease, rather than reliance on clinical observations, since a second virus, probably a parvovirus, causes a disease that presents a similar clinical picture to the coronaviral enteritis. The parvo-like virus can be distinguished by immunofluorescence with serum to feline panleukopenia virus and hemagglutination with pig erythrocytes.

Virion Characteristics

The 1-71 isolate was shown to be sensitive to chloroform, consistent with its possession of a lipid-containing envelope, and stable at pH 3 for 3 h at room temperature [9]. Replication of the virus was not significantly affected by iododeoxyuridine, indicating that the genome comprised RNA.

In the original study [9] virus particles were not examined by electron microscopy following negative staining but thin sections of infected cells were studied. These revealed round or oval virions, 59-90 nm in diameter with an inner core of 35-45 nm, in cytoplasmic vesicles. The virus appeared to mature by budding through the endoplasmic reticulum, a feature characteristic of coronaviruses. The size of the infectious particles was determined by filtration through cellulose ester membranes of varying pore size and was estimated as slightly smaller than 100 nm. Appel and his co-workers [104] published an electron micrograph of negatively stained particles, showing the characteristic morphology of a coronavirus, although the size of the virus was not recorded. We have examined the virus in our laboratory and have found it to be in no way different from TGE virus with respect to morphology and size range. The particles seen by Schnagl and Holmes [103], therefore, do not have the typical morphology expected of canine coronavirus as discussed above, and this suggests that they are of human origin.

There are no published data on the structural components of the canine coronavirus at the time of writing, but preliminary experiments in our laboratory indicate that the overall polypeptide composition of the virus closely resembles that of TGE, with minor differences in the molecular weights of the high and low molecular weight glycopolypeptides. Work is in progress to see whether these differences are significant and whether they can be used to distinguish between the two viruses.

Bovine Coronavirus Enteritis

Disease

A coronavirus was first implicated in the complex etiology of neonatal calf diarrhea in 1972 when Stair et al. detected the agent in diarrheic fecal material by electron microscopy [7]. The virus was purified from feces of experimentally infected gnotobiotic calves and was shown to have the characteristic morphology of the coronavirus group. The virus was isolated in fetal bovine kidney cells [105] and following this, was attenuated by serial passage on higher passages of fetal bovine kidney cells.

The pathology of the disease has been described in a series of reports from Mebus and his associates [105-107] and by Doughri and Storz [108]. In all the studies, the incubation period following experimental infection was 19-24 h.

Shortly after the onset of diarrhea, viral antigen was detected by immuno-fluorescence in the villous epithelium of upper, middle, and lower small intes-tine and on the surface of the colon. The villi were normal at this time, whereas in animals killed 24–48 h after the onset of diarrhea there was a pronounced shortening and fusion of the villi, particularly in the lower small intestine, resulting in a villus-to-crypt ratio of 1.0 as compared with a value of 5.3 for the uninfected control. The epithelial cells became cuboidal and vacuolated and there was a reduction in the number of goblet cells. Lesions were also seen in the mesenteric lymph nodes, and the lamina propria showed edema and in-creased cellularity. During this latter phase of the infection, virus was detected by immunofluorescence in the epithelial cells at the tip of the villi, on the sur-face, and in the crypts of the colon, and evidence of replication was obtained by electron microscopy of thin sections through infected intestine.

Epizootiology

Following its initial recognition and isolation in 1972 in the United States, bovine coronavirus has been shown to be associated with calf diarrhea in Canada [109,110], Belgium [111,112], New Zealand [113], Germany [114], Bulgaria [115], the United Kingdom, and Denmark [116]. Transmission is readily achieved by oral administration of feces from infected animals, and no other intermediate host has been implicated. There is evidence, however, that appar-ently healthy animals are infected with the virus [117], and in many parts of the world the virus is known to be enzootic. Under these conditions, newborn calves would be exposed to the virus at birth and would probably become in-fected. Whether they then go into diarrhea or stay apparently healthy would be governed by factors such as the amount and duration of specific antibody which they receive in colostrum and milk or the presence of other microorgan-isms that might influence the outcome of infection. This is an area of research in which a great deal of interest is centering, and it promises to increase our understanding of the mechanisms of resistance or protection against entero-pathogens generally.

A major problem associated with control of calf diarrhea is the complex etiology of the disease. Although the work described above has established beyond doubt that bovine coronavirus can cause severe gastroenteritis in gnoto-biotic and conventional calves, it is rare to find calves infected solely with bovine coronavirus under field conditions. Usually there is at least one more enteropathogen detected in the intestinal tract or feces, making diagnosis of the major cause of diarrhea complicated. Morin and co-workers [110], for example, examined 34 live cases of neonatal calf diarrhea and diagnosed only 2 cases in which bovine coronavirus was found alone whereas 11 further cases were associated with coronavirus and rotavirus, cryptosporidium, and/or mycotic abomasitis. In a similar study by van Opdenbosch and his associates in the Netherlands [118], coronavirus was diagnosed in 29 of 50 cases of neonatal calf diarrhea examined. The bovine coronavirus was always present with other viruses, however; with a bovine viral diarrhea (BVD)-like particle in all cases, with rotavirus as well in 16 cases, and with rotavirus and small round virus particles in 3 cases. It was of interest that the 6 cases that were fatal in this investigation each had coronavirus. It is reasonable to conclude, therefore, that bovine coronavirus is a proven enteropathogen that has been identified in association with calf diarrhea in several areas of the world. It can cause disease on its own or, more frequently, in association with other enteropathogenic viruses.

It is possible that the virus can be transmitted to Equidae, since Bass and Sharpee [10] investigated a case of gastroenteritis in three foals and found coronavirus particles in their feces. The animals died or were killed in the acute stage of disease, so antibody titers were not measurable. They came from an area in which more than 40 cases of foal diarrhea had been reported, and Bass and Sharpee examined 65 sera from horses, presumably in the same geographical area although that was not stated. They found neutralizing antibody to bovine coronavirus at titers from 0 to 181 and concluded that this added support to their belief that a coronavirus was the cause of gastroenteritis in the foals. What is not clear, however, is whether the bovine coronavirus antibody indicated an antigenically related, foal-specific virus (see Serology, below) or resulted from an epizootic of bovine coronavirus infection of horses. To date, no further information has been published about the foal coronavirus.

Serology

As with TGE and the canine coronavirus, only one serotype of bovine coronavirus has been identified. The LY-138 isolate of Hajer and Storz [119] reacted in an immunoprecipitation test with antiserum to the Mebus isolate, and bovine coronaviruses isolated in the United Kingdom and Denmark were shown to be related to each other and to the Mebus strain by immunofluorescence and hemagglutination inhibition tests [116]. It is possible, however, that more discriminatory tests, such as neutralization kinetics, might show some differences, although the relative abilities of these isolates to grow in cell culture would seriously influence the test. The LY-138 strain has not been adapted to cell culture, and it would be very expensive to provide enough calves to make meaningful tests in vivo.

The antigenic cross-reactions between the bovine coronavirus and other members of the genus are well documented. Apart from the tentative relationship to a virus infecting foals and horses described above [10], there is evidence that bovine coronavirus is a member of an antigenic subgroup of the coronaviruses. In 1975, Sharpee and Mebus reported that human serum contained neutralizing antibodies to bovine coronavirus [120]. Since they could show no cross-relationship between bovine coronavirus and the human respiratory coronavirus (HCV) prototype 229E, they concluded that this was evidence of a human enteric coronavirus. An alternative explanation was published by Kaye and his associates [121], who used serum neutralization, complement fixation, and hemagglutination inhibition tests to confirm that bovine coronavirus was not related to 229E, or to HCV strain B814, but that a good relationship existed with HCV strain OC43. Thus, they could explain the presence of bovine coronavirus-neutralizing antibodies in human serum by previous exposure to the respiratory virus OC43.

Sharpee established a cross-relationship between bovine coronavirus and hemagglutinating encephalomyelitis virus of swine [122] with a neutralization test and showed that there was no cross-reaction with TGE, avian infectious bronchitis virus, and HCV strain 229E. He observed, however, that moderately high neutralizing antibody titers were demonstrated in canine serum (Sharpee, personal communication). Since no such relationship could be shown between bovine coronavirus and the 1-71 isolate of canine coronavirus, this suggests that a second serotype of canine coronavirus, as yet unidentified, may exist.

The comprehensive study of Pedersen et al. [63], in which they compared eight coronaviruses by an immunofluorescence test, confirmed the antigenic relationships of bovine coronavirus with HCV strain OC43 and hemagglutinating encephalomyelitis virus and added a relationship to mouse hepatitis virus type 3. Immunofluorescence is a less specific test than virus neutralization, as has been shown with rotaviruses which have both type-specific and group-specific antigens; the degree of antigenic similarity within this subgroup of the coronaviruses has yet to be fully established.

Isolation, Cultivation, and Diagnosis

Primary isolation of bovine coronavirus was first achieved by Mebus and his coworkers in 1973 [105] using fetal bovine kidney cell cultures. Although several other groups attempted to isolate the virus, this was not always possible [123, 124]. This may suggest that variations exist in bovine coronavirus found in herds, since Wellemans and his associates [125] recovered the virus from field cases using calf kidney cultures, while Bridger et al. [116] could isolate virus from only one British calf using calf kidney cells but recovered virus from two British and one Danish calf by the use of fetal bovine tracheal organ cultures.

Following its isolation, the virus has been propagated in a variety of cell types. Unlike TGE, which does not readily grow in continuous cell lines, bovine coronavirus has been adapted to grow in a continuous line of bovine embryo kidney cells, BEK-1 [126], African green monkey cell line, VERO, and the bovine kidney line MDBK [117]. The usual primary cell for cultivation remains the bovine kidney, although primary and secondary calf testis cells have been used successfully (Pocock and Reynolds, personal communication). Organ cultures from fetal bovine trachea [127] and small intestine [116] have been shown to support the replication of virus, and the use of intestinal organ cultures may have application to investigation of the virus-enterocyte interaction.

Replication of bovine coronavirus in cell culture results in cytopathic changes that have been used for infectivity titration. Mebus stained the infected cell sheets and recorded the presence of syncytia [105], while subsequent workers have used cell rounding and detachment to determine end points in titration [117]. More reliable methods have been applied to the detection of monolayer infection, including specific immunofluorescence and hemadsorption [128,129]. Hemagglutination was reported by Sharpee [128] with erythrocytes from hamsters, mice, and rats but not from cats, dogs, goats, sheep, cattle, horses, turkeys, chickens, guinea pigs, rabbits, geese, pigs, and humans. Sato and others [130] confirmed these data but found that erythrocytes from some chickens would agglutinate the virus. Stott and his associates [127] used rat erythrocytes to measure the growth of bovine coronavirus in bovine tracheal organ cultures, and while this technique will not distinguish between infectious and inactivated virions it provides a rapid and reliable method for virion quantitation during procedures such as virus purification.

A contradiction appears to exist in the literature in this context. The report by Sato [130] indicated that hemagglutination would occur at 4°C, room temperature, and 37°C, whereas the hemadsorption-elution-hemagglutination assay of Ellens and co-workers [131] utilized the ability of the virus to hemagglutinate at 4°C but elute at 37°C. Of relevance to this is the recent finding (Pocock, personal communication) that the British isolate of bovine coronavirus elutes from rat erythrocytes at 37°C, whereas the vaccine strain of the Mebus isolate does not. Such differences may provide useful markers to distinguish strains, although as yet the mechanism of this elution has not been determined.

The diagnosis of bovine coronavirus infections in calves has become a routine procedure in many laboratories. Originally, the only methods available involved isolation in cell or organ cultures, as discussed above, or electron microscopy. As already stated, primary isolation in cell culture is not totally reliable and is not the method of choice. Electron microscopy of negatively stained fecal suspensions can detect the characteristic particle morphology and has been used extensively, but some problems have been encountered. At early or late stages of diarrhea, the virion titers may not be very high, making visualization of the particles on the grid difficult. This, together with the added complication of pleomorphism and possible loss of surface projections due to degradation, may help to explain the finding of Chasey and Lucas [124] that routine diagnostic electron microscopy can fail to detect coronavirus infection and supports their conclusion that examination of negatively stained preparations should be supported by electron microscopy of thin sections of infected epithelium in which virus morphogenesis can be seen. It is also possible that rapid scanning of many samples by electron microscopy might fail to distinguish particles that were of a similar size to bovine coronavirus, such as the agent detected by Mebus and his associates [132]. These fringed particles were associated with neonatal calf diarrhea but did not show coronavirus-like projections, nor were they antigenically related to bovine coronavirus.

Marsolais and others [133] have provided evidence that immunofluorescence is a more reliable diagnostic tool than electron microscopy. Of 69 cases of calf diarrhea in which bovine coronavirus was diagnosed by a combination of several methods, electron microscopy failed to detect virus in 14 cases, whereas a fluorescent antibody test applied to jejunal sections missed only 3 cases. The authors recommended that both tests be applied to achieve reliable diagnosis. Immunofluorescence of sections of small intestine was also used by Morin and others [110] to distinguish coronavirus and rotavirus infections in the presence of other enteropathogens.

Among the other diagnostic techniques that have been reported are the fluorescent virus precipitin test [134] for detecting virus in stools. This was shown to have a sensitivity as good as immune electron microscopy. Another immune precipitation technique was used by Hajer and Storz [119], who applied an agar gel precipitation test, with antigen derived from the LY-138 isolate, to detect anti-bovine coronavirus antibodies in sera from 19 herds of cattle.

Enzyme immunoassay (EIA; ELISA) has been developed for diagnosis of both bovine coronavirus particles in feces and antibodies to the virus in serum [131]. It was compared with a hemadsorption-elution-hemagglutination assay, which was found to be almost as sensitive, but enzyme immunoassay was considered to be the method of choice because of its high sensitivity, reliability, speed, and ability to handle large numbers of samples on a semiautomated basis.

Virion Characteristics

The morphology of the virus described at the time of its identification [7] has been confirmed for other isolates [116,123,124], as well as for the original isolate [128,135]. The virions have a diameter that ranges between 80 and 160 nm, with a mean diameter of 120-130 nm. They are surrounded by a fringe of surface projections of two lengths, the longer peplomers being 17-24 nm long and the shorter around 10 nm. This appearance of a double fringe seems to be a characteristic of bovine coronavirus that has not been described for other enteric coronaviruses.

In thin section, the virus particles have a diameter of 70-90 nm [7,123, 124,128], with the appearance of an electron-lucent core surrounded by a dense ring within a double-layered membrane. These particles were associated with intracytoplasmic vesicles, and it was concluded that they had formed by budding through the smooth endoplasmic reticulum.

The physicochemical properties of the virus have been examined by Sharpee [128] and Sato and co-workers [135], who agree in almost every detail. Infectivity was destroyed by treatment with ether, chloroform, and sodium deoxycholate, suggesting that the envelope contained essential lipid. The virus was also susceptible to the action of 0.5% trypsin, which was perhaps rather unexpected in an enteropathogenic virus. It is not clear from the report [135], however, whether the Mebus strain used was the calf-virulent isolate or the attenuated form produced by propagation in cell culture [105]. The virus was inactivated during incubation at 50°C for 1 h, but this was prevented if 1 M $MgCl_2$ was included in the incubation medium. Infectivity was reasonably stable at pH 3. The buoyant densities of the Mebus isolate [7,128,135] and the LY-138 strain [136] have been estimated at 1.18-1.20 g/ml in sucrose and 1.24-1.25 g/ml in CsCl solution.

There are two reports of the polypeptide structure of bovine coronavirus but they are in no way comparable. Hajer and Storz [136] purified the LY-138 strain from bovine feces and separated the polypeptides by SDS-polyacrylamide gel electrophoresis. They distinguished glycopolypeptides by PAS staining and identified seven distinct protein bands of which four were glycosylated. The molecular weights were estimated as: VP1, 110,000; VP2, 100,000; VP3, 82,000, VP4, 70,000; VP5, 53,000; VP6, 45,000; and VP7, 36,000. The glycosylated molecules were VP1, VP2, VP5, and VP6. After chloroform treatment, VP3 and VP7 were associated with a corelike structure.

These data are dissimilar to those reported by Laporte [137] for the polypeptide structure of a bovine coronavirus isolated in France. This strain also would not grow in cell culture and was therefore purified from feces and analyzed by electrophoresis. As with the LY-138 strain, seven polypeptides were detected, but their molecular weights were estimated at 125,000, 65,000, 50,000, 45,000, 36,000, 34,000, and 28,000 daltons. The two largest polypeptides were removed from the virion by the proteolytic enzyme bromelain and were considered to be structural components of the surface projection. The differences between these two studies may reflect differences in the structures of the two isolates or may confirm the inconsistencies in coronavirus polypeptide estimations that have been reported from different laboratories [138].

Guy and Brian [129] have examined the genome from the Mebus strain of the virus and have shown it to consist of single-stranded RNA of 3.8×10^6 daltons molecular weight. There was no reduction in size after heat denaturation, and there was evidence of polyadenylic acid tracts. These characteristics confirm the earlier suggestions that the genome was RNA, based on the lack of growth inhibition by iododeoxyuridine and actinomycin [128,135] and are consistent with the features found for other coronaviruses [138].

Murine Coronavirus Enteritis

Disease

Lethal intestinal virus of infant mice (LIVIM) was first described by Kraft in 1962 [139]. Like the previously recognized epizootic diarrhea of infant mice (EDIM), it affected very young animals but could be distinguished from EDIM by its pathology and clinical signs, and by serologic tests [140]. The virus was not identified at that time, but there was independent evidence from Rowe and his associates [141] that mouse hepatitis virus could be isolated from enteric infections of mice, and even though the major clinical sign in these newborn mice was not diarrhea, pathologic findings included edema and degeneration of the tips of the villus. Rowe and his associates designated this enterotropic strain S.

The following year, Biggers et al. [142] examined the pathogenesis of LIVIM in mice of different ages. In mice aged 1-3 days, inoculation of LIVIM led to a progressive enteritis. There was marked villous atrophy, and the crypt epithelium developed syncytia which regressed into "balloon cell" aggregates and were shed. The affected areas were unevenly distributed in the small intestine, whereas in animals a little older, 6-7 days, the lesions were similar but more widely distributed. There was no desquamation of the epithelium, but there was evidence of cecal involvement. After inoculation of 14-day-old mice, the virus caused less syncytial, balloon cell formation but there was a stimulation of crypt epithelium division to compensate for villous epithelium loss, resulting in a marked change in the villus-to-crypt ratio.

Reports of LIVIM and mouse enteritis ceased following the publications of the early 1960s. It was not clear at that time whether LIVIM was, in fact, a single agent or was the result of two viruses working in concert (Kraft, personal communication, 1974). The problem was resolved, however, when Broderson et al. [11] identified a coronavirus in the small intestines of mice dying of enteritis and showed that it was related antigenically to mouse hepatitis virus. The group went on to characterize the agent in more detail [143] and confirmed that LIVIM was closely related to mouse hepatitis virus strain S, could be propagated in cell culture, and would subsequently cause enteritis in newborn mice.

During that period, several other workers had recognized the relationship between LIVIM and mouse hepatitis virus. Carthew [12] in the United Kingdom showed that mouse hepatitis virus antibody could be detected by complement fixation in several mouse colonies in which lethal enteritis had broken out. Ishida and co-workers [144] isolated mouse hepatitis virus from intestinal, liver, and brain samples of suckling mice showing diarrhea, using a continuous line of mouse brain cells. The isolate produced diarrhea and hepatitis in suckling mice challenged orally or intraperitoneally. The pathological findings in the small intestine resembled those described by Biggers [142] for LIVIM, and mouse hepatitis virus was identified in the intestinal syncytial giant cells by immunofluorescence and electron microscopy of thin sections. There was also vacuolar degeneration and desquamation of epithelial cells seen in the large intestine.

Recently, Ishida and Fujiwara [145] reported a further study of their isolate. Following oral inoculation in newborn mice, the virus established a systemic infection although there were signs of enterotropism. Virus growth and syncytial formation were first detected in the intestines of mice killed 2 days after infection, and this was followed by a focal necrotic hepatitis. Virus infectivity titers were maximal at 4-5 days after infection in liver and intestine, and death occurred after day 5. Occasionally there were neurologic signs, and virus was isolated from brain. Lesions were also found in the lung and lymphoid organs.

These later reports, then, provide strong evidence that LIVIM, described by Kraft, is identified as an enteropathogenic strain of mouse hepatitis virus. There is nothing to suggest that more than one agent is involved in the disease, although other viruses can cause similar, but not identical, clinical signs. Of these, epizootic diarrhea of infant mice (EDIM) has now been identified as a murine rotavirus [146].

Epizootiology

A common feature of the reports of murine coronaviral enteritis is the highly contagious nature of the disease. Characteristically, once the infection becomes apparent in a breeding colony of mice it spreads rapidly, with very serious loss of animals. Rowe et al [141] suggested that clinically normal adult mice could act as carriers of the virus. They found antibodies to mouse hepatitis virus in these mice and showed that if healthy adults were introduced into an isolator holding a colony of weanling mice the infection was established. Feces were suggested as a major source of infecting virus, since newborn mice exposed to excrement from weanlings of various strains became infected with the disease.

Hierholzer [143] reported that the disease was readily transmitted by touching the noses of newborn mice to feces from infected mice. They controlled the epizootic at the Center for Disease Control in Atlanta, Georgia by stringent use of cage filters, disinfection, and separation of mouse colonies with physical and air barriers.

Serology

All reports subsequent to that of Rowe [141] showing isolation of the S strain of mouse hepatitis virus have established a serologic relationship between the mouse coronavirus enteritis agent and mouse hepatitis. Carthew [12] used a polyvalent antiserum to show this relationship with a complement fixation test, while the Japanese group [144] used complement fixation and immunodiffusion to relate their isolate to MHV-2 and JHM. In this latter study, the authors found a closer relationship to the JHM strain than to MHV-2 in that convalescent mice had antibodies to JHM but not to MHV-2.

A similar finding was reported by Hierholzer and his associates [143]. Using complement fixation, single radial hemolysis, and neutralization, they found that their isolate was distantly related to MHV-1, MHV-3, MHV-A59, and the human coronavirus OC43, was unilaterally related to MHV-JHM, but was most closely related to MHV-S. There have been no published reports to date of studies comparing the American and Japanese isolates of the enteritis coronavirus, so it cannot be stated whether more than one serotype of the agent exists.

Isolation, Cultivation and Diagnosis

Isolation and propagation of MHV-S was achieved by Rowe and co-workers [141] using serial passage with intracerebral or intraperitoneal inoculation in infant mice. They do report, however, a cytopathic effect, and antigen production from experimentally infected NCTC-1469 cells and this cell line was used in the investigation reported by Hierholzer [143].

Ishida and his co-workers [144] used the mouse brain tumor cell line SR-CDF$_1$-DBT for isolation and cultivation of their isolate, a cell line which had been used successfully for the cultivation of other strains of mouse hepatitis virus [147].

Diagnosis of infection and differentiation from other murine enteric viruses can be achieved by isolation in cell culture and a positive reaction by complement fixation, single radial hemolysis, neutralization, or immunofluorescence tests using a polyvalent antiserum to mouse hepatitis virus. Immunofluorescence or direct electron microscopy of infected intestinal sections has also been used successfully, but detection of antibodies to mouse hepatitis virus in sera from mice in a diseased colony could not be considered appropriate as this would not distinguish between enteric infection and the other manifestations of mouse hepatitis virus strains.

Virion Characteristics

Kraft determined that her LIVIM agent was filterable through a 300 nm filter, was destroyed by ether and deoxycholate, and would not hemagglutinate avian or mammalian erythrocytes [139]. The study of the S strain of mouse hepatitis virus [141] confirmed these characteristics but added little more. By 1976, however, the electron microscope was in routine use, and Broderson and associates [11] visualized coronavirus particles in negative-stained preparations from infected small intestine. The virions were 100-130 nm in diameter, surrounded by characteristic petal-shaped projections. This size was confirmed by their subsequent study [143], as well as by the lack of hemagglutination with erythrocytes from human, monkey, cow, sheep, goat, dog, guinea pig, hamster, gerbil, rat, mouse, chicken, turkey, or goose at 4, 23, or 37°C. They further showed that viral infectivity was destroyed by incubation with 0.5% chloroform or 0.1% deoxycholate, treatment with pH 3 buffer for 4 h, or heating at 50°C for 1 h. The virions banded at a buoyant density of 1.18-1.19 g/cm^3 in sucrose gradients.

Little information is available on the nature of the Japanese isolate except that it has the appearance of a coronavirus in thin sections examined by electron microscopy, with particles 80-120 nm in diameter.

Although the nucleic acid and structural polypeptides of other strains of mouse hepatitis virus have been examined, there are no reports of similar structural studies on LIVIM, MHV-S, or the Japanese isolate.

Turkey Coronavirus Enteritis

Disease

Blue comb in turkeys was identified as an infectious disease in 1953 [148]. Studies on the microbiology of the etiologic agent suggested that several microorganisms were associated with the disease, including *Vibrio cholerae* and viruses, but no correlation with the disease could be established. At a symposium in 1968, Wooley and Gratzek [149] reported isolation of a reovirus which could induce blue comb in experimentally inoculated 1-day-old poults, and a similar finding was reported by Fujisaki and co-workers [150]. Although these findings appeared to settle the question of blue comb etiology, some doubt was shed by the investigation of Pomeroy's group in Minnesota. Their characterization of viruses isolated from turkeys with blue comb [151] identified members of the papovavirus, enterovirus, and reovirus groups, but the blue comb infectivity had characteristics that distinguished it from the viruses recognized.

These studies suggested, therefore, that blue comb (or turkey infectious enteritis, or transmissible enteritis) was a syndrome that might be induced by more than one etiologic agent.

The first reports that a coronavirus might be involved in the disease came from two groups of workers in 1973. Pomeroy's group identified coronavirus particles in blue comb-infected turkey ceca, the bursa of Fabricius, and embryo intestines [8], while Panigrahy et al. [152] found similar particles in intestinal preparations of infected turkey poults. The previous year, Adams and his associates [153] had reported an electron microscopic study of the ultrastructural changes in intestines from blue comb-infected turkeys and had described particles that were most probably coronaviruses, although the authors did not identify them.

The agent could not be grown in cell culture but was passed in embryonated turkey eggs and 1-day-old poults. Several studies were conducted on the pathology of the virus in the turkey, and these correlated well with the clinical signs and histopathology seen in natural outbreaks of the disease. Experimental infection of poults resulted in clinical signs within 48 h, and these included chilling, anorexia, decrease in water uptake, diarrhea, dehydration, and weight loss [154]. Examination of the small intestine showed it to be gas filled and flaccid and having catarrhal enteritis, but other gross lesions were not seen. Scanning electron microscopy of intestines from poults infected at 1 day of age and examined 4 days later revealed a large number of erythrocytes and a heavy mucous exudate. Desquamation of the villous epithelium was evident, and the lamina propria was exposed in places. Viral antigen was detected by immunofluorescence in the epithelial cells. Poults infected at 3 weeks of age showed similar histopathology, but fewer erythrocytes were visible in the intestine; epithelium was flattened and became necrotic at the tips of the villi. The crypt cells showed increased mitotic figures, and the villi were shortened, resulting in markedly decreased villus-to-crypt ratios from day 2 after inoculation. The ratio started to return to normal after day 5 of infection, but it was still depressed at day 10. However, other histopathological changes had returned to normal by this time.

It had been noticed that fasting of turkeys gave rise to clinical signs that were difficult to distinguish from blue comb disease, but in a histopathological study of normal fasted and blue comb-infected intestine Deshmukh and co-workers [155] demonstrated clear differences between these two conditions. whereas fasted animals showed no intestinal lesions or changes from the normal, the infected birds had shortened villi and loss of the epithelial microvilli. The epithelial cell cytoplasm was granulated, and the nuclei showed margination of the chromatin and nucleolar accentuation.

Hematologic changes were described in a report from Warsaw of an outbreak of turkey enteritis that involved birds of 4-6 weeks of age, with 40% mortality. The small intestine showed acute catarrhal inflammation, and there was degeneration of parenchymatous organs. Blood samples revealed leukocytosis, with heterophilia and monocytosis up to 10% [156].

Turkey coronavirus enteritis constitutes, therefore, a well-defined syndrome that can be reproduced experimentally with a single agent, a coronavirus, and can be diagnosed by serologic methods in field outbreaks (see below).

Epiornithology

An extensive study of turkey coronavirus enteritis was undertaken by Pomeroy's group, involving 32 flocks (several hundred thousand birds) between 1973 and 1975 [157]. Immunofluorescence was used to detect viral antigens and specific antibodies in seven separate outbreaks. In most of the cases that they investigated it was clear that transmission of the virus had occurred following movement of infected birds to susceptible flocks or by repopulation of areas that previously housed infected birds. The recommended procedure for decontamination was complete depopulation of the infected flock, removal of all dust and litter from the house and service area, and thorough disinfection of all surfaces with saponified cresol or formaldehyde. New stock could be introduced 4 weeks after this treatment without any subsequent reinfection of the flocks.

Three outbreaks could not be accounted for by exposure to known infection, however. In two of these cases, range birds were introduced into flocks and the researchers concluded that native birds or some other local traffic might have carried the agent. In the third outbreak, neighboring flocks of turkeys were shown to be negative in the tests during and after the outbreak. The sources of infection could have been a spent breeder flock, sent to market before it could be tested, or wild turkeys that were located nearby. There have been no reports of other birds or animals acting as carriers of this disease.

Serology

The serology of turkey enteric coronavirus has not been studied as extensively as the other enteric coronaviruses, due at least in part to the lack of a cell culture assay system. Two reports, however, concern the antigenic typing of this virus. Ritchie and his associates [8] used immune electron microscopy to examine the relationship of the Minnesota isolate of turkey coronavirus to four other coronaviruses. They found no interaction of the virus with specific antisera to avian infectious bronchitis virus, porcine hemagglutinating encephalomyelitis virus, porcine TGE virus, or bovine enteric coronavirus. It should be remembered that immune electron microscopy detects only those antigens present at the surface of the virion. The possibility remains that the turkey virus could have antigenic cross-reactions with internal or nonstructural antigens of the other virus detectable by less specific tests, such as immunofluorescence.

Pomeroy's group [158] compared the original Minnesota isolate of turkey coronavirus enteritis with 13 other isolates of the agent from diverse geographical areas, using neutralization tests in poult challenge experiments. This procedure revealed that all isolates were antigenically similar, if not identical, suggesting that a single serotype of turkey coronavirus exists, in marked contrast to the serologic variation found in avian infectious bronchitis virus.

Isolation, Cultivation, and Diagnosis

Attempts had been made before 1970 to isolate the etiologic agent of turkey blue comb disease, without success. The first report that identified a coronavirus that could be cultivated in the laboratory was that of Ritchie [8] using embryonated turkey eggs. Since that time the Minnesota isolate has been serially passed and cultivated in the embryo system without apparent loss of antigen reactivity. However, multiple passage in this system may lead to lowered infectivity for poults [159].

The use of other cell systems has proven unsuccessful. Deshmukh et al. [160] measured the survival of the virus in cell cultures derived from chicken kidney, quail kidney, turkey kidney, quail intestine, and turkey embryo intestine. In all but the turkey embryo intestine cultures the virus could not be recovered after 48 h. Although virus was recoverable for 5 days in turkey embryo intestine culture, there was no evidence of increasing titer and the authors conncluded that none of the cell systems were suitable for virus propagation, recommending the use of embryonating turkey eggs.

Assay of virus infectivity has proven a major problem in research areas. Since no cytopathic effect could be demonstrated in cell cultures, due to the lack of efficient multiplication, the only reliable titration method was based upon infectivity for poults. Even propagation in embryonating turkey eggs led to no pathological changes in the embryo and relied upon subsequent challenge of poults with the harvested virus. It was of interest, therefore, that Deshmukh and Pomeroy [161] described an assay procedure based upon the interference with Newcastle disease virus in turkey enteric coronavirus-infected cells derived from infected embryonating eggs. Interference with Newcastle disease virus was not demonstrable in coronavirus-infected turkey embryos or in turkey intestinal cells inoculated in vitro with the coronavirus.

Virus infection can be diagnosed using the same method following inoculation of embryonating turkey eggs, but specific immunofluorescence has received more attention because of its applicability in field surveys. Patel and his co-workers developed a direct fluorescent antibody test for the detection of viral antigens in intestinal sections from infected birds [162]. The technique was taken one step further to measure antiviral antibodies in serum with an indirect test employing frozen sections of turkey embryo intestine infected with the Minnesota isolate [163]. Both these tests were applied to the field outbreaks described above.

Virion Characteristics

The two reports that a coronavirus was associated with turkey blue comb disease [8,152] used electron microscopy of negatively stained preparations to identify the characteristic morphology. Subsequent studies by the two groups [159,164] confirmed the original observations and furnished additional data.

The virions were described as having a diameter of 90-120 mm or approximately 135-220 nm, surrounded by pear- or club-shaped projections. Their density in aqueous sucrose was estimated at 1.16-1.17 g/ml. Infectivity was destroyed by ether and chloroform but was stable to incubation at pH 3 at 22°C for 30 min. The genome was considered to be RNA from the response of infectivity to ribonuclease and deoxyribonuclease. The virus was rapidly denatured at 50°C, but this could be prevented by the inclusion of 1M $MgCl_2$ but not of 1M $MgSO_4$. This latter finding [159] is perhaps rather surprising, since it is usually considered that divalent cations bring about the stabilization of viruses, rather than the corresponding anions. If this phenomenon has been followed up, it has not been reported.

These characteristics fully support the case for inclusion of the virus in the family Coronaviridae, and it will be interesting to compare polypeptide composition and nucleic acid configuration with the other coronaviruses when these properties of the turkey coronavirus are established.

Conclusions

The family Coronaviridae contains member viruses that cause a wide variety of diseases in a large number of animals and birds, as discussed in the introduction to this chapter. Having reviewed the published data on five of the members, it is apparent that these enteric coronaviruses share several properties.

They are morphologically similar, but this is to be expected since appearance by electron microscopy is a major feature in the taxonomy of the family. It is interesting to note that the characteristic morphology is retained by all coronaviruses even though the polypeptides that define this structure vary considerably in number and molecular weight. The significance of this is not altogether clear.

Each of the viruses discussed causes an enteritis in young animals that is characterized by necrosis and desquamation of villous epithelium, stunting of the villi with marked decreases in the villus-to-crypt ratio, and resulting in liquid scours and subsequent dehydration. These characteristics are not peculiar to coronaviruses, however, as they are also shown by rotaviruses (as described elsewhere in this volume).

It appears, then, that the common feature of the five viruses described is their ability to grow rapidly and to high titer in villous epithelium. They do not share a common antigen, although antigenic cross-reactions have been demonstrated between TGE and the canine virus and between the bovine coronavirus and mouse hepatitis virus. Detailed study of the coronaviruses since 1970 has provided a great deal of information about the group, but there are still gaps in our knowledge. The process by which replication of the virus occurs in the cell and the significance of the predominance of glycopolypeptides in virion structures are subjects which, when understood, may help to explain the success of these viruses as enteropathogens.

References

1. D. A. J. Tyrrell, D. J. Alexander, J. D. Almeida, C. H. Cunningham, B. C. Easterday, D. J. Garwes, J. C. Hierholzer, A. Z. Kapikian, M. R. Macnaughton, and K. McIntosh, Coronaviridae: Second report, *Intervirology, 10*:321-328 (1978).

2. D. A. J. Tyrrell, J. D. Almeida, D. M. Berry, C. H. Cunningham, D. Hamre, M. S. Hofstad, L. Mallucci, and K. McIntosh, Coronaviruses, *Nature (Lond.) 220*:650 (1968).

3. M. Tajima, Morphology of transmissible gastroenteritis virus of pigs, *Arch. Ges. Virusforsch., 29*:105-108 (1970).

4. J. C. Parker, S. S. Crosse, and W. P. Rowe, Rat coronavirus (RCV): A prevalent, naturally occurring pneumotropic virus of rats, *Arch. Ges. Virusforsch., 31*:293-302 (1970).

5. J. I. H. Phillip, S. F. Cartwright, and A. C. Scott, The size and morphology of transmissible gastroenteritis and vomiting and wasting disease of pigs, *Vet. Rec., 88*:311-312 (1971).

6. P. N. Bhatt, D. H. Percy, and A. M. Jonas, Characterization of the virus of sialodacryoadenitis of rats: A member of the coronavirus group, *J. Infect. Dis., 126*:123-130 (1972).

7. E. L. Stair, M. B. Rhodes, R. G. White, and C. A. Mebus, Neonatal calf diarrhea: Purification and electron microscopy of a coronavirus-like agent, *Am. J. Vet. Res., 33*:1147-1156 (1972).

8. A. E. Ritchie, D. R. Deshmukh, C. T. Larsen, and B. S. Pomeroy, Electron microscopy of coronavirus-like particles characteristic of turkey bluecomb disease, *Avian Dis., 17*:546-558 (1973).

9. L. N. Binn, E. C. Lazar, K. P. Keenan, D. L. Huxsoll, R. H. Marchwicki, and A. J. Strano, Recovery and characterization of a coronavirus from military dogs with diarrhea, *Proc. 78th Ann. Meet. U.S. Anim. Health Assoc., 359-366 (1974).*

10. E. P. Bass and R. L. Sharpee, Coronavirus and gastroenteritis in foals, *Lancet, 2*:822 (1975).

11. J. R. Broderson, F. A. Murphy, and J. C. Hierholzer, Lethal enteritis in infant mice caused by mouse hepatitis virus, *Lab. Anim. Sci., 26*:824 (1976).

12. P. Carthew, Lethal intestinal virus of infant mice is mouse hepatitis virus, *Vet. Rec., 101*:465 (1977).
13. D. Chasey and S. F. Cartwright, Virus-like particles associated with porcine epidemic diarrhea, *Res. Vet. Sci., 25*:255-256 (1978).
14. M. B. Pensaert and P. de Bouck, A new coronavirus-like particle associated with diarrhea in swine, *Arch. Virol., 58*:243-247 (1978).
15. L. P. Doyle and L. M. Hutchings, A transmissible gastroenteritis in pigs, *J. Am. Vet. Med. Assoc., 108*:257-259 (1946).
16. H. C. Smith, Advances made in swine practice. IX. Transmissible gastroenteritis, *Vet. Med., 51*:425-426, 435-440 (1956).
17. G. N. Woode, Transmissible gastroenteritis of swine, *Vet. Bull., 39*:239-248 (1969).
18. S. F. Cartwright, Recovery of virus and copro-antibody from piglets infected experimentally with transmissible gastroenteritis, *Proc. 18th World Vet. Congr. (Paris), 2*:565-568 (1967).
19. S. Konishi and R. A. Bankowski, Use of fluorescein-labelled antibody for rapid diagnosis of transmissible gastroenteritis in experimentally infected pigs, *Am. J. Vet. Res., 28*:937-942 (1967).
20. D. C. Thake, H. W. Moon, and G. Lambert, Epithelial cell dynamics in transmissible gastroenteritis in neonatal pigs, *Vet. Pathol., 10*:330-341 (1973).
21. M. B. Pensaert, Concepts and experiments on prevention and control of transmissible gastroenteritis of swine in the light of its pathogenesis, *Bull. Office Int. Epizooties, 76*:105-117 (1971).
22. D. P. Olson, G. L. Waxler, and A. W. Roberts, Small intestinal lesions of transmissible gastroenteritis in gnotobiotic pigs: A scanning electron microscope study, *Am. J. Vet. Res., 34*:1239-1245 (1973).
23. H. W. Moon, L. J. Kemeny, and G. Lambert, Effects of epithelial cell kinetics on age dependent resistance to transmissible gastroenteritis of swine, *Proc. 4th Int. Congr. Int. Pig. Vet. Soc., Ames,* K12 (1976).
24. B. E. Hooper and E. O. Haelterman, Concepts of pathogenesis and passive immunity in transmissible gastroenteritis of swine, *J. Am. Vet. Med. Assoc., 149*:1580-1586 (1966).
25. L. J. Ackerman, L. G. Morehouse, and L. D. Olson, Transmissible gastroenteritis in three-week-old pigs: Study of anemia and iron absorption, *Am. J. Vet. Res., 33*:115-120 (1972).
26. D. G. Butler, D. G. Gall, M. H. Kelly, and J. R. Hamilton, Transmissible gastroenteritis. Mechanisms responsible for diarrhea in an acute viral enteritis in piglets, *J. Clin. Invest., 53*:1335-1342 (1974).
27. Z. Prochazka, J. Hampl, M. Sedlacek, J. Masek, and J. Stepanek, Protein loss in piglets infected with transmissible gastroenteritis virus, *Zentralbl. Veterinaermed. [B], 22*:138-146 (1975).
28. L. M. Cornelius, B. E. Hooper, and E. O. Haelterman, Changes in fluid and electrolyte balance in baby pigs with transmissible gastroenteritis, *Am. J. Vet. Clin. Pathol., 2*:105-113 (1968).

29. H. W. Moon, J. O. Norman, and G. Lambert, Age dependent resistance to transmissible gastroenteritis of swine (TGE). I. Clinical signs and some mucosal dimensions in small intestine, *Can. J. Comp. Med., 37*:157–166 (1973).

30. J. O. Norman, G. Lambert, H. W. Moon, and S. L. Stark, Age dependent resistance to transmissible gastroenteritis of swine (TGE). II. Coronavirus titre in tissues of pigs after exposure, *Can. J. Comp. Med., 37*:167–170 (1973).

31. J. E. Wagner, P. D. Beamer, and M. Ristic, Electron microscopy of intestinal epithelial cells of piglets infected with a transmissible gastroenteritis virus, *Can. J. Comp. Med., 37*:177–188 (1973).

32. K. H. Witte and C. Walther, Age dependent susceptibility of pigs to infection with the virus of transmissible gastroenteritis, *Proc. 4th Int. Congr. Int. Pig Vet. Soc., Ames,* K15 (1976).

33. N. R. Underdahl, C. A. Mebus, E. L. Stair, M. B. Rhodes, L. D. McGill, and M. J. Twiehaus, Isolation of transmissible gastroenteritis virus from lungs of market-weight swine, *Am. J. Vet. Res., 35*:1209–1216 (1974).

34. N. R. Underdahl, C. A. Mebus, and A. Torres-Medina, Recovery of transmissible gastroenteritis virus from chronically infected experimental pigs, *Am. J. Vet. Res., 36*:1473–1476 (1975).

35. L. J. Kemeny, V. L. Wiltsey, and J. L. Riley, Upper respiratory infection of lactating sows with transmissible gastroenteritis virus following contact exposure to infected piglets, *Cornell Vet., 65*:352–362 (1975).

36. J. B. Derbyshire, D. M. Jessett, and G. Newman, An experimental epidemiological study of porcine transmissible gastroenteritis, *J. Comp. Pathol., 79*:445–452 (1969).

37. R. F. W. Goodwin and A. R. Jennings, Infectious gastroenteritis of pigs. I. The disease in the field, *J. Comp. Pathol., 69*:87–97 (1959).

38. L. J. Kemeny and R. D. Woods, Quantitative transmissible gastroenteritis virus shedding patterns in lactating sows, *Am. J. Vet. Res., 38*:307–310 (1977).

39. D. H. Ferris, Epizootiology of porcine transmissible gastroenteritis (TGE), *Adv. Vet. Sci. Comp. Med., 17*:57–86 (1973).

40. E. I. Pilchard, Experimental transmission of transmissible gastroenteritis virus by starlings, *Am. J. Vet. Res., 26*:1177–1179 (1965).

41. E. H. Bohl, Transmissible gastroenteritis. In *Diseases of Swine,* 3rd Ed. (H. Dunne, ed.), Iowa State University Press, Ames, Iowa, 1970, pp. 158–176.

42. D. H. Ferris, Epizootiological features of transmissible swine gastroenteritis, *J. Am. Vet. Med. Assoc., 159*:184–194 (1971).

43. E. O. Haelterman, Epidemiological studies of transmissible gastroenteritis of swine, *Proc. 66th Ann. Meeting U.S. Livestock Sanit. Assoc.,* 305–315 (1962).

44. J. O. Norman, A. W. McClurkin, and S. L. Stark, Transmissible gastroenteritis (TGE) of swine: Canine serum antibodies against an associated virus, *Can. J. Comp. Med., 34*:115–117 (1970).

45. D. J. Larson, Transmissible gastroenteritis in the neonatal dog, *Proc. 4th Int. Congr. Int. Pig Vet. Soc., Ames,* (1976).

46. R. C. Klemm and M. Ristic, The effect of propagation of transmissible gastroenteritis (TGE) virus in pups and the lungs of baby pigs on the immunological properties of the virus, *Proc. 4th Int. Congr. Int. Pig Vet. Soc., Ames,* (1976).

47. D. J. Reynolds, D. J. Garwes, and C. J. Gaskell, Detection of transmissible gastroenteritis virus neutralising antibody in cats, *Arch. Virol., 55*:77–86, (1977).

48. K. H. Witte, K. Tuch, H. Dubenkropp, and C. Walther, Antigenic relationship between the viruses of feline infectious peritonitis (FIP) and transmissible gastroenteritis (TGE) of pigs, *Berl. Munch. Tieraerztl. Wochenschr., 90*:396–401 (1977).

49. D. J. Reynolds and D. J. Garwes, Virus isolation and serum antibody responses after infection of cats with transmissible gastroenteritis virus, *Arch. Virol., 60*:161–166 (1979).

50. L. J Kemeny, Antibody response in pigs inoculated with transmissible gastroenteritis virus and cross reactions among ten isolates, *Can. J. Comp. Med., 40*:209–214 (1976).

51. A. Morilla, A. E. Ritchie, P. Sprino, and M. Ristic, Comparison of intestinal (Illinois strain) and cell culture-adapted (M-HP strain) viral populations of transmissible gastroenteritis of swine, *Am. J. Vet. Res., 38*:1491–1495 (1977).

52. J. Bohac, J. B. Derbyshire, and J. Thorsen, The detection of transmissible gastroenteritis viral antigens by immunodiffusion, *Can. J. Comp. Med., 39*: 67–75 (1975).

53. J. Bohac, Transmissible gastroenteritis virus: Growth in organ culture, and agar gel precipitation reactions, *Dissert. Abst. Int., 35*B:2501–2502 (1974).

54. S. S. Stone, L. J. Kemeny, and M. T. Jensen, Partial characterization of the principal soluble antigens associated with the coronavirus of transmissible gastroenteritis by complement fixation and immunodiffusion, *Infect. Immun., 13*:521–526 (1976).

55. D. J. Garwes, D. H. Pocock, and B. V. Pike, Isolation of subviral components from transmissible gastroenteritis virus, *J. Gen. Virol., 32*:283–294 (1976).

56. D. J. Garwes, M. H. Lucas, D. A. Higgins, B. V. Pike, and S. F. Cartwright, Antigenicity of structural components from porcine transmissible gastroenteritis virus, *Vet. Microbiol., 3*:179–190 (1979).

57. K. McIntosh, Coronaviruses: A comparative review, *Curr. Top. Microbiol. Immunol., 63*:86–129 (1974).

58. K. H. Sibinovic, M. Ristic, S. Sibinovic, and J. O. Alberts, Bentonite agglutination test for transmissible gastroenteritis of swine, *Am. J. Vet. Res., 27*:1339–1344 (1966).

59. P. J. J. Romano, E. A. Velazquez, and R. F. Olquin, Antigenic relationships of avian infectious bronchitis virus and transmissible gastroenteritis virus of pigs, *Veterinaria (Mex.), 6*:38-47 (1975).

60. S. F. Cartwright and M. H. Lucas, Vomiting and diarrhea in dogs, *Vet. Rec., 91*:571-572 (1972).

61. B. V. Pike and D. J. Garwes, The neutralizaton of transmissible gastroenteritis virus by normal heterotypic serum, *J. Gen. Virol., 41*:279-287 (1979).

62. A. D. M. E. Osterhaus, M. C. Horzinek, and D. J. Reynolds, Seroepidemiology of feline infectious peritonitis virus infections using transmissible gastroenteritis virus as antigens, *Zentralbl. Veterinaermed. [B], 24*:835-841 (1977).

63. N. C. Pedersen, J. Ward, and W. J. Mengeling, Antigenic relationship of the feline infectious peritonitis virus to coronaviruses of other species, *Arch. Virol., 58*:45-52 (1978).

64. D. J. Garwes and D. H. Pocock, The polypeptide structure of transmissible gastroenteritis virus, *J. Gen. Virol., 29*:25-34 (1975).

65. J. C. Hierholzer, Purification and biophysical properties of human coronavirus 229E, *Virology, 75*:155-165 (1976).

66. M. R. Macnaughton, The molecular structure of three coronaviruses, *Abst. 4th Int. Congr. Virol., The Hague*, 448 (1978).

67. G. C. Dulac, G. M. Ruckerbauer, and P. Boulanger, Transmissible gastroenteritis: Demonstration of the virus from field specimens by means of cell culture and pig inoculation, *Can. J. Comp. Med., 41*:357-363 (1977).

68. L. J. Kemeny and R. D. Woods, Morphology of TGE virus characteristic particles and their antigen-antibody complexes, *Proc. 4th Int. Congr. Int. Pig Vet. Soc., Ames*, K13 (1976).

69. K. H. Witte, Isolation of the virus of transmissible gastroenteritis (TGE) from naturally-infected piglets in cell culture, *Zentralbl. Veterinaermed. [B] 18*:770-778 (1971).

70. F. M. Cancellotti and A. Irsara, Isolation of transmissible gastroenteritis virus in tissue culture and its identification, *Clin. Vet., 99*:574-578 (1976).

71. L. J. Kemeny, Isolation of transmissible gastroenteritis virus from pharyngeal swabs obtained from sows at slaughter, *Am. J. Vet. Res., 39*:703-705 (1978).

72. J. Stepanek, Z. Pospisil, and E. Mesaros, Growth activity of transmissible gastroenteritis (TGE) virus in primary cultures of pig kidney cells and pig salivary gland cells, *Acta Vet. (Brno), 40*:235-240 (1971).

73. D. Rubinstein, D. A. J. Tyrrell, J. B. Derbyshire, and A. P. Collins, Growth of porcine transmissible gastroenteritis virus in organ cultures of pig tissue, *Nature (Lond.), 227*:1348-1349 (1970).

74. C. J. Welter, TGE of swine. I. Propagation of virus in cell cultures and development of a vaccine, *Vet. Med. Small Anim. Clin., 60*:1054-1058 (1965).

75. D. H. Pocock and D. J. Garwes, The influence of pH on growth and stability of transmissible gastroenteritis virus in vitro, *Arch. Virol.*, *29*:239-247 (1975).

76. S. L. Stark, A. L. Fernelius, G. D. Booth, and G. Lambert, Transmissible gastroenteritis (TGE) of swine: Effect of age of swine testes cell culture monolayers on plaque assays of TGE virus, *Can. J. Comp. Med.*, *39*:466-468 (1975).

77. C. Yen, R. F. Solorzano, and L. G. Morehouse, Studies on transmissible gastroenteritis (TGE) virus by immunopathological techniques, *Proc. 19th Ann. Meeting Am. Assoc. Vet. Lab. Diag.*, 21-46 (1977).

78. T. Sobiech, R. Bochdalek, and K. Losieczka, Transmissible gastroenteritis (TGE) of pigs and its diagnosis by the fluorescent antibody technique. I. Own investigations. II. Discussion of the results, *Med. Welt.*, *28*:328-329, 388-391 (1972).

79. A. W. Roberts, A. L. Trapp, and G. R. Carter, Laboratory diagnosis of transmissible gastroenteritis by immunofluorescence, *Vet. Med. Small Anim. Clin.*, *68*:612-614 (1973).

80. R. M. S. Wirahadiredja and J. Anakotta, Transmissible gastroenteritis of swine in the Netherlands, the application of the direct fluorescent antibody technique for diagnosis, *Tijdschr. Diergeneeskd.*, *102*:817-822 (1977).

81. M. Shimizu and Y. Shimizu, Micro-indirect hemagglutination test for detection of antibody against transmissible gastroenteritis virus of pigs, *J. Clin. Microbiol.*, *6*:91-95 (1977).

82. E. I. Skalinskii, L. A. Mel'nikova, I. I. Kasyuk, and A. A. Boiko, Diagnosis of porcine transmissible gastroenteritis, *Veterinariia*, *9*:104-106 (1977).

83. L. J. Saif, E. H. Bohl, E. M. Kohler, and J. H. Hughes, Immune electron microscopy of transmissible gastroenteritis virus and rotavirus (reovirus-like agent) of swine, *Am. J. Vet. Res.*, *38*:13-20 (1977).

84. W. Becker, P. Teufel, and W. Mields, Immune peroxidase method for detection of viral and chlamydial antigens. III. Demonstration of TGE antigen in pig thyroid cell cultures, *Zentralbl. Veterinaermed. [B]*, *21*: 59-65 (1974).

85. R. D. Woods, Leucocyte-aggregation assay for transmissible gastroenteritis of swine, *Am. J. Vet. Res.*, *37*:1405-1408 (1976).

86. N. Giles, E. D. Borland, D. E. Counter, and E. A. Gibson, Transmissible gastroenteritis in pigs: Some observations on laboratory aids to diagnosis, *Vet. Rec.*, *100*:336-337 (1977).

87. G. A. Young, R. W. Hinz, and N. R. Underdahl, Some characteristics of transmissible gastroenteritis (TGE) in disease-free antibody-devoid pigs, *Am. J. Vet. Res.*, *16*:529-535 (1955).

88. F. L. Black, Relationship between virus particle size and filterability through Gradocol membranes, *Virology*, *5*:391-392 (1958).

89. E. Caletti, M. Ristic, D. H. Ferris, and M. Abou-Youssef, Comparison of immunologic properties of a high and low cell culture passage of trans-

missible gastroenteritis (TGE) virus from a single isolant, *Proc. U.S. Livestock Sanit. Assoc., 72*:361–370 (1968).

90. K. H. Witte, M. Tajima, and B. C. Easterday, Morphological characteristics and nucleic acid type of transmissible gastroenteritis virus of pigs, *Arch. Ges. Virusforsch., 23*:53–70 (1968).

91. S. F. Cartwright, H. M. Harris, T. B. Blandford, I. Fincham, and M. Gitter, A cytopathic virus causing a transmissible gastroenteritis in swine. I. Isolation and properties, *J. Comp. Pathol., 75*:387–396 (1965).

92. A. W. McClurkin and J. O. Norman, Studies of transmissible gastroenteritis virus of swine. II. Selected characteristics of a cytopathogenic virus common to five isolates from transmissible gastroenteritis virus, *Can. J. Comp. Med., 30*:190–198 (1966).

93. S. Furuuchi, Y. Shimizu, and T. Kumagai, Comparison of properties between virulent and attenuated strains of transmissible gastroenteritis, *Natl. Inst. Anim. Health Q. (Japan), 15*:159–164 (1975).

94. H. Laude, J. Gelphi, and J. M. Aynaud, Search for in vitro markers of virulence of TGEV. In *Viral Enteritis in Humans and Animals. Colloques INSERM, 90*:213–216 (1979).

95. B. V. Pike and D. J. Garwes, Lipids of transmissible gastroenteritis virus and their relation to those of two different host cells, *J. Gen. Virol., 34*: 531–535 (1977).

96. M. C. Clarke, The effect of 5-bromodeoxyuridine and actinomycin D on the multiplication of transmissible gastroenteritis virus, *J. Gen. Virol., 3*: 267–270 (1968).

97. N. K. Mishra and W. L. Ryan, Ribonucleic acid synthesis in porcine cell cultures infected with transmissible gastroenteritis virus, *Am. J. Vet. Res., 34*:185–188 (1973).

98. D. J. Garwes, D. H. Pocock, and T. M. Wijaszka, Identification of heat-dissociable RNA complexes in two porcine coronaviruses, *Nature, 257*: 508–510 (1975).

99. D. J. Garwes, Progress in coronaviruses, *Nature, 266*, 682 (1977).

100. K. Andries, M. Pensaert, and P. Callebaut, Pathogenicity of hemagglutinating encephalomyelitis (vomiting and wasting disease) virus of pigs, using different routes of inoculation, *Zentralbl. Veterinaermed. [B], 25*:461–468 (1978).

101. K. P. Keenan, H. R. Jervis, R. H. Marchwicki, and L. N. Binn, Intestinal infection of neonatal dogs with canine coronavirus 1–71: Studies by virological, histological, histochemical and immunofluorescent techniques, *Am. J. Vet. Res., 37*:247–256 (1976).

102. G. Albrecht and W. Lupcke, Spontaneous clinical occurrence of transmissible gastroenteritis in dogs, *Monatschr. Vet., 31*:865–869 (1976).

103. R. D. Schnagl and I. H. Holmes, Coronavirus-like particles in stools from dogs, from some country areas of Australia, *Vet. Rec., 102*:528–529 (1978).

104. M. J. G. Appel, B. J. Cooper, H. Greisen, F. Scott, and L. E. Carmichael, Canine viral enteritis. I. Status report on corona- and parvo-like viral enteritides, *Cornell Vet., 69*:123–133 (1979).

105. C. A. Mebus, E. L. Stair, M. B. Rhodes, and M. J. Twiehaus, Neonatal calf diarrhea: Propagation, attenuation and characteristics of a coronavirus-like agent, *Am. J. Vet. Res., 34*:145–150 (1973).

106. C. A. Mebus, E. L. Stair, M. B. Rhodes, and M. J. Twiehaus, Pathology of neonatal calf diarrhea induced by a coronavirus-like agent, *Vet. Pathol., 10*:45–64 (1973).

107. C. A. Mebus, L. E. Newman, and E. L. Stair, Scanning electron, light, and immunofluorescent microscopy of intestine of gnotobiotic calf infection with calf diarrheal coronavirus, *Am. J. Vet. Res., 36*:1719–1725 (1975).

108. A. M. Doughri and J. Storz, Light and ultrastructural pathological changes in intestinal coronavirus infection of newborn calves, *Zentralbl. Veterinaermed. [B], 24*:367–385 (1977).

109. S. D. Acres, C. J. Laing, J. R. Saunders, and O. M. Radostits, Acute undifferentiated neonatal diarrhea in beef calves. I. Occurrence and distribution of infectious agents, *Can. J. Comp. Med., 39*:116–132 (1975).

110. M. Morin, S. Larivière, and R. Lallier, Pathological and microbiological observations made on spontaneous cases of acute neonatal calf diarrhea, Can. J. Comp. Med., 40:*228–240 (1976).*

111. N. Zygraich, A. M. Georges, and E. Vascoboinic, Aetiology of diarrhea in newborn calves. Results of a serological study relation to reo-like and corona viruses in the Belgian cattle population, *Ann. Med. Vet., 119*:105–113 (1975).

112. G. Wellemans, H. Antoine, Y. Botton, and E. van Opdenbosch, Frequency of coronaviruses in digestive disorders of the young calf in Belgium, *Ann. Med. Vet., 121*:411–420 (1977).

113. G. W. Horner, R. Hunter, and C. A. Kirkbride, A coronavirus-like agent present in faeces of cows with diarrhea, *N. Z. Vet. J., 23*:98 (1975).

114. G. Dirksen and P. A. Bachmann, Occurrence of rota- and coronavirus as a cause of neonatal calf diarrhea in the Federal Republic of Germany, *Berl. Munch. Tierarztl. Wochenschr., 90*:475–477 (1977).

115. K. Haralambiev, B. Mitov, and G. Popov, Coronavirus and rotavirus enteritis—a current problem on large farms, *Vet. Sbirka, 75*:7–11 (1977).

116. J. C. Bridger, G. N. Woode, and A. Meyling, Isolation of coronaviruses from neonatal calf diarrhea in Great Britain and Denmark, *Vet. Microbiol., 3*:101–113 (1978).

117. S. Dea, R. S. Roy, and M. E. Begin, Counterimmunoelectrophoresis for detection of neonatal calf diarrhea coronavirus: Methodology and comparison with electron microscopy, *J. Clin. Microbiol., 10*:240–244 (1979).

118. E. van Opdenbosch, D. de Kegel, R. Strobbe, and G. Wellemans, La diarrhée neonatale des bovins. Une etiologie complexe. *Report 47th Gen. Sess., Office Int. des. Epizooties, Paris* (1979).

119. I. Hajer and J. Storz, Antigens of bovine coronavirus strain LY-138 and their diagnostic properties, *Am. J. Vet. Res., 39*:441–444 (1978).

120. R. Sharpee and C. A. Mebus, Rotaviruses of man and animals, *Lancet, 1*: 639 (1975).
121. H. S. Kaye, W. B. Yarbrough, and C. J. Reed, Calf diarrhea coronavirus, *Lancet, 2*:509 (1975).
122. R. Sharpee, Characterization of a calf diarreal coronavirus, *Diss. Abst. Int., 38B*:78 (1977).
123. A. M. Doughri, J. Storz, I. Hajer, and H. S. Fernando, Morphology and morphogenesis of a coronavirus infecting intestinal epithelial cells of newborn calves, *Exp. Mol. Pathol., 25*:355–370 (1976).
124. D. Chasey and M. Lucas, A bovine coronavirus identified by thin-section electron microscopy, *Vet. Rec., 100*:530–531 (1977).
125. G. Wellemans, W. Oyaert, E. Muylle, H. Thoonen, and E. van Opdenbosch, Isolation of a coronavirus from calves, *Vlaams Dierg. Tiidschr., 46*:249–255 (1977).
126. Y. Inaba, K. Sato, H. Kurogi, E. Takahashi, Y. Ito, T. Omori, Y. Goto, and M. Matumoto, Replication of bovine coronavirus in cell line BEK-1 culture, *Arch. Virol., 50*:339–342 (1976).
127. E. J. Stott, L. H. Thomas, J. C. Bridger, and N. J. Jebbett, Replication of a bovine coronavirus in organ cultures of foetal trachea, *Vet. Microbiol., 1*:65–69 (1977).
128. R. L. Sharpee, C. A. Mebus, and E. P. Bass, Characterization of a calf diarrheal coronavirus, *Am. J. Vet. Res., 37*:1031–1041 (1976).
129. J. S. Guy and D. A. Brian, Bovine coronavirus genome, *J. Virol., 29*:293–300 (1979).
130. K. Sato, Y. Inaba, H. Kurogi, E. Takahashi, K. Satoda, T. Omori, and M. Matumoto, Haemagglutination by calf diarrhea coronavirus, *Vet. Microbiol., 2*:83–87 (1977).
131. D. J. Ellens, J. A. M. van Balken, and P. de Leeuw, Diagnosis of bovine coronavirus infections with haemadsorption-elution-haemagglutination assay (HEHA) and with enzyme linked immunosorbent assay (ELISA), *Proc. 2nd Int. Symp. Neonatal Diarrhoea, Saskatchewan*, 321–330 (1978).
132. C. A. Mebus, M. B. Rhodes, and N. R. Underdahl, Neonatal calf diarrhea caused by a virus that induces villous epithelial cell syncytia, *Am. J. Vet. Res., 39*:1223–1228 (1978).
133. G. Marsolais, R. Assaf, C. Montpetit, and P. Marois, Diagnosis of viral agent associated with neonatal calf diarrhea, *Can. J. Comp. Med., 42*: 168–171 (1978).
134. M. W. Peterson, R. S. Spendlove, and R. A. Smart, Detection of neonatal calf diarrhea virus, infant reo-virus-like diarrhea virus and a coronavirus using the fluorescent virus precipitin test, *J. Clin. Microbiol., 3*:376–377 (1976).
135. K. Sato, Y. Inaba, H. Kurogi, E. Takahashi, Y. Ito, Y. Goto, T. Omori, and M. Matumoto, Physico-chemical properties of calf diarrheal coronavirus, *Vet. Microbiol., 2*:73–81 (1977).

136. I. Hajer and J. Storz, Structural polypeptides of the enteropathogenic bovine coronavirus strain LY-138, *Arch. Virol.*, *59*:47–57 (1979).

137. J. Laporte, The polypeptide structure of neonatal calf diarrhea coronavirus (NCDCV) *Abst. 4th Int. Congr. Virol.* The Hague, 454 (1978).

138. D. J. Garwes, Structural and physicochemical properties of coronaviruses. In Viral enteritis in humans and animals, *Collogues INSERM 90*:141–162 (1979).

139. L. M. Kraft, An apparently new lethal virus disease of infant mice, *Science 137*:282–283 (1962).

140. L. M. Kraft, Epizootic diarrhea of infant mice and lethal intestinal virus infection of infant mice. *Natl. Cancer Inst. Monogr.*, *20*:55–61 (1966).

141. W. P. Rowe, J. W. Hartley, and W. I. Capps, Mouse hepatitis virus infection as a highly contagious prevalent enteric infection of mice, *Proc. Soc. Exp. Biol. Med.*, *112*:161–165 (1963).

142. D. C. Biggers, L. M. Kraft, and H. Sprinz, Lethal intestinal virus infection of mice (LIVIM), *Am. J. Pathol.*, *45*:413–422 (1964).

143. J. C. Hierholzer, J. R. Broderson, and F. A. Murphy, New strain of mouse hepatitis virus as the cause of lethal enteritis in infant mice, *Infect. Immun.*, *24*:508–522 (1979).

144. T. Ishida, F. Taguchi, Y-S. Lee, A. Yamada, T. Tamura, and K. Fujiwara, Isolation of mouse hepatitis virus from infant mice with fatal diarrhea, *Lab. Anim. Sci.*, *28*:269–276 (1978).

145. T. Ishida and K. Fujiwara, Pathology of diarrhea due to mouse hepatitis virus in the infant mouse, *Jpn. J. Exp. Med.*, *49*:33–42 (1979).

146. I. H. Holmes, B. J. Ruck, R. F. Bishop, and G. P. Davidson, Infantile enteritis viruses: Morphogenesis and morphology, *J. Virol.*, *16*:937–943 (1975).

147. N. Hirano, K. Fujiwara, S. Hino, and M. Matumoto, Replication and plaque formation of mouse hepatitis virus (MHV-2) in mouse cell line DBT culture, *Arch. Ges. Virusforsch.*, *44*:298–302 (1974).

148. B. S. Pomeroy and J. MN. Sieburth, Bluecomb disease of turkeys, *Proc. 90th Ann. meeting, Am. vet. Med. Assoc.* 321–327 (1953).

149. R. E. Wooley and J. B. Gratzek, Certain characteristics of viruses isolated from turkeys with bluecomb, *Am. J. Vet. Res.*, *30*:1027–1033 (1969).

150. Y. Fujisaki, H. Kawamura, and D. P. Anderson, Reoviruses isolated from turkeys with bluecomb, *Am. J. Vet. Res.*, *30*:1035–1043 (1969).

151. D. R. Deshmukh, C. T. Larsen, S. K. Dutta, and B. S. Pomeroy, Characterization of pathogenic filtrate and viruses isolated from turkeys with bluecomb, *Am. J. Vet. Res.*, *30*:1019–1025 (1969).

152. B. Panigrahy, S. A. Naqi, and C. F. Hall, Isolation and characterization of viruses associated with transmissible enteritis (bluecomb) of turkeys, *Avian Dis.*, *17*:430–438 (1973).

153. N. R. Adams, R. A. Ball, C. L. Annis, and M. S. Hofstad, Ultrastructural changes in the intestines of turkey poults and embryos affected with transmissible enteritis, *J. Comp. Pathol.*, *82*:187–192 (1972).

154. E. Gonder, B. L. Patel, and B. S. Pomeroy, Scanning electron, light and immunofluorescent microscopy of coronaviral enteritis of turkeys (bluecomb), *Am. J. Vet. Res., 37*:1435-1439 (1976).

155. D. R. Deshmukh, J. H. Sautter, B. L. Patel, and B. S. Pomeroy, Histopathology of fasting and bluecomb disease in turkey poults and embryos experimentally infected with bluecomb disease coronavirus, *Avian Dis., 20*:631-640 (1976).

156. W. Borzemska, K. Darmos, E. Malicka, B. Kalusinski, and W. Biernacki, Transmissible enteritis in turkeys (bluecomb disease, monocytosis), *Med. Welt, 33*:325-327 (1977).

157. B. L. Patel, E. Gonder, and B. S. Pomeroy, Detection of turkey coronaviral enteritis (bluecomb) in field epiornithics, using the direct and indirect fluorescent antibody tests, *Am. J. Vet. Res., 38*:1407-1411 (1977).

158. B. S. Pomeroy, C. T. Larsen, D. R. Deshmukh, and B. L. Patel, Immunity to transmissible (coronaviral) enteritis of turkeys (bluecomb), *Am. J. Vet. Res., 36*:553-555 (1975).

159. D. R. Deshmukh and B. S. Pomeroy, In vitro test for the detection of turkey bluecomb coronavirus-interference against Newcastle disease virus, *Am. J. Vet. Res., 35*:1553-1556 (1974).

160. D. R. Deshmukh, C. T. Larsen, and B. S. Pomeroy, Survival of bluecomb agent in embryonating turkey eggs and cell cultures, *Am. J. Vet. Res., 34*: 673-675 (1973).

161. D. R. Deshmukh and B. S. Pomeroy, Physicochemical characterization of a bluecomb coronavirus of turkeys, *Am. J. Vet. Res., 35*:1549-1552 (1974).

162. B. L. Patel, D. R. Deshmukh, and B. S. Pomeroy, Fluorescent antibody test for rapid diagnosis of coronaviral enteritis of turkeys (bluecomb), *Am. J. Vet. Res., 36*:1265-1267 (1975).

163. B. L. Patel, B. S. Pomeroy, E. Gonder, and C. E. Cronkite, Indirect fluorescent antibody test for the diagnosis of coronaviral enteritis of turkeys (bluecomb), *Am. J. Vet. Res., 37*:1111-1114 (1976).

164. S. A. Naqi, B. Panigrahy, and C. F. Hall, Purification and concentration of viruses associated with transmissible (coronaviral) enteritis of turkeys (bluecomb), *Am. J. Vet. Res., 36*:548-552 (1975).

18

Comparative Aspects of Pathogenesis and Immunity in Animals

Peter A. Bachmann and R. Guenter Hess University of Munich, Munich, Federal Republic of Germany

Pathogenetic Features of Virus-Induced Diarrheas

Before rotaviruses and coronaviruses were recognized as etiologic agents in neonatal diarrhea, transmissible gastroenteritis (TGE) in pigs had been known for years. TGE is a disease with well-defined symptoms and of economic significance for the pig industry. Many studies on its pathogenesis, pathophysiology, and immunology have been carried out using TGE virus infection in newborn piglets as a model. Since present knowledge indicates that rotavirus- and coronavirus-induced diarrheas in other animals bear a close resemblance to TGE virus infection, a comparative discussion of recent knowledge of the course of the disease and immunity in TGE may be beneficial for the understanding of similar infections in other species.

Viral Invasion, Replication Sites, and Age Susceptibility

After oronasal entry into the body, enteropathogenic viruses must survive a variety of extreme environmental conditions, i.e., low pH in the stomach, alkaline conditions, enzymatic digestion, and bile salt activity in the proximal small intestine, before they can infect susceptible enterocytes in the jejunum and ileum. We might therefore expect all pathogens to be stable to acid and bile salts, but this is not generally true. Only rotaviruses and parvoviruses are stable to these reagents. Enteropathogenic coronaviruses exhibit varying degrees of pH sensitivity. Bovine and turkey (blue comb) coronaviruses, as well as mouse hepatitis virus (MHV), are regarded as stable at pH 3 [44,45,133]. TGE virus reveals strain variations in its stability at pH 3 [64,67], like avian bronchitis virus [36]. We are able to show, however, for TGE virus that an acid-stable virus subpopulation is present in all strains and that this may initiate infection [67]. Since other agents that invade the small intestine, like avian influenza virus [168], are readily inactivated by acidic conditions, it is reasonable to assume that viruses can pass through the stomach and duodenum in a microenvironment in which they are protected by normal processes (the presence of food or reflux of intestinal alkali), or by predisposing pathophysiologic changes [104].

Infection usually begins in the proximal part of the small intestine. In some cases, like TGE, the upper duodenum and the villi-containing lymphoid tissue in the ileum remain uninfected [72,117], whereas replication of others, like turkey (blue comb) coronavirus, starts in duodenal enterocytes. Progeny virus spreads progressively to enterocytes in the jejunum and ileum as was shown for calf rotavirus [74] and canine [76] and turkey (blue comb) [61] coronaviruses. However, TGE virus ileal infection can occur almost simultaneously with invasion of jejunal enterocytes, and virus progeny from the proximal small intestine does not seem to reinfect the ileum [134]. Similar observations were made in lamb rotavirus infections [140]. Depending upon the virus species or strain involved, infection is sometimes limited to the proximal and middle part of the small intestine [72,114]. Some coronaviruses and rotaviruses also infect sites in the colon [91,140,176].

It has been generally accepted that infection sites of most of the known enteropathogenic animal viruses are strictly localized to the intestinal epithelium. There is unanimous agreement that virus does not replicate in the epithelium of the stomach, and although rotaviral and coronaviral antigen was demonstrated in the mesenteric lymph of infected pigs and dogs [76,153], there is no further evidence that rotaviruses and coronaviruses infect the submucosa and regional lymph nodes [8,61,72,91]. However, the possibility that porcine and bovine rotaviruses replicate in the lamina propria of infected animals cannot be totally excluded at present, since virions [144] and viral antigen [153] were demonstrated in the lamina propria. Whether this is virus antigen accumulated by phagocytosis or indicates viral replication is not known.

Other agents, like feline and canine parvoviruses [35,41,51,60,73] or the lethal intestinal virus of infant mice (LIVIM) which has recently been shown to be a strain of mouse hepatitis virus [70], cause an additional variety of lesions in a number of other organ systems. EDIM virus, a rotavirus responsible for the etiology of epizootic diarrhea in infant mice, rapidly spreads systematically in the body as a result of viremia [80].

There is still some uncertainty as to whether rotaviruses and coronaviruses replicate and produce lesions in the intestinal tract only, or whether they undergo an initial replication step in the upper respiratory tract. This was presumed since infants with rotavirus infection often show respiratory tract symptoms like pharyngeal erythema, reddening of the tympanic membrane, and lymphadenitis [32,46,129,150]. In animal experiments rotavirus replication was never detected in the respiratory tract epithelium. But TGE virus, also thought to be localized in the small intestine only, has been observed to replicate in lung epithelium, and virus was isolated from the respiratory tract of adult pigs with pneumonic lesions [162].

One of the main characteristics of rotavirus and coronavirus infection is the development of severe diarrhea in neonatal animals, usually between the ages of 1 and 20 days, although animals of all ages are susceptible. Whereas during infections like TGE mortality in the newborn piglets may reach 100%, in older animals less dramatic reactions with a much lower case fatality rate, milder clinical symptoms, and increasing rates of inapparent infections are observed [101]; virus production and villous atrophy of 3-week-old and adult pigs are less than in newborn pigs [99]. Similar observations were made in canine coronavirus infections [76]. This is in contrast to infectious parvovirus enteritis in cats (feline panleukopenia) and dogs, where susceptible animals of all age groups may develop severe disease after infection.

This innate, age-dependent resistance to TGE seems to be related to the rate of regeneration of villi. Normal newborn piglets replace villous epithelium in 7-10 days, whereas 3-week-old pigs do so in 2-4 days, and the normal life span of villous absorptive cells in 3-week-old pigs (2-4 days) is less than in newborn pigs (7-10 days) [96]. Adsorptive enterocytes in other species also regenerate more slowly in newborns than in older animals [98].

From these results, Moon and co-workers [99] speculate that there is a direct relationship between virus production and cell age, since virus production in the slowly replaced, comparatively old cells of newborn pigs is higher than in the relatively young cells of older pigs. This seems to be consistent with two other observations. First, TGE virus replicates in the mature, differentiated, nonproliferating villous epithelial cells, whereas juvenile epithelial cells that replace destroyed cells are relatively resistant to virus production after they have migrated to the villi [117]. Second, TGE virus enters and accumulates in the apical tubular and vacuolar system of villous absorptive cells of newborn pigs. This tubulovacuolar system is extensive in newborn pigs, but lacking or less developed in pigs older than 3 weeks [145]. It has been suggested that virus production by absorptive cells of older pigs is limited by the inadequate tubulovacuolar system, thus limiting cell damage and contributing to age resistance [166].

These conclusions were made from experiments using the TGE virus pig model. Whether similar conditions apply to intestinal coronavirus infections in other species and to rotavirus infections remains to be seen.

Morphologic Lesions and Repair Mechanisms

Morphologic lesions in the small intestine have been described in naturally occurring and experimentally induced viral diarrheal diseases in animals using light microscopy, scanning, and ultrathin section electron microscopy. These papers all show that the mature, differentiated absorptive villous epithelial cells in the small intestine are highly susceptible to rotaviruses and coronaviruses [72,76,89, 111,113,117,140,151].

Villous cells exhibit a gradient of susceptibility to infection by these viruses, increasing in sensitivity from crypt to tip of villus [5]. In contrast, enteropathogenic parvoviruses have a strong affinity to the undifferentiated cells in the crypts of Lieberkühn [8,41,148].

Lesions detected by light microscopy after infection with rotaviruses and coronaviruses are generally very similar and consist of degeneration, sometimes vacuolization, necrosis, and desquamation of infected villous cells, which lead to progressive shortening and atrophy of villi in the small intestine. The crypts elongate, and increased numbers of polymorphonuclear cells infiltrate into the thickened lamina propria and there is a temporary deficiency of mature differentiated cells in the mucosa. The microvilli become short and poorly defined, with irregular spacing and arrangement [72,151]. The microvillus (brush) border is usually altered. The ratio of the height of the villi to the depth of the crypts is drastically reduced in infected areas, to an extent which depends upon the part of the small intestine affected.

As shown for bovine and porcine rotavirus and canine coronavirus, the epithelia of adjacent villi occasionally fuse [76,82,114]. The decrease in the number and height of microvilli in the brush border reduces the amount of absorptive surface area in the lumen of the intestine, although this feature seems to be inconsistent.

Coronavirus enteritis of mice (LIVIM) is characterized in addition by the occurrence of large syncytia [70].

Usually large fat globules are seen in infected enterocytes, which may reflect the inability of the cells to transport fat to the lymphatic organs [14,76, 152].

At the height of the process of cell lysis and desquamation there are small areas where the lamina propria is completely devoid of epithelial cells and is in direct contact with the intestinal lumen [12,91,113,117]. While there is general agreement that some loss of epithelial cells from the tip of the villus is due to viral cytopathology, widespread denudation of villi, as described by some workers, may be an artefact and could be due to autolytic processes [40].

The localization of morphologic lesions in the small intestine correlates well with that of virus-specific antigens detected by fluorescent antibody techniques [76,92,114,117,151,153,176]. Sometimes the distribution of infected cells is patchy, and not all villi are infected, for example, in piglets infected with rotaviruses.

In most of the infected villi extremely brilliant fluorescent antibody (FA) staining is seen in the enterocytes on the tips of the villi [76,91,113], and in some, these cells are the only sites where virus can be demonstrated [5,140]. It was suggested that these infected cells migrated to the tips of each villus and are replaced by crypt cells [140].

The extent of epithelial damage varies from species to species and from individual to individual [5,72,99]. Cells range from those which are indistinguishable from normal to those displaying severe changes, and this may be related to the infective dose [62], virulence of the respective virus strain [68, 99], virus and host species involved, and the developmental stage of the enterocytes in the small intestine [31,99,152].

The amount of damage has been compared in studies in which samples were taken at different times after inoculation and also after the onset of diarrhea [62]. For example, only slight villous stunting was observed in calves examined 6 h after onset of diarrhea (26 h postinfection) [92], whereas very severe atrophy was found in naturally infected calves [114]. Maximum atrophy in rotavirus-infected piglets was demonstrated at 60 h postinfection [62,113]. Nevertheless, the reported variations in virus-induced lesions may be somewhat artefactual if precise time-course experiments are not available.

With respect to the severity of lesions in different species, it has been shown that in EDIM virus and sheep rotavirus infection only enterocytes at the tips of the villi are infected and sloughed [5,140]. Bovine and porcine rotavirus or canine coronavirus infect enterocytes in the upper third or half of the villus [76,91,113]. In TGE, all differentiated villous enterocytes are usually infected, leaving only crypt cells uninfected [72,117], although individual differences are possible [99]. An infection of young piglets with a bovine rotavirus strain resulted in more severe damage than an infection with a homologous rotavirus [62]. Lamb rotavirus infects the tips of villi, and slight stunting is seen. However, these morphologic lesions had gone by 72 h after infection, although crypt hypertrophy was observed for 6 days [141].

The stage of differentiation of enterocytes also influences the extent of virus infection and the development of morphologic lesions [98,99]. Enterocytes normally regenerate by a continuous process, but various stages of cellular maturity are detectable at different times, and so the number of susceptible cells at the time of inoculation may vary from animal to animal within an age group.

Furthermore, TGE virus replication can occur in the small intestine of pigs without apparent morphologic damage [31,68].

Depending upon the virulence of the virus involved, there may be differences in the extent of viral replication and the severity of morphologic changes. After infection with attenuated TGE virus strains or strains with low virulence, the uninfected proximal part of the small intestine is longer than that found in infections with virulent virus (Pensaert, personal communication, 1977). We were able to show in experiments using the same virus strain (Bl) at different levels of attenuation that the virus material with the highest degree of attenuation (after 350 tissue culture passages) infected only a small area in the middle part of the jejunum [68]. Parallel to this limited virus replication there was a quantitative difference in the degree of villous atrophy. In most experiments the middle and distal parts of the jejunum and the ileum suffered the most severe morphologic changes [68]. The results obtained with passage numbers 3, 120, 250, 300, and 350 are summarized in Fig. 1.

Persistence of virus in small intestine depends largely upon whether differentiated enterocytes are available to support virus replication. In TGE virus infection of 3- to 7-day-old piglets, virus-specific antigen can be detected first in susceptible enterocytes between 9 and 12 h postinfection and by 7 days postinfection is undetectable [117]. Rotavirus antigen can be visualized by FA techniques between 24 and 96 h postinfection in piglets and between 12 h and 96 h in lambs [140]. In canine coronavirus infection the first fluorescing cells appear between 2 and 4 days after inoculation, and virus can be recovered up to day 16 from rectal swabs [76]. In mice infected with EDIM rotavirus-specific antigen was first seen at day 2 postinfection, and intestinal infection lasted 16 days [176]. Comparable data for turkey (blue comb) coronavirus infection are 1 and 29 days, respectively [112]. Generally, as infection progresses, the number of infected cells increases, and after reaching a peak early during infection (usually between 18 and 36 h), a drop is observed that runs parallel to the desquamation and lysis of epithelial cells and usually with the appearance of villous atrophy. Infection, however, is not only limited by the reduced availability of susceptible cells in the small intestine, but also by the action of immune processes. It has been shown in pigs and calves that active local immunity develops as early as 4–8 days postinfection, resulting in the secretion of specific antibodies in the gut lumen, and this may limit infection of newly differentiated enterocytes [84,124].

Since the proliferative, secretory, immature cells in the crypts of Lieberkühn are refractory to coronavirus and rotavirus infection, damage due to viruses is rapidly repaired by replacement from the crypt. Crypt cells migrate along villi to the apical part so that the atrophic villi become covered with new, undifferentiated epithelial cells [118,151,152]. Cells covering the atrophic villi

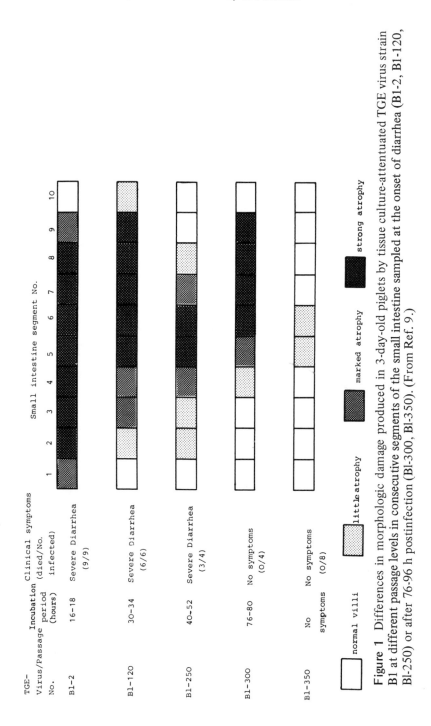

Figure 1 Differences in morphologic damage produced in 3-day-old piglets by tissue culture-attentuated TGE virus strain B1 at different passage levels in consecutive segments of the small intestine sampled at the onset of diarrhea (B1-2, B1-120, B1-250) or after 76-96 h postinfection (B1-300, B1-350). (From Ref. 9.)

in pigs with TGE or human rotavirus infection have an enzyme profile and ultra-structural characteristics similar to those of crypt cells [42,79,118,151]. Mitotic rates are high and lead to elongation and hyperplasia in the crypts [72]. In pigs with TGE the migration rates of crypt epithelial cells are accelerated and the replacement time for epithelium on atrophic villi is considerably shortened in the small intestine [99,152]. Jejunal epithelial cells migrate along the villi of 3-week-old control piglets at a rate of 13 μm/h, reaching the villous tip in about 38 h compared to 20 μm/h and 23 h in TGE virus-infected piglets [31]. In younger piglets (4 days old) these migration rates are somewhat slower, but similar to those in 3-week-old piglets, and the replacement time (2.1 days) in infected piglets is again considerably shorter than that in controls (11.9 days) [152]. In rotavirus-infected 2- to 4-day-old lambs the replacement time has been estimated to be 15 h [140,141].

These findings show that in response to infection the crypt epithelial cell generation cycle is changed so that the proliferative zone expands and the maturation zone diminishes.

Differences between the pathogenesis of enteropathic virus infection in various species may be related to species differences in the kinetics of the renewal of mature enterocytes [99,152]. In 3-week-old piglets the epithelium is replaced every 2-4 days [96], in humans every 4-6 days [139], and in 3-week-old calves and lambs every 2-3 days [98]. As has been discussed before, replacement time decreases considerably with age.

The initially flat and cuboidal cells eventually differentiate and villi are regrowing from day 3 and are restored by 7 days after infection [72,118].

Pathophysiological Changes

There are a number of functional and physiological consequences after virus replication and morphologic damage in the absorptive cells of the small intestine. In this connection, microvillus damage seems to be most important since the plasma membrane of microvilli has been reported to be the predominant site of localization of enzymes like alkaline phosphatase, aminopeptidase, β-galactosidase, maltase, sucrase, invertase, isomaltase, and trehalase. The microvillus border is viewed as a digestive-absorptive border, at which the terminal digestion of disaccharides and the absorption of monosaccharides occurs [38, 151]. Furthermore, differentiated villus cells synthesize the glucose-Na$^+$ carrier and the sodium pump (Na$^+$-K$^+$)-ATPase [58].

Studies on pathophysiological and functional changes in virus-induced diarrheas are rare. The most valuable work was done on ion transport in piglets infected with TGE virus and is discussed by Hamilton and Gall in Chap. 13. In short, following infection in 3-week-old piglets the disaccharidases, the glucose-Na$^+$ carrier, and (Na$^+$-K$^+$)-ATPase activities are greatly diminished in the jejunum and ileum, whereas adenyl cyclase and cyclic AMP levels remain normal [31]. Most important for ion transport seems to be the failure of the glucose-mediated Na^+ transport, and the defect in (Na^+-K^+)-ATPase synthesis, which result in a reduced absorption of sodium, potassium, chloride and water in the jejunum and ileum [31,79,135]. Identical or similar observations were made in rotavirus infection in piglets [42] and in calves with virus enteritis [120,173].

Defective ion transport and synthesis of disaccharidases cause a complex of symptoms in an infected animal that consists of maldigestion, malabsorption, electrolyte disturbances, and hypersecretion, which in turn lead to diarrhea, acidosis, and dehydration. Two different functional and pathophysiological concepts have been deduced from these observations. First, the deficiency in disaccharidases, especially β-galactosidase, leads to maldigestion of lactose, and the morphologic and functional changes in infected enterocytes result in malabsorption of the few monosaccharides generated from the small amount of lactose that is digested [63,97]. Due to accumulation of osmotically active lactose and other unabsorbed and undigested materials, an increase in osmotic pressure occurs in the small intestine. These nutrients may, in addition, lead to an increased accumulation of bacteria in the small intestine [47] and fermentation, with an overproduction of microbial end products. Microbial fermentation also takes place in the large intestine, and this can further add osmotically to the other intestinal solutes and to luminal acidification in the colon, causing both decreased absorption and increased secretion [15,119]. Furthermore, organic acids are produced in the intestinal lumen during the acute phase of illness and bicarbonate is lost in large amounts, leading to a systemic acidosis.

Second, hypersecretion contributes to diarrhea, as shown in TGE [31]. The undifferentiated epithelial crypt cells that replace the mature, absorptive enterocytes after desquamation lack digestive and absorptive activities, but seem to be the principal sites of intestinal secretions [97]. On the other hand, mature absorptive cells have little secretory capability. Since the undifferentiated crypt epithelium increases and expands in length, it can be assumed that the secretory capacity also increases. In addition, one must remember that at the time when the most severe diarrhea is observed most of the cells that migrated rapidly to the villus still have crypt cell characteristics and presumably retain some of their secretory functions [31,79,117,151].

This enhanced secretion may be due to a deficiency in glucose-stimulated Na^+ transport as a result of defective glucose absorption [172]. Na^+ transport from the gut lumen into the extracellular fluid is smaller than Na^+ transport in the opposite direction, and this leads to an accumulation of fluid in the small intestine and to diarrhea.

The function of the colonic mucosa in TGE is considered to be normal [31]. It remains to be seen whether this also applies to infections, such as bovine coronavirus or ovine and EDIM rotavirus diarrhea, in which the colonic epithelium is infected. There may, however, be secondary colonic malfunction even in TGE [97]. Bile salts are normally absorbed in the ileum. Since the ileal enterocytes undergo morphologic changes during infection with most coronaviruses and rotaviruses, the absorption of bile salts may be impaired. They therefore pass to the colon, where they stimulate secretion.

Complete studies of water and electrolyte balance in coronavirus-infected calves reveal that the water balance changed from a normal gain of 22 to a loss of 72 ml/kg body weight per day, which represents a daily loss of 8.5% of the calves' total body water. In addition, large amounts of Na^+, K^+, and Cl^- are lost in the feces during diarrhea [120]. These electrolyte and water losses lead to a decrease in plasma protein values. This decrease in plasma volume has a direct relationship to milk intake of calves [53]; there may, however, be considerable quantitative differences in the changes occurring in other species.

Influence of Multiple Infections

There are enough experimental data available to support the concept that coronaviruses and rotaviruses [72,76,91,140,153] are primary etiologic agents in neonatal diarrhea of animals, although differences in virulence are observed in various outbreaks [43,177]. Monoinfections with either agent lead to diarrhea in many species.

In addition to these agents, however, other enteropathogenic viruses, bacteria, and protozoa [4,19,21,49,75,103,148,165,179] may play a role in disease, and a variety of multiple infections have been described under field conditions, especially in calves. Mixed-virus infections of rotaviruses and coronaviruses are common in calves, and have been reported in a number of papers [4,43,85,100, 103,165]. The association of the two viruses occurred sometimes in up to 54% of all rotavirus cases [85]. In addition, bovine virus diarrhea virus-like viruses (BVD virus, classified as togavirus), were demonstrated frequently either combined with rotaviruses or coronaviruses or with both [4,85,165]. Other viruses, not known to cause diarrhea, that have been detected in calves with rotaviruses and/or coronaviruses were enteroviruses and infectious bovine rhinotracheitis virus, a herpesvirus [85,103]. These virus infections, furthermore, can be associated with bacteria, like enteropathogenic *Escherichia coli,* and/or protozoa, like *Cryptosporidium* and *Coccidia* [63,90,92,100,103], in various combinations.

Enteric lesions found in the intestine of calves with mixed infections usually resemble those seen in experimental monoinfections with the individual agents, e.g., villous atrophy in the jejunum for virus infections and *E. coli* infestations in the ileum [99]. In animals infected with viruses and cryptosporidia, damaged microvilli and villous atrophy were frequent in the lower jejunum and ileum [100,103].

Mixed human intestinal infection in connection with diarrhea have also been reported (rotavirus, enteropathogenic *E. coli,* salmonella, and shigella) in the Philippines and Mexico and[21,49] also in pigs (rotavirus and TGE virus) [19,154,179].

It is a matter of speculation whether the interactions in these mixed infections are additive or synergistic and increase the severity of the disease, or if they induce interference with other agents. It has been suggested that in mixed infections with rotavirus and *E. coli* in calves [92,100] there may be enhanced proliferation of *E. coli* in the intestine and predisposition to bacteremia and also accelerated damage to, and delayed regeneration of, villous epithelium. It was further postulated that, if such interactions do occur in *E. coli* and rotavirus infections, they probably occur in other mixed infections as well. In calves with diarrhea it was also shown that high susceptibility to enteropathogenic *E. coli* was longer, and this may also be induced by virus infections.

There is indirect evidence for additive and/or synergistic interactions in mixed infections in that infection with a syncytium-forming virus alone can lead to a severe illness in calves lasting 24 h only, whereas when enteropathogenic *E. coli* was also present the infection caused death [90]. In another study, mortality rates increased with the number of different viruses detected in diarrhea, being highest in infections with three or four viruses [165].

From these considerations it seems that neonatal diarrhea in the field is often complex in etiology. Field data suggest an increase in severity of disease in a few cases when more than one etiologic agent is present in calves. Experimental data are needed urgently on multiple infections in order to further evaluate the role these multiple infections play in diarrhea in calves, and whether similar situations can be encountered in other animal species.

Pathogenetic Mechanisms Contributing to Diarrhea

Diarrhea in infections with enteropathogenic viruses follows a complex chain of events. They are based mainly upon morphologic and functional alterations induced by virus replication and the inability of the neonatal host to compensate rapidly.

1. Changes begin with viral destruction of absorptive epithelial cells and alterations of microvilli leading to a decrease in disaccharidase and glucose-Na^+ carrier synthesis. Furthermore, (Na^+-K^+)-ATPase is reduced.
2. Disaccharidase deficiency induces an increase in undigested disaccharides, especially lactose, which are osmotically active and cause an influx of fluid into the gut lumen. These disaccharides and other undigested nutrients are subject to bacterial fermentation in the small and large intestines, and the fermentation end products further contribute to high osmotic pressure in

the gut lumen. The increased influx of fluid is facilitated by the greater osmotic permeability of the small intestine of newborns as compared to older animals.

3. Glucose absorption is impaired, and this results in a drastic reduction in Na^+ absorption since it is glucose dependent.

4. Replacement of absorptive villous cells by immature secretory crypt cells and crypt hypertrophy lead to an increased secretion in the gut lumen, and the net absorption of sodium, potassium, chloride, and water are significantly decreased. Some of these electrolyte imbalances can be compensated for by the colon, since Na^+ is absorbed there. However, when the capacity of the colon is exhausted, diarrhea results.

This concept is complicated by a number of events that may synergistically or antagonistically influence the pathogenesis of virus-induced diarrhea.

Glucose and Na^+ absorption are highest in the proximal and middle part of the jejunum, and it may be postulated that the severity of diarrhea must therefore depend on the location and extent of intestinal lesions. Evidence in support of this hypothesis has been presented recently [68,134].

Villous epithelial cell kinetics can influence the course and duration of diarrhea, as has been demonstrated in comparative experiments with neonatal and older animals. A more rapid turnover in epithelial cells may reduce the severity of the lesions, because dysfunctions would be repaired faster.

In this connection, also, the growth rate of the virus may be important. It was shown in piglets infected with TGE virus material of different attenuation levels that although morphologic lesions are always severe, the severity and the duration of diarrhea was directly related to the length of the incubation period [68]. This was concluded from experiments with passage number 300 of TGE strain Bl, which caused severe morphologic lesions 72-96 h after infection, but no diarrhea. Furthermore, during serial back-passages in newborn piglets of the Bl-300 attenuated strain we observed an increase in virulence that coincided with a decreasing incubation period. Compensation by other mechanisms may be more effective when the course of epithelial cell damage is slower.

In addition, the local intestinal immune response influences the course of the disease, since secretory IgA and IgM antibodies are produced and secreted 4-8 days after infection. Newly generated susceptible cells would be protected by specific IgA antibodies, thus limiting further viral replication.

An additive factor leading to more severe forms of diarrhea may be the multiple infections that occur so frequently, at least in calves.

Defense Mechanisms and Immune Prophylaxis of Gastrointestinal Virus Infections

The resorptive area of the intestine is continuously exposed to a large number of antigens, which may be toxic, allergic, or infectious in nature. Therefore, the intestinal defense mechanism is not based on one function only, but provides both nonspecific and specific immunologic barriers against these agents.

Nonspecific Defense Mechanisms

Most of the nonspecific effects have been shown to act as antibacterial barriers. Since a natural bacterial flora is one of the most effective barriers against infections with enteropathogenic agents, the mechanisms providing an intact natural flora are important. Experiments with gnotobiotic animals lacking a natural intestinal flora document this quite well. The factors involved are the mucus coat, gastric and glandular secretions, and peristaltic motility.

Mucins are the glycoproteins and glycolipids that are present on the surface of intestinal mucosae and that can act as competitive inhibitors for the receptors for microorganisms and toxins [149].

Glandular secretions from the stomach, duodenum, pancreas, and liver supply a relatively large amount of sterile fluid to the ingesta. Considering the small intestine as a continuous culture vessel these excretions assist, in cooperation with peristaltic motility, in "washing out" enteropathogenic microorganisms from the proximal part of the small intestine. The number of microorganisms is decreased when the amount of fluid is increased, and vice versa. This effect is combined with the inactivating effect of bile on some enteropathogenic viruses, such as TGE virus.

The importance of *peristaltic motility* in controlling bacterial populations has been shown in opium-treated guinea pigs [78]. Inhibition of small intestinal motility by opium treatment was a prerequisite for the experimental production of enteric forms of shigellosis and salmonellosis.

What importance these nonspecific defense mechanisms have in intestinal virus infections is not clear.

Specific Immune Response

More than 50 years ago Besredka [13] suggested a local immune mechanism in mucosal surfaces. In spite of this work the theory that serum antibodies "spilled over" into external secretions was maintained for more than 30 years. The term *coproantibodies* was proposed later for the locally produced antibodies that play an important role in the resistance to infection of the alimentary tract. The amount of antibodies found was unrelated to the level of serum antibodies.

The "spill over" theory was abandoned in 1959, when Heremans and his group [66] isolated an immunoglobulin, which was named IgA. It was found to be the most important immunoglobulin in human external secretions [34], associated with specific antibody activities to pathogenic agents [160].

Today, investigations of this local immune system have been extended to numerous animal species [30,87,163,164,175]. It seems that local immune mechanism of most mammals is based not only on immunoglobulins analogous to human sIgA [24,125] but also to sIgM [24,174]. Secretory antibodies are the predominant immunoglobulins in secretions of the alimentary, genitourinary, and respiratory tracts and of the mammary, lacrimal and salivary glands [84,167].

Cell-mediated immunity (CMI) also has a role in protection against intestinal infections. After inoculation with live poliovirus vaccine, patients with deficits in T-cell function shed virus indefinitely, and if T-cell function is reconstituted virus shedding may cease [109]. Furthermore, migration inhibition factor (MIF) and cytotoxicity have been demonstrated in splenic and lamina propria lymphocytes of pigs that had been exposed orally to TGE virus and cultured in vitro with inactivated TGE virus [55,137]. Following subcutaneous injection of TGE virus, splenic lymphocytes produced MIF, but cells from the lamina propria reacted much less. However, MIF-like activities can also be detected in the supernatant fluids of intestinal organ cultures from normal guinea pigs [57].

Pathways of Intestinal Immunoglobulin Production

Immunity against enteropathogenic agents is mediated by the antibodies secreted into the intestinal lumen. The cells which synthesize these antibodies are unusual in two aspects: they are not located in lymphoid tissue but in the lamina propria of the intestine, and they produce predominantly IgA antibodies [37]. It has been shown [121] in transfusion studies with labeled large thoracic duct lymphocytes in rats that most of the IgA-secreting plasma cells of the small intestine are derived from the thoracic duct lymph via the bloodstream. Evidence for this hypothesis comes from experiments with SPF rats in which it was shown that almost all the large and small lymphocytes of the lymph are derived from the intestinal lymphoid tissue. Since most of the immunoglobulin synthesized by these cells is IgA, it has been concluded that the large lymphocytes in the thoracic duct are the precursors of the IgA-producing plasma cells in the intestine [121].

The antibody-containing thoracic duct cells presumably originate from Peyer's patches, where sensitization by antigen takes place. The sensitized blastoid cells from Peyer's patches migrate to the regional lymph nodes and, via the lymphatic drainage, to the bloodstream [88]. They then "home" to the intestinal lamina propria, to the mammary gland, in lesser quantities also to the spleen, and perhaps to other mucosal surfaces, where they produce IgA [170]. In contrast, cells taken from popliteal lymph nodes of rabbits generally home to systemic tissues and produce predominantly IgG [167].

Immature gut-associated lymphocytes do not mature into immunocompetent cells when kept in vitro [121]. Maturation depends on exposure to antigen and possibly to contact with T lymphocytes [167].

The question of which factors influence the large lymphocytes in the bloodstream to home to the lamina propria of the small intestine is still open. Two possibilities have been discussed: first, factors intrinsic to the small intestine—possibly secretory component (SC)-containing intestinal epithelial cells—may favor the emigration of such lymphocytes into the lamina propria, or second, there may be antigen-dependent immobilization of these cells [25]. Present evidence supports the second hypothesis because SC fails to bind to large lymphocytes in suspension, and moreover, migration of large lymphocytes into the intestine was not disturbed by pretreatment of animals with antibodies directed against either SC or IgA.

In addition, IgM is produced locally and exhibits properties similar to those of secretory IgA [110,155]. Recent studies in humans and animals demonstrated that 19S pentamers of IgM also contain SC. However, compared to SC in IgA, the binding of SC in IgM is less stable [24].

A model of the transport of IgA and IgM in glands has been suggested by Brandtzaeg and Baklien and is shown in Fig. 2 [25]. An epithelial membrane receptor specific for IgA and IgM is postulated to be identical with SC in this model. However, there may be species differences, since in the bovine mammary gland a specific epithelial receptor for IgG exists which is responsible for the transmission of intact IgG_1 molecules from serum to colostrum [77].

IgA dimers and IgM pentamers are stabilized by the incorporation of J (joining) chains in immunocytes. In contrast, SC is produced in epithelial cells and secreted into the intestinal lumen or incorporated into the epithelial cell membrane. The immunoglobulins released from immunocytes are bound by noncovalent interaction to the membrane-associated SC. Ig-SC complexes are then taken up by the epithelial cells through pinocytosis, and completed secretory polymers are secreted into the intestinal lumen. The ratio of free SC in the intestinal lumen to bound SC is important for the stability of secretory immunoglobulins, but secretory IgM is more dependent on an excess of free SC than is secretory IgA [24].

Secretory IgA, and similarly sIgM, protect the epithelial surfaces of the young pig [22] and human infant [161]. Calves may be an exception, since IgG_1 is postulated to be the predominant immunoglobulin secreted into the intestinal lumen [83,107]. But antibody activity in the intestine is not necessarily limited to IgA. Sometimes the role of sIgA in intestinal protection may be taken over by sIgM, as in cases with IgA deficiency [26]. The question of whether there is a "memory" in the secretory system of the intestine remains unanswered. In some cases an anamnestic response of IgM was found in serum after oral reinfection [127]. In other cases tolerance against repeatedly given antigen was recognized [25].

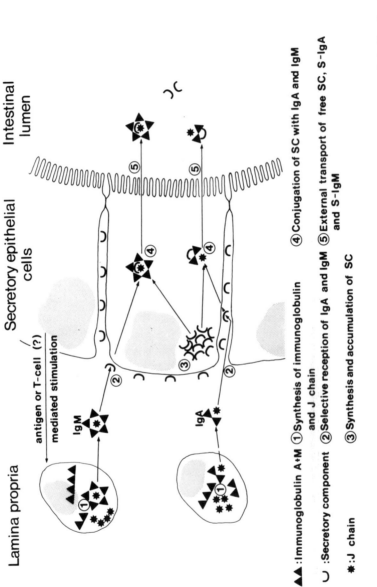

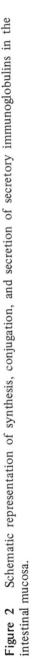

Figure 2 Schematic representation of synthesis, conjugation, and secretion of secretory immunoglobulins in the intestinal mucosa.

Passage of circulating serum antibodies into the intestinal lumen is also possibly, mainly of IgG and IgM. The amount is small compared with locally produced antibodies [39,65]. Although usually the presence of preexisting specific serum antibody to enteropathogenic viruses does not correlate with resistance to infection [94,115,180], some protective effect may be elicited when antibody is present in large amounts [142].

Pathways of Lacteal Immunoglobulin Production

Secretory IgA is the predominant antibody in postcolostral milk of most mammalian species and protects the intestine of nursing neonates by local action. It is produced in plasma cells underlying the glandular epithelium of the mammary organ. As has been discussed before, IgA-producing plasma cells orig- inate from lymphocytes in the gut-associated lymphoid tissue [130]. These cells presumably are also involved in lacteal Ig secretion since thoracic duct lympho- cytes were also shown to home to the mammary gland. This homing takes place only in the terminal stages of pregnancy and during lactation [130]. It does not occur in virgins, in early pregnancy, or after weaning. The cells homing to the mammary gland are probably members of the same population which regularly homes to the small intestine throughout adult life, because both plasma cell pop- ulations have similar characteristics. Whereas homing to the intestine is a con- tinuous process, homing to the mammary gland occurs only in pregnancy and is probably hormone induced [130].

Not all the immunoglobulins present in lacteal secretions are locally pro- duced. Part of the colostrum and milk antibodies are derived from the blood. The proportions depend on the species. In sow colostrum all IgG and about 80% of IgM are derived from blood. However, only 40% of colostral IgA comes from the blood and within 6 h after the onset of suckling this proportion de- clines to 11% [23]. Thus it appears that sow colostrum is mainly a transudate, and in this respect is similar to colostrum in the cow, goat, sheep [30], and horse [87], in which IgG_1 is always the most important globulin (Table 1). In species where maternal IgG passes the placenta in utero, such as human [7], monkey, and rabbit [164], the major immunoglobulin of colostrum is sIgA. In cow colostrum, 81% of the whole immunoglobulin content is IgG_1 [30]. A specific receptor for IgG_1 is responsible for the selective transfer of this im- munoglobulin from the plasma to the udder during colostrum formation [77]. In the IgA and IgM fractions of bovine colostrum, about equal amounts are plasma derived and locally produced [108]. In canine colostrum there are 100 times as much sIgA as sIgM.

There are striking differences in the proportion of immunoglobulin classes in milk of different species. After the rapid decrease of Ig content during early lactation the major immunoglobulin of milk in sows and horses is IgA (70%). Cow milk, however, contains IgG_1 in an amount of 73% of the whole Ig. In addition, a large amount of free, unbound SC is present in cow milk [83].

Table 1 Transmission of Maternal Immunoglobulins in Different Species Depending on Placentation and Predominance of Immunoglobulin Classes in Serum, Colostrum, and Milk

	Epitheliochorial placenta			Endotheliochorial placenta	Hemochorial placenta		
	Ruminants	Horse	Pig	Carnivores	Primates	Rodents	Rabbit, guinea pig
Route of transmission	Colostral	Colostral	Colostral	Transplantal, colostral	Trans-placental	Trans-placental colostral	Yolksack
Predominance of Ig classes							
Serum	$IgG_1 > IgG_2$ [30]	$IgG > IgG(T) \gg IgA$ [87]	$IgG \gg IgA$ [163]	$IgG_2 > IgG_1 > IgM$ [163]	$IgG \gg IgA$ [7]	$IgG > IgA$ [175]	$IgG_2 \gg IgG_1 > IgM$ [164]
Colostrum	$IgG_1 \gg IgA$ [30]	$IgG \gg IgG(T)$ [87]	$IgG \gg IgA$ [163]	$IgG > IgA \gg IgM$ [163]	$IgA \gg IgM$ [7]	$IgA > IgG$ [175]	$IgA > IgG$ [164]
Milk	$IgG_1 > IgA$ [30]	$IgA > IgG$ [87]	$IgA > IgG$ [163]	$IgA > IgM \gg IgG$ [163]	$IgA \gg IgM$ [7]	$IgA > IgG$ [175]	$IgA > IgG_2 > IgG_1$ [164]
Intestinal resorption within	24-36 h	24-36 h	24-56 h	10 days	None	16-20 days	None

Localization and Distribution of Antibody-Containing Cells in the Intestinal Tract

In a newborn mammal the number of lymphoid cells in the intestinal lamina propria is small. In response to the development of the intestinal microflora the lamina propria is infiltrated with lymphocytes and plasma cells. In newborn piglets IgM-containing cells outnumber those containing IgA and IgG [6]. In the lymphoid tissue of Peyer's patches of piglets the first IgA- and IgM-containing cells can be demonstrated at 3 days of age. In the intestine of pigs older than 1 month there is a slight predominance of IgA- over IgM-containing cells [28].

IgA- and IgM-containing plasma cells are most numerous in intestinal crypt epithelium, indicating that both immunoglobulins are secreted by a similar intracellular pathway. However, IgG-producing plasma cells are present in a considerable number, too. Immunoglobulin-bearing plasma cells have never been described in the stomach or the large intestine of pigs [29], and compared with the lamina propria of the intestinal tract the spleen and mesenteric lymph nodes of young and adult pigs contain relatively few mature plasma cells.

In the preruminant calf, IgA was demonstrated in the apical cytoplasm of epithelial cells in the lower region of the crypts in all regions of the small intestine, but less so in the duodenum. The localization of IgM was very similar to that described for IgA. IgG was seen in extravascular deposits throughout the connective tissue of the lamina propria in all regions of the small intestine [29].

In the lamina propria, IgA-bearing plasma cells were mainly present in the crypt regions of the small intestine, but very few were seen in the ileum [126].

Role of Secretory and Humoral Antibodies in Immunity

Neonatal animals are usually infected with enteropathogenic rotaviruses and coronaviruses within the first few hours or days of life [9,177]. One of the most important problems in these infections, therefore, is their prevention. Since the period between birth and infection is generally too short for an immunity to develop before infection, and uptake of colostral antibodies can interfere with the development of an active immunity [3], passive, "lactogenic" immunity seems to be relatively important in the prevention of neonatal viral gastroenteritis. In addition, active immunity is less important because susceptibility to these viruses decreases with age, and older animals usually undergo subclinical infections [99,177].

Passive, Lactogenic Immunity

Mechanisms by which immunity to a neonatal virus enteritis can be transmitted from dam to offspring have been studied extensively in TGE of pigs [10, 17,20,71,146]. The term *lactogenic immunity* was used to describe the protection conferred by the continuing presence of antibody in the intestine. It is assumed that immunity depends on the neutralization of virus in the lumen of the alimentary tract by antibody in colostrum or milk [71]. The newborn animal nursing from an immune mother, therefore, is protected against infection with enteropathogenic viruses only while lacteal antibodies are excreted. The duration of this period is species dependent and lasts from a few days in ruminants [2,50,171,180] to several weeks in pigs [10,18]. The most effective protection is provided by continued secretion of sIgA [17,18,20,66] although IgG has been shown to be protective when present in high concentration [20, 146].

In naturally infected pigs, TGE-specific IgG titers drop within 3-4 days after parturition to one-tenth of those in early colostrum. IgA shows a two- to threefold decrease within the first week of lactation and is secreted for 3-4 weeks thereafter with only slow reduction in titer.

Preliminary results indicate that the situation is similar in rotavirus infection in pigs. High specific rotavirus antibody titers have been demonstrated in colostrum and milk from naturally infected sows, and antibodies were associated with both IgA and IgG fractions [16].

Furthermore, the stability of purified porcine colostral immunoglobulin classes is variable. Secretory IgA is more resistant to trypsin, pepsin, and gastric juice than IgG, IgG being more stable than IgM [147].

In contrast, immunoglobulin levels in cow's milk decrease rapidly within 2-3 days after parturition, independently of the initial amount in colostrum [123]. Investigations determining the amount and duration of specific rotavirus antibodies in bovine colostrum and milk confirm these results [2,50,180]. Rotavirus antibody titers sank rapidly during the first 48 h after parturition and could not be demonstrated for longer than 3-4 days. Specific rotavirus antibody titers in bovine colostrum, however, vary to a large extent [50]. Similar observations were made in sheep [142,171].

In spite of these species differences, it seems clear that IgA colostral and milk antibodies can be effectively stimulated only after an intestinal infection of the dam [17,20]. Other inoculation routes gave variable results in experiments with TGE in pigs. Oral application of virulent TGE virus always results in the secretion of high IgA antibody titers in colostrum and milk [10,18]. Similarly, high specific milk IgA antibody titers can be induced with certain attenuated TGE virus strains when given orally in acid-stable capsules [10] or intranasally [138] to pregnant sows. Experiments with different attenuated TGE virus strains, however, revealed differences in their capacity to induce lacteal IgA or protection [116,181]. If virus is given by mouth, strains propagated in swine kidney cells may not stimulate sufficient lacteal IgA production [20, 102]; whereas those propagated in thyroid cells induce large amounts of lacteal

IgA and give good passive protection of newborn piglets [10,69]. In addition, a TGE virus variant propagated in a leukocyte cell line induces enough passive immunity in sows' milk to protect newborn piglets against a virulent oral challenge infection [181].

Intramuscular application of attenuated [20,128] or inactivated [156, 157] TGE virus does not stimulate any protective effect in the colostrum and milk of treated sows. After separation and purification it was shown that the immunoglobulin class present in the lacteal secretions of these immunized sows was almost entirely IgG, which rapidly disappeared after a few days of lactation [16,20]. Also, purified TGE virus components do not induce lactogenic immunity when given to pregnant sows [59]. In cases where virulent virus was given parenterally some of the recipients developed diseases, and these amounts produced sufficient lacteal antibodies to protect piglets [17,20].

After intramammary application to pregnant sows of virulent TGE virus [48], the results are contradictory. In some investigations sIgA stimulation has been reported [1], while others found only IgG [20,132]. But in all reports challenged piglets were protected. Specific antibody activity was found not only in the mammary glands that were vaccinated but also in nonvaccinated glands [48,156]. However, when attenuated TGE virus was given intramammarily, specific antibody activity was always associated with IgG and declined rapidly shortly after parturition [132,136]. There is no proper explanation for these findings, which invite speculation, and at the moment they cannot be applied in the field.

With respect to lactogenic immunity, the situation in the ruminant is not so favorable. As was discussed earlier, specific rotavirus antibody is present in high titer in day 1 colostrum, and a rapid decline is observed within 2-3 days [171,180]. This is associated with a drastic decrease in total immunoglobulins in cow's colostrum and milk [123].

Inactivated calf rotavirus has been given to cows, and a reduced incidence of diarrhea in their calves was observed, but milk antibody estimates are not available [94]. More detailed studies were made in which ewes were inoculated prior to mating with inactivated lamb rotavirus [142,171]. Nonimmunized control ewes had moderate titers of antibody in day 1 colostrum, but these were undetectable by day 4. The immunized ewes had high antibody titers in colostrum, and these remained higher, compared to controls, for the 10 day sampling period. The antibody activity in both groups, however, was associated largely with IgG.

Another approach to stimulation of high antibody titers in colostrum and milk was taken by Wellemans et al. [169], who applied a mixture of aluminum hydroxide and oil adjuvant parenterally to pregnant cows 15 days prior to, and at the day of, parturition. Since almost all cattle have antibodies to rotavirus from previous infections, it was possible to stimulate prolonged secretion of specific antibodies against bovine rotavirus and coronavirus as well as against BVD virus. During the whole sampling period of 20 days, specific IgG and IgA was detectable, although in a considerably reduced amount. In untreated controls, antibodies were absent from 4 days after parturition. The treatment resulted in a lower incidence of virus-induced diarrheas in calves [169].

In addition, the question has been raised whether circulating antibodies absorbed from colostrum can protect neonates. Although passage of circulating IgM and IgG antibodies into the gut lumen has been reported [39,65], there is little evidence that they protect against intestinal virus infection. It seems, however, from limited experiments that antibodies in the intestinal lumen of sheep originating from serum can interfere with the development of diarrhea, when present in large amounts [14].

There appear to be two ways in which colostrum can be used to confer protection against virus diarrhea. The first is to ensure that large amounts of colostrum and, later, milk are ingested, and one has to keep in mind that there are considerable species differences. This may be the method of choice in pigs [18], but is only of limited value in ruminants [142] or humans [158], since antibody titers decline rapidly a few days after parturition. Second, and possibly more effectively, smaller amounts of colostrum can be fed in the diet, and this probably protects for as long as it is continued. Antibody-containing serum has also been fed with encouraging results [27,52,142]. The regular feeding of either colostrum, serum, or gammaglobulin to lambs or pigs resulted in the alleviation of clinical signs [82,142]. In addition to specific antibodies in colostrum and milk, nonspecific viral inhibitors may also be present. Antiviral activity in a glycoprotein fraction of human and bovine milk not containing antibody has been reported [86]. This same glycoprotein fraction from cow milk was shown to exhibit anti-rotaviral action [158]. Its role in vivo, however, has not been assessed.

Active Immune Response

Earlier studies involving inoculation with polioviruses suggested that individuals with a history of natural infection or oral inoculation with live virus had a local intestinal immunity against poliovirus infection. On challenge of such persons the virus replicated more slowly and was excreted for longer than in susceptible individuals [131]. These results support the concept that active immunity against enteropathogenic virus infections largely depends on locally produced antibodies, or is mediated by a combination of B- and T-cell-mediated immune mechanisms.

Natural infection of 5-month-old pigs with TGE virus protects the affected animal against reinfection for 9-12 months [18]. Virus-binding and neutralizing activities were detected in intestinal extracts between 7 and 56 days after infection. The concentration of binding antibodies (measured by complexing with labeled specific antibody and TGE virus) reached a peak 21 days after infection and declined thereafter. Neutralizing antibody increased up to day 56. Both antibody populations consisted predominantly of IgA [143].

These results, however, may not be representative for young piglets since TGE virus replication was delayed. Antigen was demonstrated in the intestinal epithelium for 14-21 days after infection. The course of infection runs much faster in newborn piglets, and the development of active immunity may show a different pattern. There is evidence that newborn piglets develop effective active local immunity as early as 3-4 days of age, when immunized with an attenuated TGE virus strain [56,138].

Very interesting results were obtained in turkey poults infected with (blue comb) coronavirus. Specific IgA antibodies were found in the intestine and bile throughout the sampling period of between 10 days and 6 months, whereas in recovered birds specific serum antibodies were undetectable for 30 days after infection [106]. These results fit in with observations that birds that have recovered from natural infection have lifelong immunity in spite of very low virus-neutralizing capacity in serum [122], and show once more that the presence or absence of serum antibodies is of little use as a parameter of immunity in intestinal infection.

Early experiments with bovine rotavirus and coronavirus infection revealed that gnotobiotic calves are protected within 2-3 days after they are inoculated with an attenuated rotavirus [93,94]. It was suggested that this protection was due to interference, since local immunity in the calf intestine only develops between 4 and 8 days after infection [123]. In a more recent study of calves inoculated with the same attenuated rotavirus strain, followed by a different challenge virus, protection was detected between 7 and 21 days after inoculation [178]. It was suggested that these differences result from the greater virulence of the challenge virus strain; however, they do illustrate the complexity of such studies and show the preliminary state of recent investigations.

Contradictory results have also been reported from experiments on the protection of calves or pigs by rotaviruses isolated from different species. These investigations were made on the assumption that all rotaviruses share a common antigen, and that at least some rotavirus strains can induce disease in heterologous species.

Calves were immunized in utero 3-5 weeks before delivery with bovine rotavirus and at birth were fully protected against a challenge with human rotavirus type 2 (Wyatt and Mebus, unpublished data, 1978). However, in another study, only one of three calves inoculated with foal rotavirus, and one of three given human rotavirus, were protected against bovine rotavirus challenge [180].

Furthermore, a tissue culture-attenuated bovine rotavirus strain did not protect piglets against infection with porcine rotavirus [81]. Some of these differences are due to the inability of the immunizing strains to replicate and induce local immunity in a heterologous host [81], but probably they are also due to antigenic differences since different serotypes of human rotavirus have been demonstrated recently [183]. Observations made during longitudinal surveillance of infants and young children indicate that infection with human rotavirus type 1 does not protect against disease caused by type 2 [54]. A similar situation may also exist among animal rotavirus strains, and this would explain these conflicting results.

The effect of the uptake of specific colostrum and milk antibodies on the development of a local immune response has an important effect on the development of active immunity in the neonate. Field investigations with a bovine rotavirus vaccine given to calves on the day of birth show that lacteal antibodies can interfere with the induction of a specific, active local immune response [3, 43]. Apparently the mechanisms that prevent an early infection with wild virus also prevent the replication of vaccine virus.

Aspects of Immune Prophylaxis

It is well established that the route of administration of an antigen determines the site and nature of the immunoglobulin produced. The local administration of an antigen stimulates a local immune response predominantly of secretory IgA, although a systemic response may also occur. Conversely, following parenteral administration of an antigen, the immune response is systemic and predominantly of IgG [105]. In principal, either live or inactivated vaccines can be used. It has been convincingly shown that heat-inactivated *E. coli* bacteria induce a local immunity in newborn calves and pigs, when given orally [11]. Since, however, the effective dose of inactivated antigen needed for stimulation is about 100 times higher than that of living bacteria, it is likely that live, attenuated viral vaccines given orally will be more effective than inactivated vaccines administered orally or parenterally.

A number of theoretical considerations have to be taken into account before a vaccine effective against neonatal diarrhea is developed. First, rotaviruses and coronaviruses are difficult to grow to high titers in tissue culture, a prerequisite for attenuating and producing virus antigen for vaccination. This problem has only been adequately solved for a bovine rota-coronavirus vaccine and for TGE virus vaccine strains. Rotaviruses or coronaviruses of many species, including the human, do not replicate well. In addition, the possibility of antigenic variation has been inadequately studied so far. There is evidence that there are different serotypes of human rotaviruses [183], but for animal rotaviruses the question is still unanswered.

Heterospecific vaccines have been discussed for the prevention of rotavirus disease [33]. Rotaviruses from certain species may be close enough antigenically to be useful in other species. Nevertheless the preliminary results available so far do not show whether attenuated rotaviruses replicate well enough in the heterologous vaccinee to stimulate a solid local immunity. With one exception, in which bovine rotavirus protected calves against diarrhea induced by human rotavirus (Wyatt and Mebus, unpublished data, 1978), the results reported have been negative. Piglets could not be protected with bovine rotavirus vaccine against porcine rotavirus [81], and calves inoculated orally with human and foal rotavirus were only partly protected against bovine rotavirus challenge [178].

Furthermore, immunologic obstacles have to be overcome. Neonates may show an inadequate or transient immune response to rotavirus vaccination. It is known from studies in humans that immunity from prior natural infection is not completely protective although reinfection is usually subclinical [33]. Also, as discussed earlier, local IgA immune response is possibly deficient in immunologic memory and difficult to boost.

Whether active or passive immunization would be more useful depends on the species involved.

Animal species that secrete IgA antibodies with colostrum and milk for some weeks after parturition are likely to be candidates for a passive immunization method. This applied to pigs, and after a considerable number of failures using attenuated TGE virus strains for oral or parenteral applications [17,69, 116], a small number of tissue culture-attenuated virus strains has been developed that stimulate lacteal IgA antibodies in the sow. These vaccines are still in an experimental stage, but are at present being tested in the field. They are applied orally to pregnant sows usually twice at about 6 and 2 weeks before parturition, and the piglets of these sows survive well after challenge [69,95]. We have used the TGE virus strain Bl after 300 passages in thyroid cell cultures [68] for oral vaccination of sows, and were able to stimulate high proportions of specific IgA antibodies in colostrum and milk [10]; 90% of the piglets survived when challenged with 100–500 lethal doses of a standard dose of a virulent field strain [69]. Limited field experiments confirmed the encouraging results obtained in the laboratory. The routine use of this vaccine, however, is limited at present by technical problems, such as the production of the vaccine in thyroid cell cultures and the administration of the vaccine by mouth.

In species in which IgA antibodies are secreted for only a short period after parturition, active immunization would be more promising. Ruminants are an example of such species, and several attempts have been made to actively vaccinate against rotaviruses and coronaviruses in calves. A commercially available tissue culture-attenuated rota-coronavirus combination vaccine induces immunity to challenge in gnotobiotic calves between 3 [94] and 7-21 [178] days, depending on the virulence of the challenge virus strain. The vaccine is administered orally immediately after birth and a few hours before first colostrum intake. Although the mechanism of early protection is uncertain, a considerable decrease in the incidence of viral enteritis was observed in herds in which all calves were vaccinated [159]. However, the efficacy of this vaccine in the field has been questioned. Two well-controlled double-blind studies [3, 43] did not reveal significant differences among the immunization groups in the incidence and severity of diarrhea. The failure may have been due to concomitant infections with other enteropathogenic agents [75], or because colostral antibodies interfered with the development of an effective local immunity.

A similar approach was made with an attenuated TGE virus strain (TO), and vaccination of newborn piglets resulted in immunity to challenge 4–5 days later [56]. In these experiments vaccinal virus replication was reduced if animals were fed colostrum before oral administration of the vaccine. However, recent investigations show that proper immunologic engineering could activate the enormous immunologic potentials at mucous surfaces. For example, IgA antibody induced by a previous infection is stimulated by parenteral administration of virus antigen. This approach has been used successfully to increase an already existing IgA immunity to cholera [33]. In addition, prolonged secretion of IgA antibodies was induced by stimulating nonspecifically the defense mechanisms of pregnant cows with an adjuvant [169].

References

1. M. H. Abou-Youssef and M. Ristic, Protective effect of immunoglobulins in serum and milk of sows exposed to transmissible gastroenteritis virus, Can. J. Comp. Med., 35:41 (1975).
2. S. D. Acres and L. A. Babiuk, Studies on rotaviral antibody in bovine serum and lacteal secretions, using radioimmunoassay, J. Am. Vet. Med. Assoc., 173:555 (1978).
3. S.D. Acres and O. M. Radostits, The efficacy of a modified live reo-like virus vaccine and an E. coli bacterin for prevention of acute undifferentiated neonatal diarrhea of beef calves, Can. Vet. J., 17:197 (1976).
4. S. D. Acres, C. J. Laing, J. R. Saunders, and O. M. Radostits, Acute undifferentiated neonatal diarrhea in beef calves. I. Occurrence and distribution of infectious agents, Can. J. Comp. Med., 39:116 (1975).
5. W. R. Adams and L. M. Kraft, Electron-microscopic study of the intestinal epithelium of mice infected with the agent of epizootic diarrhea of infant mice (EDIM virus), Am. J. Pathol., 51:39 (1967).
6. W. D. Allen and P. Porter, The relative distribution of IgM and IgA cells in intestinal mucosa and lymphoid tissue of the young unweaned pig and their significance in ontogenesis of secretory immunity, Immunology, 24: 493 (1973).
7. A. J. Ammann and E. R. Stiehm, Immune globulin levels in colostrum and breast milk, and serum from formula- and breast-fed newborns, Proc. Soc. Exp. Biol. Med., 122:1098 (1966).

8. M. J. G. Appel, B. J. Cooper, H. Greisen, F. Scott, and L. E. Carmichael, Canine viral enteritis. I. Status report on corona- and parvo-like viral enteritides, *Cornell Vet., 69*:123 (1979).

9. P. A. Bachmann, Pathogenetic features of intestinal coronavirus infections, Proc. 4th Munich Symp. Microbiol. Munich, 1979.

10. P. A. Bachmann and R. G. Hess, Versuche zur Entwicklung einer Immunprophylaxe gegen die Übertragbare Gastroenteritis (TGE) der Schweine. II. Immunogenität des Stammes Bl im Verlauf von Serienpassagen, *Zentralbl. Veterinaermed. [B], 25*:52 (1978).

11. G. Baljer, Possibilities and limitations of oral immunization against *Escherichia coli* in piglets and calves, *Fortschr. Vet. Med.*, in press (1979).

12. W. Bay, W. Doyle and L. M. Hutchings, The pathology and symptomatology of transmissible gastroenteritis, *Am. J. Vet. Res., 12*:215 (1951).

13. A. Besredka, *Local Immunization*, Williams & Wilkins, Baltimore, 1927.

14. D. C. Biggers, L. M. Kraft, and H. Sprintz, Lethal-intestinal virus infection of mice (LIVIM): An important new model for study of the response of the intestinal mucosa to injury, *Am. J. Pathol., 45*:413 (1964).

15. K. L. Blaxter and W. A. Wood, Some observations on the biochemical and physiological events associated with diarrhea in calves, *Vet. Rec., 65*:889 (1953).

16. E. H. Bohl, Comments on passive immunity in rotaviral infections, *J. Am. Vet. Med. Assoc., 173*:568 (1978).

17. E. H. Bohl, G. T. Frederick, and L. J. Saif, Passive immunity in transmissible gastroenteritis of swine: Intramuscular injection of pregnant swine with a modified live virus vaccine, *Am. J. Vet. Res., 36*:267 (1975).

18. E. H. Bohl, R. K. P. Gupta, F. M. W. Olquin, and L. J. Saif, Antibody responses in serum, colostrum and milk of swine after infection or vaccination with transmissible gastroenteritis virus, *Infect. Immun., 6*:289 (1972).

19. E. H. Bohl, E. M. Kohler, L. J. Saif, R. F. Cross, A. G. Agnes, and K. W. Theil, Rotavirus as a cause of diarrhoea in pigs, *J. Am. Vet. Med. Assoc., 172*:458 (1978).

20. E. H. Bohl and L. J. Saif, Passive immunity in transmissible gastroenteritis of swine: Immunoglobulin characteristics of antibodies in milk after inoculating virus by different routes, *Infect. Immun., 11*:23 (1975).

21. R. Bolivar, R. H. Conklin, J. J. Vollett, L. K. Pickering, H. L. Dupont, D. L. Walters, and S. Kohl. Rotavirus in Traveler's diarrhea: study of an adult student population in Mexico, *J. Infect. Dis., 137*:324 (1978).

22. J. F. Bourne, Structural features of pig IgA, *Immunol. Commun., 3*:157 (1974).

23. F. J. Bourne and J. Curtis, The transfer of immunoglobulins IgG, IgA and IgM from serum to colostrum and milk in the sow, *Immunology, 24*:157 (1973).

24. P. Brandtzaeg, Human secretory immunoglobulin M. An immunochemical and immunohistochemical study, *Immunology, 29*:559 (1975).

25. P. Brandtzaeg and K. Baklien, Intestinal secretion of IgA and IgM: A hypothetical model. In *Immunology of the gut*, Ciba Found. Symposium No. 46 Elsevier/Excerpta Medica/North Holland, Amsterdam, 1977, p. 77.

26. P. Brandtzaeg, I. Fjellanger, and S. T. Gjeruldsen, Local synthesis and selective secretion in patients with IgA deficiency, *Science, 160*:789 (1968).

27. J. C. Bridger and G. N. Woode, Neonatal calf diarrhoea: Identification of a reovirus-like (rotavirus) agent in faeces by immunofluorescence and immune electron microscopy, *Br. Vet. J., 131*:528 (1975).

28. P. J. Brown and F. J. Bourne, Distribution of immunoglobulin-containing cells in alimentary tract, spleen and mesenteric lymph node of the pig demonstrated by peroxidase-conjugated antiserums to porcine immunoglobulins G, A, and M, *Am. J. Vet. Res., 37*:9 (1976).

29. P. J. Brown and F. J. Bourne, Development of immunoglobulin-containing cell populations in intestine, spleen, and mesenteric lymph node of the young pig, as demonstrated by peroxidase-conjugated antiserums, *Am. J. Vet. Res., 37*:1309 (1976).

30. J. E. Butler, Synthesis and distribution of immunoglobulins, *J. Am. Vet. Med. Assoc., 163*:795 (1973).

31. D. G. Butler, D. G. Gall, M. H. Kelly, and J. R. Hamilton, Transmissible gastroenteritis. Mechanisms responsible for diarrhea in an acute enteritis in piglets, *J. Clin. Invest., 53*:1335 (1974).

32. M. E. Carr, D. W. McKendrick, and T. Spyridakis, The clinical features of infantile gastroenteritis due to rotavirus, *Scand. J. Infect. Dis., 8*:241 (1976).

33. R. M. Chanock, R. G. Wyatt, and A. Z. Kapikian, Immunization of infants and young children against rotaviral gastroenteritis—prospects and problems, *J. Am. Vet. Med. Assoc., 173*:570 (1978).

34. W. Chodirker and T. B. Tomasi, Gamma globulins: Quantitative relationships in human serum and nonvascular fluids, *Science, 142*:1080 (1963).

35. B. J. Cooper, L. E. Carmichael, M. J. G. Appel, and H. Greisen, Canine viral enteritis. II. Morphologic lesions in naturally occurring parvovirus infection, *Cornell Vet., 69*:134 (1979).

36. B. S. Cowan and S. B. Hitchner, pH stability studies with avian infectious bronchitis virus (coronavirus) strains, *J. Virol., 16*:430 (1975).

37. P. A. Crabbé, A. O. Carbonara, and J. F. Heremans, The normal human intestinal mucosa as a major source of plasma cells containing γ_A-immunoglobulins, *Lab. Invest., 14*:235 (1965).

38. R. K. Crane, Enzymes and malabsorption: A concept of brush border membrane disease, *Gastroenterology, 50*:254 (1966).

39. A. W. Cripps, A. J. Husband, and A. K. Lacelles, The origin of immunoglobulins in intestinal secretion of sheep, *Aust. J. Exp. Biol. Med. Sci., 52*:711 (1974).

40. R. F. Cross and E. M. Kohler, Autolytic changes in the digestive system of germfree, *Escherichia coli* contaminated, and conventional baby pigs, *Can. J. Comp. Med., 33*:108 (1969).

41. C. K. Czisa, A. de Lahunta, F. W. Scott, and J. H. Gillespie, Pathogenesis of feline panleukopenia virus in susceptible newborn kittens. II. Pathology and immunofluorescence, *Infect. Immun., 3*:838 (1971).

42. G. P. Davidson, D. G. Gall, M. Petric, D. G. Butler, and J. R. Hamilton. Human rotavirus enteritis induced in conventional piglets, *J. Clin. Invest., 60*:1402 (1977).
43. P. W. De Leeuw, D. J. Ellens, P. J. Straver, and J. A. M. van Balken, Rotavirus and coronavirus infections in dairy calves in the Netherlands, *Bull. Off. Int. Epizootics* (1979).
44. D. R. Desmukh and B. S. Pomeroy, Physicochemical characterization of a bluecomb coronavirus of turkeys, *Am. J. Vet. Res., 35*:1549 (1974).
45. G. W. A. Dick, J. S. F. Niven, and A. W. Gledhill, A virus related to that causing hepatitis in mice (MHV), *Br. J. Exp. Pathol., 137*:90 (1956).
46. H. C. Dominick and G. Maass, Rotavirusinfektionen im Kindesalter, *Klin. Paediatr., 191*:33 (1979).
47. R. M. Donaldson, Role of enteric microorganisms in malabsorption, *Fed. Proc., 26*:1426 (1967).
48. S. Djurickovic and J. Thorsen, Experimental immunization of sows against transmissible gastroenteritis. I. Immunization with a bacteria-free suspension of transmissible gastroenteritis virus prepared from the intestines of infected pigs, *Vet. Rec., 87*:62 (1970).
49. P. Eccheverria, N. R. Blacklow, J. L. Vollet, C. V. Ulyangco, G. Cukor, V. B. Soriano, H. L. DuPont, J. H. Cross, F. Ørskov and I. Ørskov, Reovirus-like agent and enterotoxigenic *Escherichia coli* infections in pediatric diarrhea in the Phillipines, *J. Infect. Dis., 138*:326 (1978).
50. D. J. Ellens, P. W. de Leeuw, and P. J. Straver, The detection of rotavirus specific antibody in colostrum and milk by Elisa, *Ann. Rech. Vet., 9*: 337 (1978).
51. A. K. Eugster and C. Nairn, Diarrhea in puppies: Parvovirus-like particles demonstrated in their feces, *Southwest Vet., 30*:59 (1977).
52. M. Eskildsen, Examination of field material with a view to isolating transmissible gastroenteritis virus in Denmark and experimental testing of prophylactic immune serum treatment, *Bull. Off. Int. Epizootics, 76*:257 (1971).
53. E. W. Fisher and A. A. Martinez, Aspects of body fluid dynamics of neonatal calf diarrhoea, *Res. Vet. Sci., 20*:302 (1976).
54. J. Fonteyne, G. Zissis, and J. P. Lambert, Recurrent rotavirus gastroenteritis, *Lancet, 1*:983 (1978).
55. G. T. Frederick and E. H. Bohl, Local and systemic cell-mediated immunity against transmissible gastroenteritis: An intestinal viral infection of swine, *J. Immunol., 116*:1000 (1976).
56. S. Furuuchi, Y. Shimizu, and T. Kumagai, Vaccination of newborn pigs with an attenuated strain of transmissible gastroenteritis virus, *Am. J. Vet. Res., 37*:1401 (1976).
57. N. Gadol, R. H. Waldman, and L. W. Clem, Inhibition of macrophage migration by normal guinea pig intestinal secretions, *Proc. Soc. Exp. Biol. Med., 151*:654 (1976).
58. D. G. Gall, D. Chapman, M. Kelly, and J. R. Hamilton, Sodium transport in jejunal crypt cells, *Gastroenterology, 72*:452 (1977).

59. D. J. Garwes, M. H. Lucas, D. E. Higgins, B. V. Pike, and S. F. Cartwright, Antigenicity of structural components from porcine transmissible gastro-enteritis virus, *Vet. Microbiol., 3*:179 (1978/79).

60. J. H. Gillespie and F. W. Scott, Feline viral infections, *Adv. Vet. Sci. Comp. Med., 17*:164 (1973).

61. E. Gonder, B. L. Patel, and B. S. Pomeroy, Scanning electron, light and immunofluorescent microscopy of coronaviral enteritis of turkeys (blue-comb), *Am. J. Vet. Res., 37*:1435 (1976).

62. G. A. Hall, J. C. Bridger, R. L. Chandler, and G. N. Woode, Gnotobiotic piglets experimentally infected with neonatal calf diarrhoea reovirus-like agent (rotavirus), *Vet. Pathol., 13*:197 (1976).

63. C. G. Halpin and I. W. Caple, Changes in intestinal structure and function of neonatal calves infected with reovirus-like agent and *Escherichia coli, Aust. Vet. J., 52*:438 (1976).

64. K. Harada, T. Kaji, T. Kumagai, and J. Sasahara, Studies on transmissible gastroenteritis in pigs. IV. Physicochemical and biological properties of TGE virus, *Natl. Inst. Anim. Health. Q., 8*:140 (1968).

65. R. J. Heddle and D. Rowley, The source of IgM and IgG in the dog intes-tine, *Aust. J. Exp. Biol. Med. Sci., 56*:713 (1978).

66. J. F. Heremans, H. T. Heremans, and H. E. Schultze, Isolation and descrip-tion of a few properties of β_{2A}-globulin of human serum, *Clin. Chim. Acta, 4*:96 (1959).

67. R. G. Hess and P. A. Bachmann, In vitro differentiation and pH sensitivity of field and cell culture attenuated strains of transmissible gastroenteritis virus (TGE), *Infect. Immun., 13*:1642 (1976).

68. R. G. Hess, P. A. Bachmann, and T. Hänichen, Versuche zur Entwicklung einer Immunprophylaxe gegen die Übertragbare Gastroenteritis (TGE) der Schweine. I. Pathogenität des Stammes Bl im Verlaufe von Serien-passagen, *Zentralbl. Veterinaermed. [B]24*:753 (1977).

69. R. G. Hess, P. A. Bachmann, and A. Mayr, Versuche zur Entwicklung einer Immunprophylaxe gegen die Übertragbare Gastroenteritis (TGE) der Schweine. III. Passiver Immuntransfer nach oraler Impfung trächtiger Sauen mit dem attenuierten TGE-Virusstamm Bl, *Zentralbl. Veterin-aermed. [B] 25*:308 (1978).

70. J. C. Hierholzer, J. R. Broderson, and F. A. Murphy, A new strain of mouse hepatitis virus as the cause of lethal enteritis (LIVIM) infection in infant mice, *Infect. Immun., 24*:508 (1979).

71. B. E. Hooper and E. O. Haelterman, Concepts of pathogenesis and passive immunity in transmissible gastroenteritis of swine, *J. Am. Vet. Med. Assoc., 149*:1580 (1966).

72. B. E. Hooper and E. O. Haelterman, Lesions of the gastrointestinal tract of pigs infected with transmissible gastroenteritis, *Can. J. Comp. Med., 33*:29 (1969).

73. D. E. Kahn, Pathogenesis of feline panleukopenia, *J. Am. Vet. Med. Assoc., 173*:628 (1978).

74. A. Z. Kapikian, R. G. Wyatt, A. R. Kalica, R. M. Chanock, and C. A. Mebus, Rotaviruses, Norwalk and Norwalk-like viruses: Experimental animals and "in vitro" systems, *Proc. 2. Munich Symp. Microbiol.*, Munich, 1977.

75. A. Z. Kapikian, R. H. Yolken, R. G. Wyatt, A. R. Kalica, R. M. Chanock, and H. W. Kim, Viral diarrhea. Etiology and control, *Am. J. Clin. Nutr., 31*:2219 (1978).

76. K. P. Keenan, H. R. Jervis, R. H. Marchwicki, and L. N. Binn, Intestinal infection of neonatal dogs with canine coronavirus 1-71: Studies by virologic, histologic, histochemical, and immunfluorescent techniques, *Am. J. Vet. Res., 37*:247 (1976).

77. R. Kemler, H. Mosmann, K. Strohmaier, B. Kickhöfer, and D. K. Hammer, In vitro studies on the selective binding of IgG from different species to tissue sections of the bovine mammary gland, *Eur. J. Immunol., 5*:603 (1975).

78. T. H. Kent, S. B. Formal, E. H. LaBrec, and A. Takeuchi, Diffuse enteritis due to *S. typhimurium* in opium-treated guinea pigs, *Fed. Proc. 25*:1494 (1966).

79. B. Kerzner, M. H. Kelly, D. G. Gall, D. G. Butler, and J. R. Hamilton, Transmissible gastroenteritis: sodium transport and the intestinal epithelium during the course of viral enteritis, *Gastroenterology, 72*:457 (1977).

80. L. M. Kraft, Observations on the control and natural history of epidemic diarrhoea of infant mice (EDIM), *Yale J. Biol. Med., 31*:121 (1958).

81. J. G. Lecce and M. W. King, The calf reo-like virus (rotavirus) vaccine: An ineffective immunization agent for rotaviral diarrhoea of piglets, *Can. J. Comp. Med., 43*:90 (1979).

82. J. G. Lecce, M. W. King, and R. Mock, Reovirus-like agent associated with fatal diarrhea in neonatal pigs, *Infect. Immun., 14*:816 (1976).

83. J. P. Mach and J. J. Pahud, Secretory IgA, a major immunoglobulin in most bovine external excretions, *J. Immunol., 106*:552 (1971).

84. J. P. Mach, J. J. Pahud, and H. Isliker, IgA with secretory piece in bovine colostrum and saliva, *Nature, 223*:952 (1969).

85. G. Marsolais, R. Assaf, C. Montpetit, and P. Marois, Diagnosis of viral agents associated with neonatal calf diarrhea, *Can. J. Comp. Med., 42*:168 (1978).

86. T. H. J. Matthews, C. D. G. Nair, M. K. Lawrenc, and D. A. J. Tyrrell, Antiviral activity in milk of possible clinical importance, *Lancet, 2*:1387 (1976).

87. T. C. McGuire and T. B. Crawford, Identification and quantitation of equine serum and secretory IgA, *Infect. Immun., 6*:610 (1972).

88. A. F. McWilliams and J. L. Gowans, The presence of IgA on the surface of rat thoracic duct lymphocytes which contain internal IgA, *J. Exp. Med., 141*:335 (1975).

89. C. A. Mebus and L. E. Newman, Scanning electron, light and immunofluorescent microscopy of intestine of gnotobiotic calf infected with reovirus-like agent, *Am. J. Vet. Res., 38*:553 (1977).

90. C. A. Mebus, M. B. Rhodes, and N. R. Underdahl, Neonatal calf diarrhea caused by a virus that induces epithelial cell syncytia, *Am. J. Vet. Res.*, *39*:1223 (1978).

91. C. A. Mebus, E. L. Stair, M. B. Rhodes, and M. J. Twiehaus, Pathology of neonatal calf diarrhea induced by a coronavirus-like agent, *Vet. Pathol.*, *10*:45 (1973).

92. C. A. Mebus, E. L. Stair, N. R. Underdahl, and M. J. Twiehaus, Pathology of neonatal calf diarrhoea induced by a reolike virus, *Vet. Pathol.*, *8*: 490 (1971).

93. C. A. Mebus, A. Torres-Medina, M. J. Twiehaus, and E. P. Bass, Immune response to orally administered calf reovirus-like agent and coronavirus vaccine, *Dev. Biol. Stand.*, *33*:346 (1976).

94. C. A. Mebus, R. G. White, E. P. Bass, and M. J. Twiehaus, Immunity to neonatal calf diarrhoea virus, *J. Am. Vet. Med. Assoc.*, *163*:880 (1973).

95. E. Mocsari, J. Benyeda, and E. Haghy, Vaccination experiments against transmissible gastroenteritis (TGE) of swine, *Acta Vet. Acad. Sci. Hung.*, *25*:37 (1975).

96. H. W. Moon, Epithelial cell migration in the alimentary mucosa of the suckling pig, *Proc. Soc. Exp. Biol. Med.*, *137*:151 (1971).

97. H. W. Moon, Mechanisms in the pathogenesis of diarrhea: A review, *J. Am. Vet. Med. Assoc.*, *172*:443 (1978).

98. H. W. Moon and D. D. Joel, Epithelial cell migration in the small intestine of sheep and calves, *Am. J. Vet. Res.*, *36*:187 (1975).

99. H. W. Moon, L. J. Kemeny, G. L. Lambert, S. L. Stark, and G. D. Booth, Age-dependent resistence to transmissible gastroenteritis of swine. III. Effects of epithelial cell kinetics on coronavirus production and atrophy of intestinal villi, *Vet. Pathol.*, *12*:434 (1975).

100. H. W. Moon, A. W. McClurkin, R. E. Isaacson, J. Pohlenz, S. M. Skartvedt, K. G. Gilette, and A. L. Baetz, Pathogenic relationships of rotavirus *Escherichia coli*, and other agents in mixed infections in calves, *J. Am. Vet. Med. Assoc.*, *173*:577 (1978).

101. H. W. Moon, J. O. Norman, and G. Lambert, Age dependent resistance to transmissible gastroenteritis of swine (TGE). I. Clinical signs and some mucosal dimensions in small intestine, *Can. J. Comp. Med.*, *37*:157 (1973).

102. A. Morilla, R. C. Klemm, P. Sprino, and M. Ristic, Neutralization of a transmissible gastroenteritis virus of swine by colostral antibodies elicited by intestine- and cell culture-propagated virus, *Am. J. Vet. Res.*, *37*:1011 (1976).

103. M. Morin, S. Lariviére, and R. Lallier, Pathological and microbiological observations made on spontaneous cases of acute neonatal calf diarrhea, *Can. J. Comp. Med.*, *40*:228 (1976).

104. F. A. Murphy, Viral pathogenetic mechanisms, Proc. 4. Munich Symp. Microbiol. Munich, 1979.

105. M. Murray, Local immunity and its role in vaccination, *Vet. Rec.*, *93*: 500 (1973).

106. K. V. Nagaraja and B. S. Pomeroy, Secretory antibodies against turkey coronaviral enteritis, *Am. J. Vet. Res., 39*:1463 (1978).
107. T. J. Newby and F. J. Bourne, The nature of the local immune system of the bovine small intestine, *Immunology, 31*:475 (1976).
108. T. J. Newby and F. J. Bourne, The nature of the local immune system of the bovine mammary gland, *J. Immunol., 118*:461 (1977).
109. P. L. Ogra, P. R. Coppola, M. H. MacGillivray, and J. L. Dzierba, Mechanisms of mucosal immunity to viral infections in β_A-immunoglobulin-deficiency syndrome, *Proc. Soc. Exp. Biol. Med., 145*:811 (1974).
110. P. L. Ogra, R. B. Wallace, G. Umana, S. S. Ogra, D. Kerrgrant, and A. Morag, Implications of secretory immune system in viral infections, *Adv. Exp. Med. Biol., 45*:271 (1974).
111. D. P. Olson, G. L. Wachsler, and A. W. Roberts, Small intestinal lesions of transmissible gastroenteritis in gnotobiotic pigs: A scanning electron microscopic study, *Am. J. Vet. Res., 34*:1239 (1973).
112. B. L. Patel, D. R. Deshmukh, and B. S. Pomeroy, Fluorescent antibody test for rapid diagnosis of coronaviral enteritis of turkeys (bluecomb), *Am. J. Vet. Res., 37*:1111 (1975).
113. G. R. Pearson and M. S. McNulty, Pathological changes in the small intestine of neonatal pigs infected with a pig reovirus-like agent (rotavirus), *J. Comp. Pathol., 87*:363 (1977).
114. G. R. Pearson and M. S. McNulty, Pathological changes in the small intestine of neonatal calves naturally infected with reo-like virus (rotavirus), *Vet. Rec., 102*:454 (1978).
115. M. Pensaert, Concepts and experiments on prevention and control of transmissible gastroenteritis of swine in the light of its pathogenesis, *Bull. Off. Int. Epizootics, 76*:105 (1971).
116. M. Pensaert, K. Andries, and P. De Roose, Vaccination trials in experimental and field sows using an attenuated transmissible gastroenteritis virus, *Bull. Off. Int. Epizootics* (1978).
117. M. Pensaert, E. O. Haelterman, and T. Burnstein, Transmissible gastroenteritis of swine: Virus-intestinal cell interactions. I. Immunofluorescence, histopathology and virus production in the small intestine through the course of infection, *Arch. Ges. Virusforsch., 31*:321 (1970).
118. M. Pensaert, E. O. Haelterman, and E. J. Hinsman, Transmissible gastroenteritis of swine: Virus-intestinal cell interactions. II. Electron microscopy of the epithelium in isolated jejunal loops, *Arch. Ges. Virusforsch., 31*:335 (1970).
119. S. F. Phillips, Diarrhoea: a current view of the pathophysiology, *Gastroenterology, 63*:495 (1972).
120. R. W. Phillips and L. D. Lewis, Viral induced changes in intestinal transport and resultant body fluid alterations in neonatal calves, *Ann. Rech. Vet., 4*:87 (1973).
121. N. P. Pierce and J. L. Gowans, Cellular kinetics of the intestinal immune response to cholera toxoid in rats, *J. Exp. Med., 142*:1550 (1975).

122. B. S. Pomeroy, C. T. Larsen, D. R. Deshmukh, and B. L. Patel, Immunity to transmissible (coronaviral) enteritis of turkeys (bluecomb), *Am. J. Vet. Res., 36*:553 (1975).

123. P. Porter, Immunoglobulins in bovine mammary secretions: Quantitative changes in early lactation and absorption by the neonatal calf, *Immunology, 23*:225 (1972).

124. P. Porter, Intestinal defence in the young pig—a review of the secretory antibody system and their possible role in oral immunization, *Vet. Rec., 92*:658 (1973).

125. P. Porter and W. D. Allen, Immunoglobulin A in the urine of conventional and colostrum-deprived hypogammaglobulinaemic pigs, *Immunology, 17*: 789 (1969).

126. P. Porter, D. E. Noakes, and W. D. Allen, Intestinal secretion of immunoglobulins in the preruminant calf, *Immunology, 23*:299 (1972).

127. P. Porter, S. H. Parry, and W. D. Allen, Significance of immune mechanisms in relation to enteric infections of the gastrointestinal tract in animals. In *Immunology of the Gut,* Ciba Foundation Symposium No. 46 Elsevier/Excerpta Medica/North Holland, Amsterdam, 1977, p. 77.

128. M. Ristic and M. H. Abou-Youssef, Comments on the immunology of transmissible gastroenteritis, *J. Am. Vet. Med. Assoc., 160*:549 (1972).

129. W. J. Rodriguez, H. W. Kim, J. O. Arrobio, C. D. Brandt, R. M. Chanock, A. Z. Kapikian, R. G. Wyatt, and R. H. Parrott, Clinical features of acute gastroenteritis associated with human reovirus-like agent in infants and young children, *J. Pediatr., 91*:188 (1977).

130. M. E. Roux, M. McWilliams, J. M. Phillips-Quagliata, P. Weisz-Carrington, and M. E. Lamm, Origin of IgA-secreting plasma cells in the mammary gland, *J. Exp. Med., 146*:1311 (1977).

131. A. B. Sabin, M. Ramos-Alvarez, J. Alvarez-Amezquita, H. W. Pelon, R. H. Michaels, J. Spigland, M. A. Koch, and J. M. Barnes, Live, orally given, poliovaccine, *JAMA, 173*:1521 (1960).

132. L. J. Saif, E. H. Bohl, and R. G. P. Gupta, Isolation of porcine immunoglobulins and determination of immunoglobulin classes of transmissible gastroenteritis viral antibodies, *Infect. Immun., 6*:600 (1972).

133. R. L. Sharpee, C. A. Mebus, and E. P. Bass, Characterization of a calf diarrhea coronavirus, *Am. J. Vet. Res., 37*:1031 (1976).

134. R. W. Shepherd, D. G. Butler, E. Cutz, D. G. Gall, and J. R. Hamilton, The mucosal lesion in viral enteritis: Extent and dynamics of the epithelial response to virus invasion in transmissible gastroenteritis in piglets, *Gastroenterology 76*:770 (1979).

135. M. B. Shepherd, D. G. Gall, D. G. Butler, and J. R. Hamilton, Determinants of diarrhoea in viral enteritis. The role of ion transport and epithelial changes in the ileum in transmissible gastroenteritis in piglets, *Gastroenterology, 76*:20 (1979).

136. G. P. Shibley, D. L. Salsbury, S. M. Djurickovic, and S. Johnson, Application of an intramammary role of vaccination against transmissible gastroenteritis in swine, *Vet. Med. Small Anim. Clin., 68*:59 (1973).

137. M. Shimizu and Y. Shimizu, Demonstration of cytotoxic lymphocytes to virus-infected target-cells in pigs inoculated with TGE virus, *Am. J. Vet. Res., 40*:208 (1979).

138. Y. Shimizu, M. Shimizu, and S. Furuuchi, Recent progress in research on prevention and diagnosis of transmissible gastroenteritis of pigs in Japan, *Bull. Off. Int. Epizootics* (1979).

139. R. G. Shorter, C. G. Moertel, J. L. Titus, and R. G. Reitemeier, Cell kinetics in the jejunum and rectum of man, *Am. J. Dig. Dis., 9*:760 (1964).

140. D. R. Snodgrass, K. W. Angus, and E. W. Gray, Rotavirus infection in lambs: Pathogenesis and pathology, *Arch. Virol., 55*:263 (1977).

141. D. R. Snodgrass, A. Ferguson, F. Allan, K. W. Angus, and B. Mitchel, Small intestinal morphology and epithelial cell kinetics in lamb rotavirus infections, *Gastroenterology, 76*:477 (1979).

142. D. R. Snodgrass and P. W. Wells, Passive immunity in rotaviral infections, *J. Am. Vet. Med. Assoc., 173*:565 (1978).

143. P. J. Sprino, A. Morilla, and M. Ristic, Intestinal immune response of feeder pigs to infection with transmissible gastroenteritis virus, *Am. J. Vet. Res., 37*:171 (1976).

144. E. L. Stair, C. A. Mebus, M. J. Twiehaus, and N. J. Underdahl, Neonatal calf diarrhoea. Electron microscopy of intestines infected with a reovirus-like agent, *Vet. Pathol., 10*:155 (1973).

145. T. E. Staley, E. W. Jones, and A. E. Marshall, The jejunal absorptive cell of the newborn pig: An electron microscopic study, *Anat. Rec., 161*: 497 (1968).

146. S. S. Stone, L. J. Kemeny, R. D. Woods, and M. T. Jensen, Efficacy of isolated colostral IgA, IgG and IgM (A) to protect neonatal pigs against the coronavirus of transmissible gastroenteritis, *Am. J. Vet. Res., 38*:1285 (1977).

147. S. S. Stone, M. Phillips, and L. J. Kemeny, Stability of porcine colostral immunoglobulins IgA, IgG2 and IgM to proteolytic enzymes, *Am. J. Vet. Res., 40*:607 (1979).

148. J. Storz, J. J. Leary, J. H. Carlson, and R. C. Bates, Parvoviruses associated with diarrhea in calves, *J. Am. Vet. Med. Assoc., 173*:624 (1978).

149. D. R. Strombeck and D. Harrold, Binding of cholera toxin to mucins and inhibition by gastric mucin, *Infect. Immun., 10*:1266 (1974).

150. S. Tallett, C. Mackenzie, P. Middleton, B. Kerzner, and R. J. Hamilton, Clinical, laboratory, and epidemiologic features of a viral gastroenteritis in infants and children, *Pediatrics, 60*:217 (1977).

151. D. C. Thake, Jejunal epithelium in transmissible gastroenteritis of swine. An electron microscopic and histochemical study, *Am. J. Pathol., 53*:149 (1968).

152. D. C. Thake, H. W. Moon, and G. Lambert, Epithelial cell dynamics in transmissible gastroenteritis of neonatal pigs, *Vet. Pathol., 10*:330 (1973).

153. K. W. Theil, E. H. Bohl, R. F. Cross, E. M. Kohler, and A. G. Agnes, Pathogenesis of porcine rotaviral infection in experimentally inoculated pigs, *Am. J. Vet. Res., 39*:213 (1978).

154. K. W. Theil, L. J. Saif, E. H. Bohl, A. G. Agnes, and E. M. Kohler, Concurrent porcine rotaviral and transmissible gastroenteritis viral infections in a three-day-old piglet, *J. Am. Vet. Med. Assoc., 40*:719 (1979).

155. R. E. Thompson and H. Y. Reynolds, Isolation and characterization of canine secretory immunoglobulin M, *J. Immunol., 117*:323 (1977).

156. J. Thorsen and S. Djurickovic, Experimental immunization of sows with cell-cultured TGE virus, *Can. J. Comp. Med., 34*:177 (1970).

157. J. Thorsen and S. Djurickovic, Experimental immunization of sows with inactivated transmissible gastroenteritis (TGE) virus, *Can. J. Comp. Med., 35*:99 (1972).

158. M. E. Thouless, A. S. Bryden, and T. H. Flewett, Rotavirus neutralization by human milk, *Br. Med. J., 2*:1390 (1977).

159. E. T. Thurber, E. P. Bass, and W. H. Beckenhauer, Field trial evaluation of a reo-coronavirus calf diarrhoea vaccine, *Can. J. Comp. Med., 41*:131 (1977).

160. T. B. Tomasi and J. Bienenstock, Secretory immunoglobulins, *Adv. Immunol., 9*:1 (1968).

161. D. R. Tourville, R.H. Adler, J. Bienenstock, and T. B. Tomasi, The human secretory immunoglobulin system: immunohistological localisation of β-A, secretory piece, and lactoferrin in normal tissues, *J. Exp. Med., 129*:411 (1969).

162. N. R. Underdahl, C. A. Mebus, E. L. Stair, M. B. Rhodes, L. D. McGill, and M. J. Twiehaus, Isolation of transmissible gastroenteritis virus from lungs of market swine, *Am. J. Vet. Res., 35*:1209 (1974).

163. J. P. Vaerman, Comparison between several mammalian IgA's, including the bovine, *J. Dairy Sci., 54*:1317 (1971).

164. J. P. Vaerman and J. F. Heremans, The IgA system of the guinea pig, *J. Immunol., 108*:637 (1972).

165. E. Van Opdenbosch, D. de Kegel, R. Strobbe, and G. Wellemans, La diarrhee neonatale des bovins: Une etiologie complexe, *Bull. Off. Int. Epizootics* (1979).

166. J. E. Wagner, P. D. Beamer, and M. Ristic, Electron microscopy of intestinal epithelial cells of piglets infected with transmissible gastroenteritis virus, *Can. J. Comp. Med., 37*:177 (1973).

167. W. A. Walker and K. J. Isselbacher, Intestinal antibodies, *N. Engl. J. Med., 297*:767 (1977).

168. R. G. Webster, M. Yakhno, V. S. Hinshaw, W. J. Bean, and K. G. Murti, Intestinal influenza: Replication and characterization of influenza viruses in duck, *Virology, 84*:268 (1978).

169. G. Wellemans, E. V. Opdenbosch, D. L. De Brabander, and C. V. Boucque, Prevention de la diarrhee neonatale des veaux par la prolongation de la secretion d'anticorps a un haut niveau dans le lait maternel, *Bull. Off. Int. Epizootics* (1979).

170. R. C. Welliver and P. L. Ogra, Importance of local immunity in enteric infection, *J. Am. Vet. Med. Assoc., 173*:560 (1978).

171. P. W. Wells, D. R. Snodgrass, J. A. Herring, and A. M. Dawson, Antibody titres to lamb rotavirus in colostrum and milk of vaccinated ewes, *Vet. Rec., 103*:46 (1978).
172. S. C. Whipp, Physiology of diarrhea-small intestine, *J. Am. Vet. Med. Assoc., 173*:662 (1978).
173. E. H. Whitten and R. W. Phillips, In vitro intestinal exchanges of Na^+K^+, Cl^-, $3H_2O$ in experimental bovine neonatal enteritis, *Am. J. Dig. Dis., 16*: 891 (1971).
174. M. D. Willard, J. E. Cook, L. S. Rodkey, A. D. Dayton, and N. V. Anderson, Morphologic evaluaction of IgM cells of the canine small intestine by fluorescence microscopy, *Am. J. Vet. Res., 39*:1502 (1978).
175. J. T. Willerson, R. Asofsky, and W. F. Barth, Experimental murine amyloid. IV. Amyloidosis and immunoglobulins, *J. Immunol., 103*:741 (1969).
176. R. E. Wilsnack, J. H. Blackwell, and J. C. Parker, Identification of an agent of epizootic diarrhoea of infant mice by immunofluorescent and complement-fixation tests, *Am. J. Vet. Res., 30*:1195 (1969).
177. G. N. Woode, Pathogenic rotaviruses isolated from pigs and calves. In *Diarrhoea in Childhood*, Ciba Foundation Symposium No. 42, Elsevier/ Excerpta Medica/North Holland, Amsterdam, 1976, p. 251.
178. G. N. Woode, M. E. Bew, and M. J. Dennis, Studies on cross protection induced in calves by rotaviruses of calves, children and foals, *Vet. Rec., 103*:32 (1978).
179. G. N. Woode and C. F. Crouch, Naturally occurring and experimentally induced rotaviral infection of domestic and laboratory animals, *J. Am. Vet. Med. Assoc., 173*:522 (1978).
180. G. N. Woode, J. M. Jones, and J. C. Bridger, Levels of colostral antibodies against neonatal calf diarrhoea virus, *Vet. Rec., 97*:148 (1975).
181. R. D. Woods, Small plaque variant transmissible gastroenteritis virus, *J. Am. Vet. Med. Assoc., 173*:643 (1978).
182. G. Zissis and J. P. Lambert, Different serotypes of human rotaviruses, *Lancet, 1*:38 (1978).

19

An Update on Viral Gastroenteritis

Albert Z. Kapikian, M.D. National Institute of Allergy and Infectious Diseases, Bethesda, Maryland

The purpose of this update is to review some of the major research advances in viral gastroenteritis which occurred too late to be included in the chapters submitted for publication in this book. The field of rotavirus research has moved especially fast and has yielded numerous major advances which need to be reviewed, including: (1) the rescue of noncultivatable human rotaviruses by genetic reassortment, (2) a redefinition of the term "rotavirus serotype," (3) the distribution of rotavirus serotypes, and (4) the efficient cell culture propagation and characterization of human rotavirus strains. In addition, some notes on rotavirus vaccines are added as concluding remarks.

Rescue of Noncultivatable Human Rotaviruses by Genetic Reassortment with Cultivatable Bovine ts Rotavirus

Human rotaviruses are extremely fastidious agents [1]. As noted previously, human rotavirus strain Wa (previously designated a type 2 human rotavirus) was propagated in primary African green monkey kidney cell cultures following prior serial passages in gnotobiotic piglets [2]. Since the DS-1 strain (previously designated type 1 human rotavirus) could not be serially passaged in piglets, another strategy for propagation of this distinct strain was adopted which took advantage of the well-known characteristic of the reoviridae—which have a

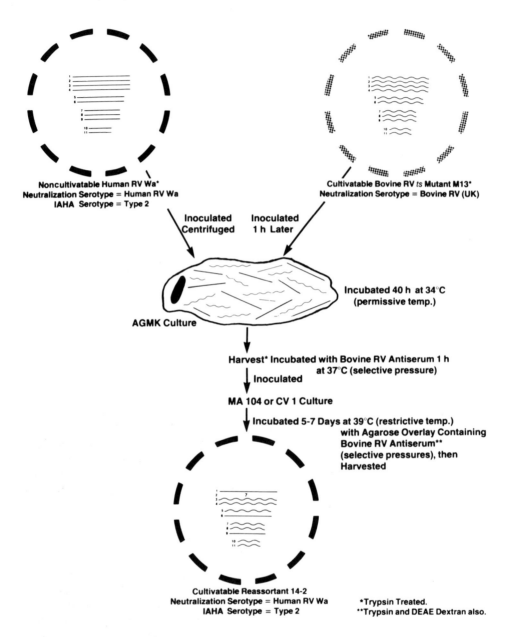

Figure 1 Rescue of noncultivatable human rotavirus (RV) Wa (type 2) by gene reassortment during mixed infection with a cultivatable *ts* mutant of bovine RV UK. (From Ref. 9.)

segmented genome—to genetically reassort with efficiency during mixed infection in cell culture [3-7]. [Previously, a reassortant from two cultivatable animal rotaviruses, SA-11 and Nebraska calf diarrhea virus (NCDV), had been obtained following mixed infection of cells with NCDV and UV-irradiated SA-11 in the presence of anti-NCDV serum; the reassortant progeny had the neutralization specificity of SA-11] [8]. With such an approach, it was hoped that coinfection of cell cultures with a noncultivatable human rotavirus and a cultivatable bovine *ts* mutant would yield a cultivatable reassortant with the neutralization specificity of the human rotavirus parent [4].

Two types of selective pressure were employed to favor the selection of reassortants: (1) *ts* mutants of bovine rotavirus were used for coinfection at permissive temperature, but were selected against when the mixed infection yield was examined at restrictive temperature; and (2) high-titered antibovine rotavirus serum was employed to neutralize virus with bovine rotavirus neutralization specificity [4]. Initially, such "rescue" experiments were carried out with noncultivatable Wa virus and later with noncultivatable DS-1 virus [4]. In each instance, the reassortants grew well in tissue culture, produced plaques at 39°C, and had the neutralization specificity of the human Wa or DS-1 virus [4]. The rescue of Wa strain by this method is shown schematically in Fig. 1 [9].

In this way, previously noncultivatable strains could be rescued. Rescue of noncultivatable human rotaviruses as reassortants has yielded important information on (1) the antigenic specificity of rotaviruses, (2) the genes which code for these specificities, (3) the gene responsible for restriction of growth in cell culture, and (4) the distribution of human rotavirus serotypes—all of which are outlined below. In addition, it may also yield important information on the genetic determinants of virulence, a major consideration in vaccine development [4-6].

Redefinition of the Term "Serotype" and Proposal for the Term "Subgroup" As An Additional Designation for Rotaviruses

Human rotaviruses have been analyzed for serotypic differences by various techniques including specific complement fixation (CF), immune electron microscopy (IEM), enzyme-linked immunosorbent assay (ELISA), and neutralization of immunofluorescent foci (NIFF) [10-15a,b]. A large number of strains obtained from epidemiologic studies have been examined serologically by the ELISA technique and have been classified into two distinct serotypes designated types 1 and 2 as originally described by specific CF [10,14]. In addition, rotaviruses have been classified by the NIFF technique, with at least three serotypes being described [13]. Such serotype designations have been employed in this book and in current literature until very recently. However, recent studies indicate that the serotype designations as heretofore employed need to be clarified as

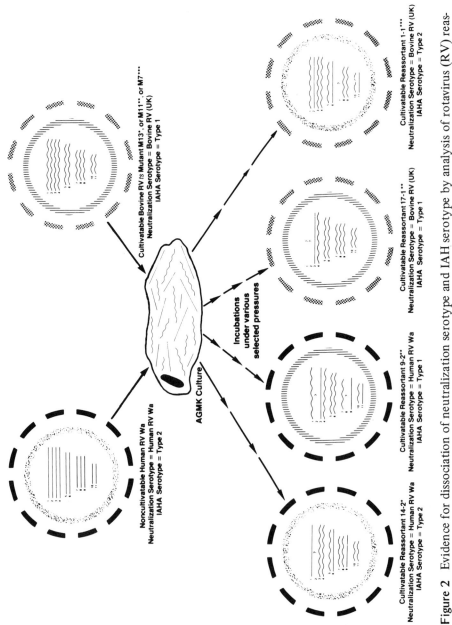

Figure 2 Evidence for dissociation of neutralization serotype and IAH serotype by analysis of rotavirus (RV) reassortants produced by mixed infection with human and bovine rotaviruses. (From Ref. 9.)

outlined below, with the introduction of an additional term—"subgroup"—to denote an antigenic specificity distinct from the neutralization serotype [16].

It has generally been assumed that the various assays outlined above were measuring the same or similar antigenic specificities and that once these fastidious human rotaviruses were propagated in cell culture, the differentiation into various serotypes would be confirmed by conventional neutralization assay. In addition, animal rotaviruses have been considered to be outside the realm of human rotavirus serotypes since by neutralization tests most animal rotaviruses are distinct from one another [2,4,17–19]. However, with a newly developed immune adherence hemagglutination assay (IAHA) in which infection sera from a gnotobiotic calf infected with a type 1 or 2 human rotavirus were employed, the calf rotavirus (UK or NCDV), the O agent, and two rhesus rotaviruses were found to share IAHA specificity with human rotavirus type 1 and thus these animal viruses could clearly be classified as type 1 rotaviruses [16]. Absence of reactivity with human rotavirus type 2 was striking. This finding raised some rather perplexing questions about the meaning of the term "rotavirus serotype" since, as noted above, most animal rotaviruses were distinct from each other by neutralization and yet most of them shared a type 1 specificity with each other and with the human rotavirus as well.

This dilemma was resolved when reassortants of human rotavirus Wa and bovine rotavirus UK were analyzed for neutralization and IAHA specificities [16,20]. Such studies revealed that the neutralization and IAHA specificities segregated independently. For example, as shown in Fig. 2, in experiments with or without selective pressure in which one parent was noncultivatable rotavirus Wa (cultivatable Wa is an IAHA type 2 virus) and the other parent was a bovine rotavirus *ts* mutant UK (an IAHA type 1 virus), it was found that the cultivatable progeny reassortants fell into four different categories: (1) human rotavirus Wa by neutralization and type 2 by IAHA; (2) human rotavirus Wa by neutralization and type 1 by IAHA; (3) bovine rotavirus by neutralization and type 1 by IAHA; and (4) bovine rotavirus by neutralization and type 2 by IAHA [9,16,20]. Thus from such studies it was clear that the IAHA and neutralization specificities segregated independently and were coded for by different genes [20]. With the typing of animal rotaviruses and the dissociation of neutralization and IAHA specificities, it is clear that the term "serotype" as previously applied to rotaviruses must be redefined. It was therefore suggested that (1) the term "serotype" be reserved to identify the antigen that reacts with neutralizing antibody, as is the fashion for other viruses, and (2) the term "subgroup" be employed to identify the antigen that had previously been defined by type-specific CF, IEM, ELISA, and now IAHA [16]. In studies with Wa-UK reassortants, it was shown that gene 9 coded for the neutralization protein of Wa virus and gene 6 code for the subgroup protein of both Wa and UK viruses (and that gene 4 was associated with restriction of growth in tissue culture) [20,21a,b]. Thus when rotaviruses are numbered in the future by their neutralization specificity, the strain could be referred to as human rotavirus type 1, subgroup 1, or human rotavirus type 2, subgroup 2, etc., with the type designation referring to the neutralization specificity and the subgroup designation to the reactivity related to the 6th gene segment which has been shown to code for the major internal structure protein [16,22].

Recent studies have also shown an association between the electrophoretic mobility of the 10th and 11th RNA segments of human rotavirus and classification according to subgroup: Subgroup 1 human rotaviruses have slower moving RNA segments 10 and 11 than do subgroup 2 human rotaviruses [23–26]. Thus, human rotaviruses belonging to either of these subgroups can be classified according to subgroup by the electrophoretic mobility of their 10th and 11th gene segments in polyacrylamide gels. However, it is important to note that studies have also shown that viruses with "long" 10 and 11 segments (i.e., faster-moving) can have different neutralization specificities and thus can belong to different serotypes [27–29]. The association of electrophoretic mobility of the 10th and 11th RNA segments with subgroup does not hold for animal rotaviruses as they display the long RNA pattern, yet most animal strains tested belong to the subgroup 1 classification [4,7,11,16,24,27,30,31]. It should also be noted that a third subgroup of human rotavirus has been reported recently [11].

Serotypic Distribution of Rotaviruses as Determined From Rescue Experiments

The rescue of human rotavirus strains by reassortment technology has enabled the delineation of the epidemiology of various strains from different parts of the world. Thirty-three strains of human rotavirus were successfully rescued by genetic reassortment as described above [4,28a,b,32]. Twenty of these strains were studied serologically by plaque reduction assay [28a,b]. It was noteworthy that 14 of the 20 were Wa-like and 2 were similar to DS-1, whereas 4 appeared to be distinct from the Wa and DS-1 viruses in tests with hyperimmune guinea pig serum prepared against these 2 distinct serotypes. These four strains were found to belong to a third distinct serotype which was serologically related to rhesus rotavirus [28a,b]. The ability to type such a high percentage of strains was encouraging and may indicate that the number of distinct serotypes is limited, an important consideration in vaccine development.

Efficient Propagation of Human Rotavirus Directly From Clinical Specimens

As various chapters in this book have indicated, human rotaviruses are extremely fastidious, a factor which has limited efforts (1) to study the epidemiology of rotavirus serotypes, (2) to examine the mechanism of immunity by conventional neutralization assay, (3) to select strains for potential candidate vaccines, and (4) to move forward in the development of a vaccine. However, important strides have been made recently in the cell culture propagation of rotaviruses from human clinical material [33-37]. A very recent major advance has been the efficient cell culture propagation and characterization of human rotavirus strains [35-37].

In these studies, numerous human rotavirus strains have been efficiently propagated directly from clinical specimens into cell cultures and selected strains have been characterized by cross-neutralization studies in cell culture and by RNA gel electrophoresis [35-37]. The cultivation of three human rotavirus strains which induced a definite cytopathic effect (CPE) in MA104 cell cultures, a cell line derived from embryonic rhesus monkey kidney, was reported [35]. The virus was pretreated with trypsin (10 μg/ml) and, in addition, 1 μg/ml trypsin was added to the maintenance medium; tube cultures were rolled at 37°C [35]. The CPE was so clear cut in later passages that tube culture neutralization assays could be carried out with CPE as the indicator of virus growth. The isolation of three additional rotavirus strains directly from clinical specimens by similar methods was also reported [36]. These strains were later not only propagated in stationary cell cultures but also produced plaques in overlay medium containing 0.6% purified agar, 3 μg/ml acetylated trypsin, and 50 μg/ml DEAE dextran. More recently the successful cell culture cultivation of 20 of 24 rotavirus-containing human stool specimens was reported [37]. The efficient propagation of human rotavirus is a major breakthrough in rotavirus research and it should have wide-ranging implications, not only in the understanding of rotavirus infection but also in attempts to develop methods of immunoprophylaxis.

Control of Rotavirus Illness

With respect to the control of rotavirus illnesses, it is clear from various studies that an effective rotavirus vaccine would make a major contribution in reducing morbidity from gastroenteritis in both the developed and developing countries [38-40]. In addition, in developing countries which experience a staggering mortality from diarrheal illnesses in infants and young children, it appears that an effective rotavirus vaccine would reduce an as yet unknown portion of the mortality from such disease as well [38].

Recent reviews [5,6,19,38] of approaches to immunization against rotavirus gastroenteritis have defined some of the strategies that are being considered for vaccine development. Among them: a live attenuated human rotavirus vaccine; an attenuated reassortant rotavirus vaccine; a vaccine made from an animal rotavirus strain if such a strain is able to infect humans without causing illness but induce protection; a rotavirus vaccine intended for expectant mothers in order to boost breast milk antibodies for increasing protection for the infant; cloning of the human rotavirus genome by DNA technology for vaccine preparation purposes; production of synthetic vaccines derived from the specific amino acid sequences responsible for the induction of protective antibodies [41–48].

In addition, there has been a recent surge of interest in passive immunization against rotavirus disease [49–64]. With this approach rotavirus antibody would be produced by one of several methods, and such antibody would be added to the diet of the infant in an attempt to prevent or modify rotaviral illness. Human milk containing rotavirus antibody has been employed as a therapeutic measure for immunodeficient patients with rotavirus infection [65].

Hopefully the stage has been set for a very exciting period in which a major pathogen of infants and young children may be controlled.

References

1. R. G. Wyatt and W. D. James. Methods of virus culture of gastroenteritis viruses in vivo and in vitro. In *Virus Infections of the Gastrointestinal Tract.* (D. A. J. Tyrrell and A. Z. Kapikian, eds.), Marcel Dekker, New York, 1982, pp. 13–36.

2. R. G. Wyatt, W. D. James, E. H. Bohl, K. W. Theil, L. J. Saif, A. R. Kalica, H. B. Greenberg, A. Z. Kapikian, and R. M. Chanock. Human rotavirus type 2: cultivation *in vitro. Science 207*:189-191 (1980).

3. R. K. Cross and B. N. Fields. Genetics of reovirus. In *Comprehensive virology, Vol. 9* (H. Fraenkel-Conrat and R. R. Wagner, eds.), Plenum, New York, 1970, pp. 291-340.

4. H. B. Greenberg, A. R. Kalica, R. G. Wyatt, R. W. Jones, A. Z. Kapikian, and R. M. Chanock. Rescue of noncultivatable human rotavirus by gene reassortment during mixed infection with *ts* mutants of a cultivatable bovine rotavirus. *Proc. Natl. Acad. Sci. USA 78*:420-424 (1981).

5. R. M. Chanock, R. G. Wyatt, and A. Z. Kapikian. Immunization of infants and young children against rotaviral gastroenteritis—prospects and problems. *JA VMA 173*:570-572 (1978).

6. R. M. Chanock. Strategy for development of respiratory and gastrointestinal viral vaccines in the 1980s. Joseph E. Smadel Memorial Lecture. *J. Inf. Dis. 143*:364-374 (1981).

7. H. B. Greenberg, R. G. Wyatt, A. R. Kalica, R. H. Yolken, R. Black, A. Z. Kapikian, and R. M. Chanock. New insights in viral gastroenteritis. In *Perspectives in virology* (M. Pollard, ed.), *11*:163-187 (1980).

8. S. Matsuno, A. Hasegawa, A. R. Kalica, and R. Kono. Isolation of a recombinant between simian and bovine rotaviruses. *J. Gen. Virol. 48*: 253-256 (1980).

9. A. Z. Kapikian, H. B. Greenberg, A. R. Kalica, R. G. Wyatt, H. W. Kim, C. D. Brandt, W. J. Rodriguez, J. Flores, N. Singh, R. H. Parrott, and R. M. Chanock. New developments in viral gastroenteritis. In *Acute Enteric Infections in Children. New Prospects for Treatment and Pre-*

vention (T. Holme, J. Holmgren, M. H. Merson, and R. Mollby, eds.), Elsevier/North Holland Biomedical Press, 1981, pp. 9-57.

10. G. Zissis and J. P. Lambert. Different serotypes of human rotaviruses. *Lancet 1*:38-39 (1978).

11. G. Zissis, J. P. Lambert, J. G. Kapsenberg, G. Enders, and L. N. Mutanda. Human rotavirus serotypes. *Lancet 1*:944-945 (1981).

12. G. Zissis and J. P. Lambert. Enzyme-linked immunosorbent assays adapted for serotyping of human rotavirus strains. *J. Clin. Micro. 11*:1-5 (1980).

13. G. M. Beards, J. N. Pilfold, M. E. Thouless, and T. H. Flewett. Rotavirus serotypes by serum neutralization. *J. Med. Virol. 5*:231-237 (1980).

14. R. H. Yolken, R. G. Wyatt, G. Zissis, C. D. Brandt, W. J. Rodriguez, H. W. Kim, R. H. Parrott, J. J. Urrutia, L. Mata, H. B. Greenberg, A. Z. Kapikian, and R. M. Chanock. Epidemiology of human rotavirus types 1 and 2 as studied by enzyme-linked immunosorbent assay. *N. Engl. J. Med. 299*: 1156-1161 (1978).

15a. W. J. Rodriguez, H. W. Kim, C. D. Brandt, R. H. Yolken, J. O. Arrobio, A. Z. Kapikian, R. M. Chanock, and R. H. Parrott. Sequential enteric illnesses associated with different rotavirus serotypes. *Lancet 2*:37 (1978).

15b. F. R. Bishai, L. Spence, D. Goodwin, and R. Petro. Use of antisera against bovine (NCDV) and simian (SA11) rotaviruses in ELISA to detect different types of human rotavirus. *Can. J. Microbiol. 25*:1118-1124 (1979).

16. A. Z. Kapikian, W. L. Cline, H. B. Greenberg, R. G. Wyatt, A. R. Kalica, C. E. Banks, H. D. James, Jr., J. Flores, and R. M. Chanock. Antigenic characterization of human and animal rotaviruses by immune adherence hemagglutination assay (IAHA): evidence for distinctness of IAHA and neutralization antigens. *Infect. Immun. 33*:415-425 (1981).

17. G. N. Woode, J. C. Bridger, J. M. Jones, T. H. Flewett, A. S. Bryden, H. Davies, and G. B. B. White. Morphological and antigenic relationships between viruses (rotaviruses) from acute gastroenteritis of children, calves, piglets, mice, and foals. *Infect. Immun. 14*:804-810 (1976).

18. M. E. Thouless, A. S. Bryden, T. H. Flewett, G. N. Woode, J. C. Bridger, D. R. Snodgrass, and J. A. Herring. Serological relationships between rotaviruses from different species as studied by complement fixation and neutralization. *Arch. Virol. 53*:287-289 (1977).

19. R. G. Wyatt, A. Z. Kapikian, H. B. Greenberg, A. R. Kalica, and R. M. Chanock. Prospects for immunization against rotaviral disease. In *Nobel Conference 3. Acute enteric infections in children. New prospects for treatment and prevention* (T. Holme, J. Holmgren, M. H. Merson, and R. Molby, eds.), Elsevier/North Holland Biomedical Press, 1981, pp. 505-522.

20. A. R. Kalica, H. B. Greenberg, R. G. Wyatt, J. Flores, M. M. Sereno, A. Z. Kapikian, and R. M. Chanock. Genes of human (strain Wa) and bovine (strain UK) rotaviruses that code for neutralization and subgroup antigens. *Virology 112*:385-390 (1981).

21a. J. Flores, H. B. Greenberg, J. Myslinski, I. Perez, L. White, R. Marquina, A. Kalica, R. G. Wyatt, A. Z. Kapikian, and R. M. Chanock. Use of transcription probes in genotyping rotavirus. Fifteenth Joint Working Conference on Diarrheal Diseases. United States–Japan Cooperative Medical Science Program, Bethesda, Maryland, November, 1981, p. 31 (Abstr.)

21b. H. Greenberg, A. R. Kalica, R. G. Wyatt, J. Flores, A. Kapikian, and R. Chanock. Rescue of noncultivatable human rotavirus by gene reassortment in tissue culture. Fifth International Congress of Virology, Strasbourg, France, August 1981, W47/10, p. 426 (Abstr.)

22. M. L. Smith, I. Lazdins, and I. H. Holmes. Coding assignments of double-stranded RNA segments of SA11 virus established by *in vitro* translation. *J. Virol. 33*:976-982 (1980).

23. S. M. Rodger, R. F. Bishop, C. Birch, B. McLean, and I. H. Holmes. Molecular epidemiology of human rotaviruses in Melbourne, Australia from 1973 to 1979 as determined by electrophoresis of genome ribonucleic acid. *J. Clin. Micro 13*:272-278 (1981).

24. A. R. Kalica, H. B. Greenberg, R. T. Espejo, J. Flores, R. G. Wyatt, A. Z. Kapikian, and R. M. Chanock. Distinctive ribonucleic acid patterns of human rotavirus subgroups 1 and 2. *Infect. Immun. 33*:958-961 (1981).

25. T. Kutsuzawa, T. Konno, H. Suzuki, T. Ebina, and N. Ishida. Two distinct RNA patterns of human rotavirus prevalent in Japan. Fifth International Congress of Virology, Strasbourg, France, August, 1981, p. 16/13, p. 195.

26. T. Konno, T. Kutsuzawa, H. Suzuki, and N. Ishida. Further study on the epidemiology of human rotavirus: genomic variations among rotaviruses obtained from hospitalized children during a 7-year period. Fifteenth Joint Working Conference on Diarrheal Diseases. United States–Japan Cooperative Medical Science Program, Bethesda, Maryland, November, 1981, p. 27. (Abstr.).

27. A. R. Kalica, M. M. Sereno, R. G. Wyatt, C. A. Mebus, R. M. Chanock, and A. Z. Kapikian. Comparison of human and animal rotavirus strains by gel electrophoresis of viral RNA. *Virology 87*:247-255 (1978).

28a. R. G. Wyatt, H. B. Greenberg, A. R. Kalica, Y. Hoshino, J. Flores, and A. Z. Kapikian. Definition of human rotavirus serotypes by plaque reduction assay. (Abstr.) Fifteenth Joint Working Conference on Viral Diseases. United States–Japan Cooperative Medical Science Program, Bethesda, Maryland, November, 1981, p. 30.

28b. R. G. Wyatt, H. B. Greenberg, W. D. James, A. L. Pittman, A. R. Kalica, J. Flores, R. M. Chanock, and A. Z. Kapikian. Definition of human rotavirus serotypes by plaque reduction assay. Infect. Immun. (in press) 1982.

29. R. G. Wyatt, A. R. Kalica, et al., unpublished studies.

30. R. G. Wyatt, A. R. Kalica, C. A. Mebus, H. W. Kim, W. T. London, R. M. Chanock, and A. Z. Kapikian. Reovirus-like agents (rotaviruses) associated with diarrheal illnesses in animals and man. In *Perspectives in Virology* (M. Pollard, ed.), *10*:121-145 (1978).

31. R. T. Espejo, O. Munoz, F. Serafin, and P. Romero. Shift in the prevalent human rotavirus detected by ribonucleic acid segment differences. *Infect. Immun. 27*:351-354 (1980).

32. H. B. Greenberg, R. G. Wyatt, A. Z. Kapikian, A. R. Kalica, J. Flores, and R. Jones. Rescue of thirty-three strains of noncultivatable human rotavirus by gene reassortment. *Infect. Immun.* (in press) 1982.

33. S. G. Drozdov, L. A. Shekoian, M. B. Korolev, and A. G. Andzhaparidze. Human rotavirus in cell culture: isolation and passaging. *Vopr. Virusol. 4*: 389-392 (1979).

34. S. G. Drozdov, M. B. Korolev, L. A. Shekoyan, and V. I. Haustov. Human rotavirus in tissue cultures: morphogenenesis and hemagglutinating activity. (Abstr.) Fifth International Congress of Virology, Strasbourg, France, August, 1981, p 16/05, p. 193 (Abstr.).

35. K. Sato, Y. Inaba, T. Shinozaki, R. Fujii, and M. Matumoto. Isolation of human rotavirus in cell cultures. Brief Report. *Arch. Virol. 69*:155-160 (1981).

36. T. Urasawa, S. Urasawa, and K. Taniguchi. Sequential passages of human rotavirus in MA-104 cells. *Microbiol. Immunol. 25(10)*:1025-1035 (1981).

37. S. Urasawa, T. Urasawa, and K. Taniguchi. Sequential passages of human rotavirus in cell culture. Fifteenth Joint Working Conference on Viral Diseases. United States–Japan Cooperative Medical Science Program, Bethesda, Maryland, 1981, p. 29 (Abstr.).

38. A. Z. Kapikian, R. G. Wyatt, H. B. Greenberg, A. R. Kalica, H. W. Kim, C. D. Brandt, W. J. Rodriguez, R. H. Parrott, and R. M. Chanock. Approaches to the immunization of infants and young children against gastroenteritis due to rotaviruses. *Rev. Inf. Dis. 2*:459-469 (1980).

39. J. A. K. Carlson, P. J. Middleton, M. Szymanski, J. Huber, and M. Petric. Fatal rotavirus gastroenteritis. An analysis of 21 cases. *Am. J. Dis. Child. 132*:477-479 (1978).

40. R. E. Black, M. M. Merson, A. S. M. M. Rahman, M. Yunus, A. R. M. A. Alim, I. Huq, R. H. Yolken, and G. T. Curlin. A two-year study of bacterial, viral, and parasitic agents associated with diarrhea in rural Bangladesh. *J. Inf. Dis. 142*:660-664 (1980).

41. R. G. Wyatt, C. A. Mebus, R. H. Yolken, A. R. Kalica, H. D. James, Jr., A. Z. Kapikian, and R. M. Chanock. Rotaviral immunity in gnotobiotic calves: heterologous resistance to human virus induced by bovine virus. *Science 203*:548-550 (1979).

42. M. Lobmann, P. Charlier, A. Delem, N. Zygraich, J. P. Lambert, and G. Zissis. Challenge experiments in colostrum-deprived piglets previously immunized with human type 2 and bovine RIT 4237 rotavirus strains: evidence of homologous and heterologous protection. Fifth International Congress of Virology, Strasbourg, France. August, 1981, p 16/15, p. 195 (Abstr.).

43. M. Lobmann, P. Charlier, A. Delem, N. Zygraich, J. P. Lambert, and G. Zissis. Cross-protection studies in piglets artificially infected with the bovine rotavirus strain RIT 4237 and challenged with human rotavirus type 2 and type 3. Proceedings, International Symposium, Recent Advances in Enteric Infections, Brugge, Belgium, September, 1981, p. 37. (Abstr.).

44. G. N. Woode, M. E. Bew, and M. J. Dennis. Studies on cross protection induced in calves by rotaviruses of calves, children, and foals. *Vet. Rec. 102*:32-34 (1978).

45. C. R. Bartz, R. H. Conklin, C. B. Tunstall, and J. H. Steele. Prevention of murine rotavirus infection with chicken egg yolk immunoglobulins. *J. Inf. Dis. 142*:439-441 (1980).

46. J. Flores et al., unpublished studies.

47. R. A. Lerner, N. Green, A. Olson, T. Shinnick, and J. G. Sutcliffe. The development of synthetic vaccines. *Hosp. Pract. 16*:55-62 (1981).

48. A. Z. Zuckerman. Developing synthetic vaccines. *Nature 295*:98-99 (1982).

49. C. A. Mebus, R. G. White, E. P. Bass, and M. J. Twiehaus. Immunity to neonatal calf diarrhea virus. *JA VMA 163*:880-883 (1973).

50. G. N. Woode, J. Jones, and J. Bridger. Levels of colostral antibodies against neonatal calf diarrhea virus. *Vet. Rec. 97*:148-149 (1975).

51. J. C. Bridger and G. N. Woode. Neonatal calf diarrhoea: identification of a reovirus-like (rotavirus) agent in faeces by immunofluorescence and immune electron microscopy. *Br. Vet. J. 131*:528-535 (1975).

52. D. R. Snodgrass and P. W. Wells. Rotavirus infection in lambs: studies on passive protection. *Arch. Virol. 52*:201-205 (1976).

53. J. G. Lecce, M. W. King, and R. Mock. Reovirus-like agent associated with fatal diarrhea in neonatal pigs. *Infect. Immun. 14*:816-825 (1976).

54. D. R. Snodgrass, C. R. Madeley, P. W. Wells, and K. W. Angus. Human rotavirus in lambs: infection and passive protection. *Infect. Immun. 16*: 268-270 (1977).

55. D. R. Snodgrass and P. W. Wells. Passive immunity in rotaviral infections. *J. Am. Vet. Med. Assoc. 173*:565-569 (1978).

56. D. R. Snodgrass and P. W. Wells. The immunoprophylaxis of rotavirus infections in lambs. *Vet. Rec. 102*:146-148 (1978).

57. C. Mietens, H. Keinhorst, H. Hilpert, H. Gerber, H. Amster, and J. J. Pahud. Treatment of infantile *E. coli* gastroenteritis with specific bovine anti-*E. coli* milk immunoglobulins. *European J. Pediatr. 132*:239-252 (1979).

58. J. C. Bridger and J. F. Brown. Protection of piglets from disease caused by porcine rotavirus by feeding bovine colostrum. Les Colloques de l'INSERM. Viral Enteritis. *INSERM 90*:373-376 (1979).

59. G. Wellemans and E. van Opdenbosch. Prevention of neonatal calf diarrhea by prolongation of secretion of antibodies in the milk at a high level. Les Colloques de l'INSERM. Viral Enteritis. *INSERM 90*:369-372 (1979).

60. D. R. Snodgrass, K. H. Fahey, and P. W. Wells. Rotavirus infections in calves from vaccinated and normal cows. Les Colloques de l'INSERM. Viral Enteritis. *INSERM 90*:365-368 (1979).

61. B. McLean and I. H. Holmes. Transfer of antirotaviral antibodies from mothers to their infants. *J. Clin. Microbiol. 12*:320-325 (1980).

62. B. S. McLean and I. H. Holmes. Effects of antibodies, trypsin, and trypsin inhibitors on susceptibility of neonates to rotavirus infection. *J. Clin. Microbiol. 13*:22-29 (1981).

63. L. J. Saif, D. R. Redman, K. L. Smith, and K. W. Theil. Passive immunity to rotavirus in colostrum-deprived newborn calves. 62nd Annual Confer-

ence of Research Workers on Animal Disease, Chicago, November, 1981, p. 34. (Abstr. 194)

64. L. J. Saif, K. L. Smith, B. L. Landmeier, E. H. Bohl, and K. W. Theil. Immunization of pregnant cows with bovine rotavirus. 62nd Annual Conference of Research Workers on Animal Disease, Chicago, November, 1981, p. 34. (Abstr. 194)

65. F. T. Saulsbury, J. A. Winkelstein, and R. H. Yolken. Chronic rotavirus infection in immunodeficiency. *J. Ped. 97*:61-65 (1980).

Author Index

Numbers in brackets are reference numbers and indicate that an author's work is referred to although the name is not cited in the text. Numbers in parentheses give the page on which the complete reference is listed.

A

Aas, K., 90[6], (102)
Abbott, G. D., 51[8], (71), 112
[52], (121), 126[63], 127[63],
132[63], (143), 212[35], (223),
229[11], 235[11], (237)
Abdo, J. A. 264[166], (282)
Abou-Gareeb, A. H. 268[192], (284)
Abou-Youssef, M. H., 381[1,128],
(386,394)
Abraham, A. A. 133[1], (139)
Ackerman, L. J. 318[25], (350)
Ackerman, P. B., 264[156], (281)
Acres, S. D., 300[1], (307), 335
[109], (356), 370[4], 379[3],
380[2], 384[3], 386[3], (386)
Adachi, M., 78[34], (85), 128[48],
127[48], 134[48], 136[49], 138
[48], (142), 213[41], (223)
Adams, N. R., 345[153], (358)
Adams, W. R., 113[1], (118), 364
[5], 365[5], (386)
Adler, I., 148[1], 158[1], (172)
Adler, R. H., 375[161], (396)

Agarwal, S. K., 253[90], 262[90],
(277)
Agnes, A. G., 18[46], 20[46],
[46], 25[46], (34), 111[69], 117
[69], (122), 298[72], 299[4,72],
302[72], 303[71], (307,311)
Agus, S. G., 139[2], (139), 161[2],
162[2], (172)
Ahlstedt, S., 96[77], (106)
Ahmed, A. 261[121], 268[195],
(279, 284)
Ahmed, Q. S., 249[228], 254[278],
(286,289)
Akagi, K., 148[21], (173)
Akhter, M. H., 264[162], (282)
Akihara, M., 135[19], 138[19],
(140), 154[10], (172)
Alam, A. K. M. J., 259[102], (278)
Alam, S. A., 258[99], (278)
Alauddin Chowdhury, A. K. M., 268
[195], (284)
Albert, M. J. 112[27], (120), 133
[58], (142)
Alberts, J. O., 322[58], (352)
Albrecht, G., 331[102], (355)

413

K

L

Q

R

Radostits, O. M., 300[1], (307), 335
[109], (356), 379[3], 384[3],
386[3], (386)
Radovanovic, M. L., 268[198],
(284)
Rafiqul, Islam, A. F. M., 262[130],
(279)
Rahaman, M. M., 254[278], 256
[94], 259[106], 262[136], 263
[94,141], 265[179], (277,278,
280,283,289)
Rahman, A. S. M. M., 132[76],
133[76], 138[76], (144), 265
[169], 267[169], (282), 405
[40], (409)
Ramia, S., 22[37], 23[37], 25[37],
(34)
Ramos-Alvarez, M., 382[131],
(394)
Rebhun, L. I., 251[73], (276)
Redman, D. R., 406[23], (410)
Reed, C. J., 337[121], (357)
Reed, D. E., 296[55], (307,310)
Reed, S. E., 31[23], (33), 131[21],
138[52], (140,142) 148[12], 150
[12], 152[12], 159[12], 171
[12], (173), 200[20], (207,222)
Rees, R. J. W., 81[40,41], (85)
Reichmann, R. C., 165[19], (173)
Reid, N., 37[31], (47)
Reimann, H. A., 148[59], (176)
Reller, L. B., 265[178], 267[180],
(283)
Remmer, E., 265[174], (282)
Retter, M., 31[38], (34)
Reynolds, D. J., 321[47,49], 323
[47,62], 332[47], (352)
Reynolds, H. Y., 269[203], (284,
395)
Reynolds, J., 98[92], (107)
Rhode, J. E., 264[51], (281)
Rhodes, A. J., 37[22,23], (46)
Rhodes, M. B., 31[33], (34), 292
[1], (293), 296[47], 297[47],
(310), 315[7], 318[23], 325[33],
334[7,105,106], 337[105], 338

[Rhodes, M. B.], [105], 339[7,
132], 340[7,105], (349,351,356,
357), 362[91], 364[91], 365[91],
370[90,91], 371[90], (391)
Richards, R. L., 249[226], (286)
Richardson, L. S., 213[37], (223)
Richardson, S. H., 249[37], 251
[68], (273)
Richerson, H. B., 99[104], (108)
Richman, L. K., 99[109], (108)
Richmond, S. J., 138[70], (143)
Rifkin, G. D., 260[118], 268[189],
(279,283)
Riggs, J. L., 149[57], 151[57], 154
[57], 156[57], 160[57], 171
[57], (176)
Righthand, F., 98[93], (107)
Riley, J. L., 318[35], (351)
Riou, Y., 300[21], 301[21], (308)
Rische, H., 249[252], (288)
Ristic, M., 318[31], 320[46], 321
[51], 322[58], 326[51,89], 328
[89], (351,352,352,354), 363
[166], 381[1,128], 383[143],
(385,394,395,396)
Ritchie, A. E., 22[15], (33), 293[3],
[3], (293), 316[8], 321[51], 326
[51], 344[8], 348[8], (349,352)
Rivas, E. N., 265[178], (283)
Roberts, A. W., 317[22], 325[79],
(350,354), 364[111], (393)
Robertson, D. C., 246[39,40], 247
[55,58], (273,274,275)
Robertson, S. M., 95[61], (105)
Robins-Brown, R. M., 249[260],
(288)
Robinson, N. M., 147[75], (177),
198[51], (209)
Roche, J. K., 82[49], (86)
Rodrigot, M., 54[31], (72)
Rodger, S. M., 114[57,58,59], 115
[57], 116[28,58], 118[57], (120,
122), 218[69], (225), 296[56],
304[57], (310,311), 404[23],
(408)
Rodkey, L. S., 374[174], (396)

Subject Index